TEXTBOOK AND COLOR ATLAS OF SALIVARY GLAND PATHOLOGY

DIAGNOSIS AND MANAGEMENT

TEXTBOOK AND COLOR ATLAS OF SALIVARY GLAND PATHOLOGY
DIAGNOSIS AND MANAGEMENT

By

Eric R. Carlson

Robert A. Ord

WILEY-BLACKWELL

A John Wiley & Sons, Inc., Publication

Edition first published 2008
© 2008 Wiley-Blackwell

Blackwell Munksgaard, formerly an imprint of Blackwell Publishing was acquired by John Wiley & Sons in February 2007. Blackwell's publishing programme has been merged with Wiley's global Scientific, Technical, and Medical business to form Wiley-Blackwell.

Editorial Office
2121 State Avenue, Ames, Iowa 50014-8300, USA

For details of our global editorial offices, for customer services and for information about how to apply for permission to reuse the copyright material in this book please see our website at www.wiley.com/wiley-blackwell.

Library of Congress Cataloguing-in-Publication Data

Textbook and color atlas of salivary gland pathology :
diagnosis and management / edited by Eric Carlson, Robert Ord.
     p. ; cm.
  Includes bibliographical references and index.
  ISBN-13: 978-0-8138-0262-6 (alk. paper)
  ISBN-10: 0-8138-0262-8 (alk. paper)
  1. Salivary glands–Diseases–Textbooks. 2. Salivary glands–Diseases–Atlases. I. Carlson, Eric R. II. Ord, Robert A.
  [DNLM: 1. Salivary Gland Diseases–diagnosis–Atlases. 2. Salivary Gland Diseases–surgery–Atlases. 3. Salivary Glands–anatomy & histology–Atlases. WI 17 T355 2008]
  RC815.5.T49 2008
  616.3′16–dc22
                          2008006941
A catalogue record for this book is available from the U.S. Library of Congress.

Set in 10.5/12pt ITC Slimbach by SNP Best-set Typesetter Ltd., Hong Kong
Printed in Singapore by Markono Print Media Pte Ltd

1 2008

Disclaimer

Contents

Foreword

The mention of "head and neck cancer" immediately connotes the sobering realities and potentials of oral squamous cell carcinoma. Left to secondary recollection and awareness is the significance of salivary gland malignancy. The same can be said for the general perception of benign salivary neoplasia. In this brilliant new textbook, authors Carlson and Ord correct these notions, focusing proper emphasis on the group of diseases which, in their malignant form, represent some three percent of all North American head and neck tumors, affecting a minimum of twenty-five hundred victims per year.

One marvels at the dedication, energies, and resources—to say nothing of the expertise—mustered to produce a volume of this depth and expanse. While almost forty percent of the effort is directed toward the vitally significant elements of classification, diagnosis, and clinical care of neoplasia, there is more—much more—here, for both the training and practicing readerships. The whole array of salivary gland dysfunctions is marvelously displayed in meaningful clinical color, in easily grasped sketches and graphs, and in well-chosen descriptive imaging. From the mandatory fundaments for such an undertaking—John Langdon's discourse on macro- and microanatomy, Pradeep Jacob's presentation on imaging diagnostics (forty-five pages!), John Sauk's explanations of current classification and staging of tumors—to the surgical demonstrations of pathology, anatomy, and technique, the visual material is extraordinary.

What are the vagaries in defining the SMAS layer, can cell type be distinguished on the basis of imaging alone, what influence do genomics and biomarkers have in clinical classification, does contemporary understanding explain the etiology of mucous escape phenomena? Up-to-date propositions on such topics occupy these chapters. Clinical challenges, traditional and new, e.g., transection of ducts and nerves, intraductal micromanipulations, salivary diagnostics—they're all here, presented in clear, expansive, prose (twenty-eight pages of information on sialolithiasis alone!). The detriments of age and metabolic disorder on gland function, the genesis of non-salivary tumors inside the glands, and the lodging of metastatic disease within their confines receive emphasis in these pages. So do the presence of aberrant glands and the esoteric transplantation of salivary tissue in the management of xerophthalmia.

The Textbook and Color Atlas of Salivary Gland Pathology is authoritative. Its authors do not write anecdotally, but from the combined experience of decades which has elevated them both to international recognition in the field of head and neck neoplasia. Their clinical material here presented represents volumes in the operating room, and the comprehensive bibliographies in each of the text's chapters testify to the authors' awareness of their topic and their world-views. Eric Carlson displays the fruits of his earlier endeavors in Pittsburgh, Detroit, and Miami, and speaks now from his position as Professor and Chairman in the Department of Oral and Maxillofacial Surgery at the University of Tennessee Graduate School of Medicine in Knoxville. Robert Ord established his worthy reputation in Britain before resettling himself in Baltimore on the western shores of the Atlantic some twenty years ago, where he now serves as Professor and Chairman of the Department of Oral and Maxillofacial Surgery at the University of Maryland. Theirs is the first tome in this domain engineered authoritatively by oral and maxillofacial surgeons, and does honor to their colleagues and forebears in the specialty who have toiled in the vineyards of salivary gland pathology. Neither in design nor execution, however, is their marvelous achievement directed to a parochial audience. Rather, surgeons or clinicians of whatever ilk will offer the authors a nod of appreciation in benefitting from this text.

Probably, one day, an expansion of this work will be written; and, undoubtedly, Carlson and Ord will write it.

R. Bruce MacIntosh, DDS
Detroit

Preface

The concept of this book devoted to the diagnosis and management of salivary gland pathology arose from our long-standing friendship and professional relationship, when we first collaborated in the early 1990s. This led to a trip to India with the Health Volunteers Overseas in 1996, where we operated on numerous complex cancer cases, including salivary gland malignancies. Dr. Carlson's interest in benign and malignant tumor surgery was fostered by the expert surgical tutelage of Dr. Robert E. Marx at the University of Miami Miller School of Medicine/Jackson Memorial Hospital in Miami, Florida. It was the training by Professor John Langdon who nurtured Dr. Ord's love of the parotidectomy. Over the years, following the publication of several papers and book chapters devoted to salivary gland surgery, we realized that a textbook and atlas related to this discipline should be produced. It was believed that a work written by two surgeons who shared similar surgical philosophies would be a unique addition to the current literature. This has been a project that we have approached with energy and enthusiasm, which hopefully is evident to the reader.

The diagnosis and management of salivary gland pathology is an exciting and thought-provoking discipline in medicine, dentistry, and surgery. It is incumbent on the clinician examining a patient with a suspected developmental, neoplastic, or non-neoplastic lesion of the major or minor salivary glands to obtain a comprehensive history and physical examination, after which time a differential diagnosis is established. A definitive diagnosis is provided with either an excisional or incisional biopsy, depending on the gland involved and the differential diagnosis established preoperatively. A complete understanding of the anatomic barriers surrounding a salivary gland lesion is paramount when performing surgery for a salivary gland neoplasm.

It is the purpose of this *Textbook and Color Atlas of Salivary Gland Pathology* to provide both text and clinical images, thereby making this a singular work. The reader interested in the science and evidence-based medicine associated with the management of salivary gland pathology will be attracted to our text. The reader interested in how to perform salivary gland surgery as a function of diagnosis and anatomic site will find the real-time images useful. To that end, artist sketches are limited in this book. Where appropriate, algorithms have been included as a guide for diagnosis and management. It is our hope that this text and atlas will find a home on the bookshelves of those surgeons who share our fascination with the diagnosis and management of salivary gland disease.

Acknowledgments

I would like to thank the loves of my life, Susan, Katie, and Kristen Carlson, for excusing me during the time required to write this book. I also thank my father, Reinhold Carlson, who has always reminded me that the goal of education is not to give you all the answers, but to provide resources where you can find them. I hope this book represents a resource for answers to your questions regarding the diagnosis and management of salivary gland pathology.

ERC

To my wife, Sue.
RAO

We thank Sophia Joyce, Senior Commissioning Editor; Shelby Hayes, Editorial Assistant; Erin Magnani, Production Editor; and Sarah Brown, Copy Editor for their valuable and insightful editorial support, without whom this book would not have been possible.

ERC, RAO

Contributors

Eric R. Carlson, DMD, MD, FACS
Professor and Chairman
Department of Oral and Maxillofacial Surgery
Director, Oral and Maxillofacial Surgery Residency
  Program
University of Tennessee Medical Center and the
  University of Tennessee Cancer Institute
Knoxville, Tennessee

Robert A. Ord, DDS, MD, FRCS, FACS, MS
Professor and Chairman
Department of Oral and Maxillofacial Surgery
University of Maryland Medical Center and the
  Greenbaum Cancer Institute
Baltimore, Maryland

Pradeep Jacob, MD, MBA
Clinical Assistant Professor
Department of Radiology
The University of Tennessee at Chattanooga
College of Medicine
Chattanooga, Tennessee

John D. Langdon, FKC, MB BS, BDS, MDS, FDSRCS,
  FRCS, FMedSCi
Emeritus Professor of Maxillofacial Surgery
King's College
London, England

John J. Sauk, DDS, MS, FAAAS, FAHNS
Dean and Professor
School of Dentistry
University of Louisville
Louisville, Kentucky

TEXTBOOK AND COLOR ATLAS OF SALIVARY GLAND PATHOLOGY

DIAGNOSIS AND MANAGEMENT

Chapter 1

Surgical Anatomy, Embryology, and Physiology of the Salivary Glands

John D. Langdon, FKC, MB BS, BDS, MDS, FDSRCS, FRCS, FMedSCi

Outline

Introduction

There are three pairs of major salivary glands consisting of the parotid, submandibular, and sublingual glands. In addition there are numerous minor glands distributed throughout the oral cavity within the mucosa and submucosa.

On average about 0.5 liters of saliva are produced each day but the rate varies throughout the day. At rest, about 0.3 ml/min are produced, but this rises to 2.0 ml/min with stimulation. The contribution from each gland also varies. At rest, the parotid produces 20%, the submandibular gland 65%, and the sublingual and minor glands 15%. On stimulation, the parotid secretion rises to 50%. The nature of the secretion also varies from gland to gland. Parotid secretions are almost exclusively serous, the submandibular secretions are mixed, and the sublingual and minor gland secretions are predominantly mucinous.

Saliva is essential for mucosal lubrication, speech, and swallowing. It also performs an essential buffering role that influences demineralization of teeth as part of the carious process. When there is a marked deficiency in saliva production, xero-stomia, rampant caries, and destructive periodontal disease ensue. Various digestive enzymes—salivary amylase—and antimicrobial agents—IgA, lysozyme, and lactoferrin—are also secreted with the saliva.

The Parotid Gland

EMBRYOLOGY

The parotid gland develops as a thickening of the epithelium in the cheek of the oral cavity in the 15 mm Crown Rump length embryo. This thickening extends backward toward the ear in a plane superficial to the developing facial nerve. The deep aspect of the developing parotid gland produces bud-like projections between the branches of the facial nerve in the third month of intra-uterine life. These projections then merge to form the deep

3

lobe of the parotid gland. By the sixth month of intra-uterine life the gland is completely canalized. Although not embryologically a bilobed structure, the parotid comes to form a larger (80%) superficial lobe and a smaller (20%) deep lobe joined by an isthmus between the two major divisions of the facial nerve. The branches of the nerve lie between these lobes invested in loose connective tissue. This observation is vital in the understanding of the anatomy of the facial nerve and surgery in this region (Berkovitz, Langdon, and Moxham 2003).

ANATOMY

The parotid is the largest of the major salivary glands. It is a compound, tubuloacinar, merocrine, exocrine gland. In the adult, the gland is composed entirely of serous acini.

The gland is situated in the space between the posterior border of the mandibular ramus and the mastoid process of the temporal bone. The external acoustic meatus and the glenoid fossa lie above together with the zygomatic process of the temporal bone (Figure 1.1). On its deep (medial) aspect lies the styloid process of the temporal bone. Inferiorly, the parotid frequently overlaps the angle of the mandible and its deep surface overlies the transverse process of the atlas vertebra.

The shape of the parotid gland is variable. Often it is triangular with the apex directed inferiorly. However, on occasion it is more or less of even width and occasionally it is triangular with the apex superiorly. On average, the gland is 6 cm in length with a maximum of 3.3 cm in width. In 20% of subjects a smaller accessory lobe arises from the upper border of the parotid duct approximately 6 mm in front of the main gland. This accessory lobe overlies the zygomatic arch.

The gland is surrounded by a fibrous capsule previously thought to be formed from the investing layer of deep cervical fascia. This fascia passes up from the neck and was thought to split to enclose the gland. The deep layer is attached to the mandible and the temporal bone at the tympanic plate and styloid and mastoid processes (Berkovitz and Moxham 1988; Ellis 1997; McMinn, Hutchings, and Logan 1984; Williams 1995). Recent investigations suggest that the superficial layer of the parotid capsule is not formed in this way but is part of the superficial musculo-aponeurotic system (SMAS) (Flatau and Mills 1995; Gosain, Yousif, and Madiedo et al. 1993; Jost and Levet 1983; Mitz and Peyronie 1976; Thaller, Kim, and Patterson et al. 1989; Wassef 1987; Zigiotti, Liverani, and Ghibellini 1991). Anteriorly the superficial layer of the parotid capsule is thick and fibrous but more posteriorly it becomes a thin translucent membrane. Within this fascia are scant muscle fibers running parallel with those of the platysma. This superficial layer of the parotid capsule appears to be continuous with the fascia overlying the platysma muscle. Anteriorly it forms a separate layer overlying the

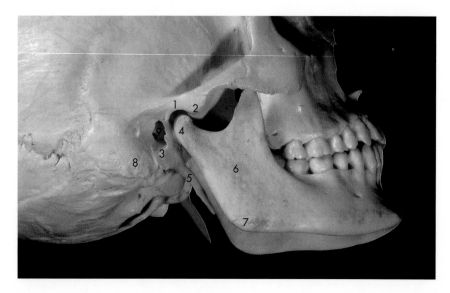

Figure 1.1. A lateral view of the skull showing some of the bony features related to the bed of the parotid gland. 1: Mandibular fossa; 2: Articular eminence; 3: Tympanic plate; 4: Mandibular condyle; 5: Styloid process; 6: Ramus of mandible; 7: Angle of mandible; 8: Mastoid process; 9: External acoustic meatus. Published with permission, Martin Dunitz, London, Langdon JD, Berkowitz BKB, Moxham BJ, editors, Surgical Anatomy of the Infratemporal Fossa.

masseteric fascia, which is itself an extension of the deep cervical fascia. The peripheral branches of the facial nerve and the parotid duct lie within a loose cellular layer between these two sheets of fascia. This observation is important in parotid surgery. When operating on the parotid gland, the skin flap can either be raised in the subcutaneous fat layer or deep to the SMAS layer. The SMAS layer itself can be mobilized as a separate flap and can be used to mask the cosmetic defect following parotidectomy by reattaching it firmly to the anterior border of the sternocleidomastoid muscle as an advancement flap (Meningaud, Bertolus, and Bertrand 2006).

The superior border of the parotid gland (usually the base of the triangle) is closely molded around the external acoustic meatus and the temporomandibular joint. An avascular plane exists between the gland capsule and the cartilaginous and bony acoustic meatus (Figure 1.2). The inferior border (usually the apex) is at the angle of the mandible and often extends beyond this to overlap the digastric triangle, where it may lie very close to the posterior pole of the submandibular salivary

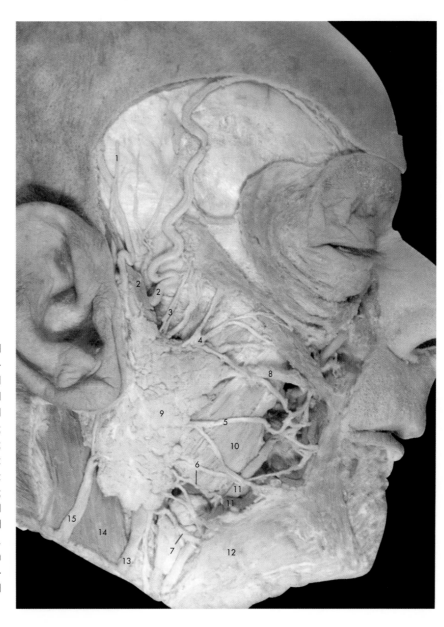

Figure 1.2. The parotid gland and associated structures. 1: Auriculotemporal nerve; 2: Superficial temporal vessels; 3: Temporal branch of facial nerve; 4: Zygomatic branch of facial nerve; 5: Buccal branch of facial nerve; 6: Mandibular branch of facial nerve; 7: Cervical branch of facial nerve; 8: Parotid duct; 9: Parotid gland; 10: Masseter muscle; 11: Facial vessels; 12: Platysma muscle; 13: External jugular vein; 14: Sternocleidomastoid muscle; 15: Great auricular nerve. Published with permission, Martin Dunitz, London, Langdon JD, Berkowitz BKB, Moxham BJ, editors, Surgical Anatomy of the Infratemporal Fossa.

gland. The anterior border just overlaps the posterior border of the masseter muscle and the posterior border overlaps the anterior border of the sternocleidomastoid muscle.

The superficial surface of the gland is covered by skin and platysma muscle. Some terminal branches of the great auricular nerve also lie superficial to the gland. At the superior border of the parotid lie the superficial temporal vessels with the artery in front of the vein. The auriculotemporal branch of the mandibular nerve runs at a deeper level just behind the superficial temporal vessels.

The branches of the facial nerve emerge from the anterior border of the gland. The parotid duct also emerges to run horizontally across the masseter muscle before piercing the buccinator muscle anteriorly to end at the parotid papilla. The transverse facial artery (a branch of the superficial temporal artery) runs across the area parallel to and approximately 1 cm above the parotid duct. The anterior and posterior branches of the facial vein emerge from the inferior border.

The deep (medial) surface of the parotid gland lies on those structures forming the parotid bed. Anteriorly the gland lies over the masseter muscle and the posterior border of the mandibular ramus from the angle up to the condyle. As the gland wraps itself around the ramus it is related to the medial pterygoid muscle at its insertion on to the deep aspect of the angle. More posteriorly, the parotid is molded around the styloid process and the styloglossus, stylohyoid, and stylopharyngeus muscles from below upward. Behind this, the parotid lies on the posterior belly of the digastric muscle and the sternocleidomastoid muscle. The digastric and the styloid muscles separate the gland from the underlying internal jugular vein, the external and internal carotid arteries and the glossopharyngeal, vagus, accessory, and hypoglossal nerves and the sympathetic trunk.

The fascia that covers the muscles in the parotid bed thickens to form two named ligaments (Figure 1.3). The stylomandibular ligament passes from the styloid process to the angle of the mandible. The mandibulostylohyoid ligament (the angular tract) passes between the angle of the mandible and the stylohyoid ligament. Inferiorly it usually extends down to the hyoid bone. These ligaments are all that separates the parotid gland anteriorly from the posterior pole of the superficial lobe of the submandibular gland.

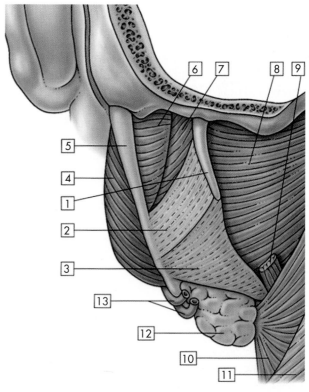

Figure 1.3. The mandibulostylohyoid ligament. 1: Styloid process; 2: Stylomandibular ligament; 3: Mandibulostylohyoid ligament; 4: Masseter muscle; 5: Posterior border of ramus; 6: Lateral pterygoid muscle; 7: Medial pterygoid muscle; 8: Superior pharyngeal constrictor muscle; 9: Stylopharyngeus muscle; 10: Middle pharyngeal constrictor muscle; 11: Inferior pharyngeal constrictor muscle; 12: Submandibular gland; 13: Facial vein and artery. Published with permission, Martin Dunitz, London, Langdon JD, Berkowitz BKB, Moxham BJ, editors, Surgical Anatomy of the Infratemporal Fossa.

CONTENTS OF THE PAROTID GLAND

The Facial Nerve

From superficial to deep, the facial nerve, the auriculotemporal nerve, the retromandibular vein, and the external carotid artery pass through the substance of the parotid gland.

The facial nerve exits the skull base at the stylomastoid foramen. The surgical landmarks are important (Figure 1.4). To expose the trunk of the facial nerve at the stylomastoid foramen the dissection passes down the avascular plane between the parotid gland and the external acoustic canal until the junction of the cartilaginous and bony canals can be palpated. A small triangular extension of the cartilage points toward the facial nerve as it exits

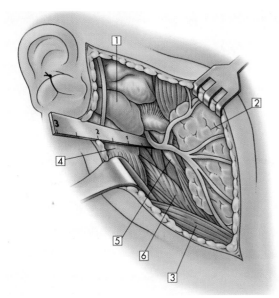

Figure 1.4. Anatomical landmarks of the extratemporal facial nerve. 1: Cartilaginous external acoustic meatus; 2: Parotid gland; 3: Sternocleidomastoid muscle; 4: Tip of the mastoid process; 5: Styloid process; 6: Posterior belly of digastric muscle. Published with permission, Martin Dunitz, London, Langdon JD, Berkowitz BKB, Moxham BJ, editors, Surgical Anatomy of the Infratemporal Fossa.

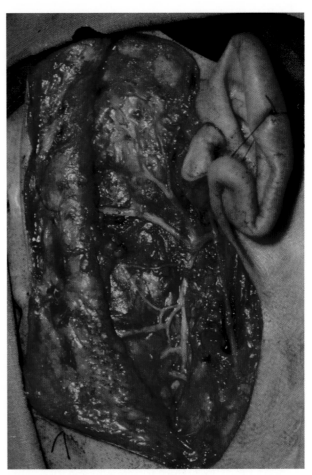

Figure 1.5. Clinical photograph of dissected facial nerve following superficial parotidectomy.

the foramen (Langdon 1998b). The nerve lies about 9 mm from the posterior belly of the digastric muscle and 11 mm from the bony external meatus (Holt 1996). The facial nerve then passes downward and forward over the styloid process and associated muscles for about 1.3 cm before entering the substance of the parotid gland (Hawthorn and Flatau 1990). The first part of the facial nerve gives off the posterior auricular nerve supplying the auricular muscles and also branches to the posterior belly of the digastric and stylohyoid muscles.

On entering the parotid gland the facial nerve separates into two divisions, temporofacial and cervicofacial, the former being the larger. The division of the facial nerve is sometimes called the "pes anserinus" due to its resemblance to the foot of a goose. From the temporofacial and cervicofacial divisions, the facial nerve gives rise to five named branches—temporal, zygomatic, buccal, mandibular, and cervical (Figure 1.5). The peripheral branches of the facial nerve form anastomotic arcades between adjacent branches to form the parotid plexus. These anastomoses are important during facial nerve dissection, as accidental damage to a small branch often fails to result in any facial

weakness due to dual innervation from adjacent branches. Davis et al. (1956) studied these patterns following the dissection of 350 facial nerves in cadavers. The anastomotic relationships between adjacent branches fell into six patterns (Figure 1.6). They showed that in only 6% of cases (type VI) is there any anastomosis between the mandibular branch and adjacent branches. This explains why, when transient facial weakness follows facial nerve dissection, it is usually the mandibular branch that is affected.

Auriculotemporal Nerve

The auriculotemporal nerve arises from the posterior division of the mandibular division of the trigeminal nerve in the infratemporal fossa. It runs backward beneath the lateral pterygoid muscle between the medial aspect of the condylar neck and the sphenomandibular ligament. It enters the

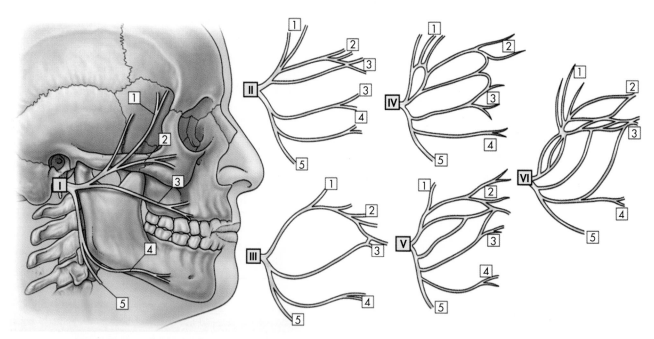

Figure 1.6. The branching patterns of the facial nerve. I: Type I, 13%; II: Type II, 20%; III: Type III, 28%; IV: Type IV, 24%; V: Type V, 9%; VI: Type VI, 6%; 1: Temporal branch; 2: Zygomatic branch; 3: Buccal branch; 4: Mandibular branch; 5: Cervical branch. Published with permission, Martin Dunitz, London, Langdon JD, Berkowitz BKB, Moxham BJ, editors, Surgical Anatomy of the Infratemporal Fossa.

anteromedial surface of the parotid gland passing upward and outward to emerge at the superior border of the gland between the temporomandibular joint and the external acoustic meatus. This nerve communicates widely with the temporofacial division of the facial nerve and limits the mobility of the facial nerve during surgery (Flatau and Mills 1995). Further communications with the temporal and zygomatic branches loop around the transverse facial and superficial temporal vessels (Bernstein and Nelson 1984).

Retromandibular Vein

The vein is formed within the parotid gland by the union of the superficial temporal vein and the maxillary vein. The retromandibular vein passes downward and close to the lower pole of the parotid, where it often divides into two branches passing out of the gland. The posterior branch passes backward to unite with the posterior auricular vein on the surface of the sternocleidomastoid muscle to form the external jugular vein. The anterior branch passes forward to join the facial vein.

The retromandibular vein is an important landmark during parotid gland surgery. The division of the facial nerve into its temporofacial and cervicofacial divisions occurs just behind the retromandibular vein (Figure 1.7). The two divisions lie just superficial to the vein in contact with it. It is all too easy to tear the vein while exposing the division of the facial nerve!

External Carotid Artery

The external carotid artery runs deeply within the parotid gland. It appears from behind the posterior belly of the digastric muscle and grooves the parotid before entering it. It gives off the posterior auricular artery before ascending and dividing into its terminal branches, the superficial temporal and maxillary arteries at the level of the condyle. The superficial temporal artery continues vertically to emerge at the superior border of the gland and crosses the zygomatic arch. Within the substance of the parotid it gives off the transverse facial artery, which emerges at the anterior border of the gland to run across the face above the parotid duct. The maxillary artery emerges from the deep aspect of the gland anteriorly to enter the infratemporal fossa. The maxillary artery gives off the deep auricular artery and the anterior tympanic artery within the substance of the parotid. All these branches from the external carotid also give off numerous

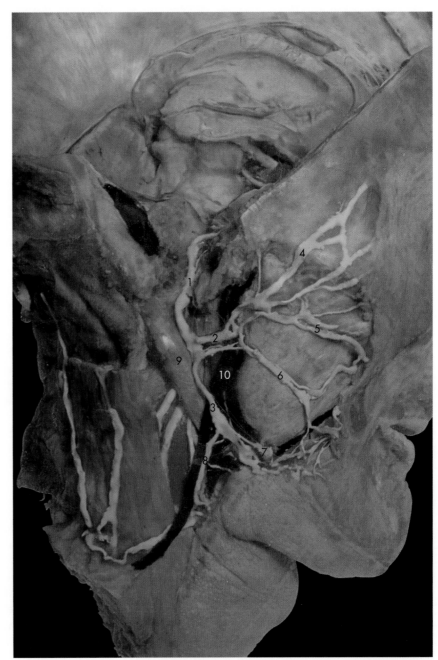

Figure 1.7. The facial nerve and its relationship to the retromandibular vein within the parotid gland. 1: Facial nerve at stylomastoid foramen; 2: Temporofacial branch of facial nerve; 3: Cervicofacial branch of facial nerve; 4: Temporal branch of facial nerve; 5: Zygomatic branch of facial nerve; 6: Buccal branch of facial nerve; 7: Mandibular branch of facial nerve; 8: Cervical branch of facial nerve; 9: Posterior belly of digastric muscle; 10: Retromandibular vein and external carotid artery. Published with permission, Martin Dunitz, London, Langdon JD, Berkowitz BKB, Moxham BJ, editors, Surgical Anatomy of the Infratemporal Fossa.

small branches within the parotid to supply the gland itself.

Parotid Lymph Nodes

Lymph nodes are found within the subcutaneous tissues overlying the parotid to form the preauricular nodes and also within the substance of the gland. There are typically ten nodes within the substance of the gland, the majority being within the superficial lobe and therefore superficial to the plane of the facial nerve. Only one or two nodes lie within the deep lobe (Garetea-Crelgo et al. 1993; Marks 1984; McKean, Lee, and McGregor 1985). All the parotid nodes drain into the upper deep cervical chain.

Parotid Duct

The parotid duct emerges from the anterior border of the parotid gland and passes horizontally across the masseter muscle. The surface markings of the duct are obtained by drawing a line from the lowest point of the alar cartilage to the angle of the mouth (Figure 1.8). This line is bisected and its midpoint is joined with a straight line to the most anterior point of the tragus. This line is divided into three equal parts and the middle section corresponds to the position of the parotid duct. The duct lies approximately 1 cm below the transverse facial vessels. The accessory lobe of the parotid gland, when present, drains into its upper border via one or two tributaries. Anastomosing branches

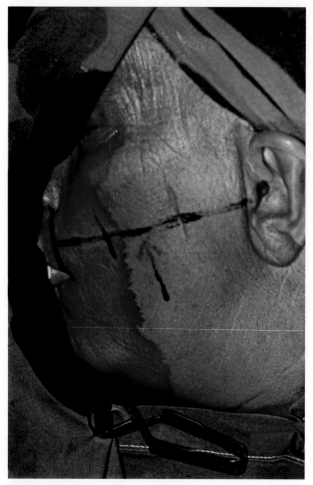

Figure 1.8. The surface markings for the parotid duct.

between the buccal and zygomatic branches of the facial nerve cross the duct. At the anterior border of the masseter, the duct bends sharply to perforate the buccal pad of fat and the buccinator muscle at the level of the upper molar teeth. The duct then bends again to pass forward for a short distance before entering the oral cavity at the parotid papilla.

Nerve Supply to the Parotid

The parasympathetic secretomotor nerve supply comes from the inferior salivatory nucleus in the brain stem (Figure 1.9). From there the fibers run in the tympanic branch of the glossopharyngeal nerve contributing to the tympanic plexus in the middle ear. The lesser petrosal nerve arises from the tympanic plexus leaving the middle ear and running in a groove on the petrous temporal bone in the middle cranial fossa. From here it exits through the foramen ovale to the otic ganglion, which lies on the medial aspect of the mandibular branch of the trigeminal nerve. Postsynaptic postganglionic fibers leave the ganglion to join the auriculotemporal nerve, which distributes the parasympathetic secretomotor fibers throughout the parotid gland. Some authorities suggest that there are also some parasympathetic innervations to the parotid from the chorda tympani branch of the facial nerve.

The sympathetic nerve supply to the parotid arises from the superior cervical sympathetic ganglion. The sympathetic fibers reach the gland via the plexus around the middle meningeal artery. They then pass through the otic ganglion without synapsing and innervate the gland through the auriculotemporal nerve. There is also sympathetic innervation to the gland arising from the plexuses that accompany the blood vessels supplying the gland.

Sensory fibers arising from the connective tissue within the parotid gland merge into the auriculotemporal nerve and pass proximally through the otic ganglion without synapsing. From there the fibers join the mandibular division of the trigeminal nerve. The sensory innervation of the parotid capsule is via the great auricular nerve.

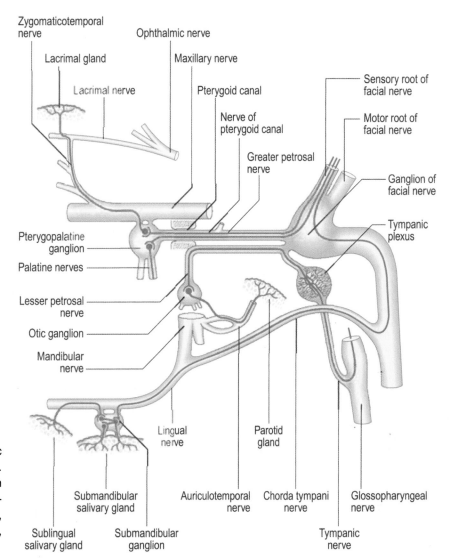

Figure 1.9. The parasympathetic innervations of the salivary glands. The parasympathetic fibers are shown as blue lines. Published with permission, Elsevier Churchill Livingstone, Oxford, Standring S, Editor in Chief, Gray's Anatomy. 39th edition.

The Submandibular Gland

EMBRYOLOGY

The submandibular gland begins to form at the 13 mm stage as an epithelial outgrowth into the mesenchyme forming the floor of the mouth in the linguogingival groove. This proliferates rapidly, giving off numerous branching processes that eventually develop lumina. Initially the developing gland opens into the floor of the mouth posteriorly, lateral to the tongue. The walls of the groove into which it drains come together to form the submandibular duct. This process commences posteriorly and moves forward so that ultimately the orifice of the duct comes to lie anteriorly below the tip of the tongue close to the midline.

ANATOMY

The submandibular gland consists of a larger superficial lobe lying within the digastric triangle in the neck and a smaller deep lobe lying within the floor of the mouth posteriorly (Figure 1.10). The two lobes are continuous with each other around the posterior border of the mylohyoid muscle. As in the parotid gland, the two "lobes" are not true lobes embryologically, as the gland arises as a single epithelial outgrowth. However, surgically it consists of the two lobes as described above. It is a mixed seromucinous gland.

The Superficial Lobe

The superficial lobe lies within the digastric triangle. Its anterior pole reaches the anterior belly of

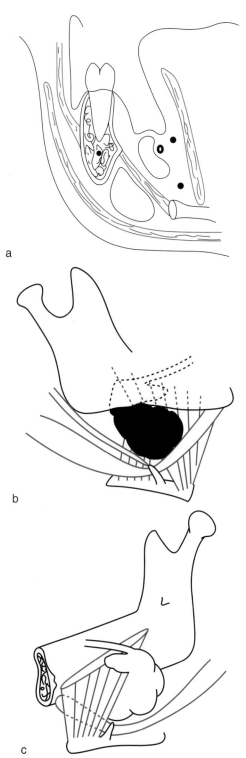

the digastric muscle and the posterior pole reaches the stylomandibular ligament. This structure is all that separates the superficial lobe of the sub-mandibular gland from the parotid gland. It is important to realize just how close the lower pole of the parotid is to the posterior pole of the sub-mandibular gland, as confusion can arise if a mass in the region is incorrectly ascribed to the wrong anatomical structure (Figure 1.2). Superiorly, the superficial lobe lies medial to the body of the mandible. Inferiorly it often overlaps the intermediate tendon of the digastric muscles and the insertion of the stylohyoid. The lobe is partially enclosed between the two layers of the deep cervical fascia that arise from the greater cornu of the hyoid bone and is in intimate proximity of the facial vein and artery (Figure 1.11). The superficial layer of the fascia is attached to the lower border of the mandible and covers the inferior surface of the superficial lobe. The deep layer of fascia is attached to the mylohyoid line on the inner aspect of the mandible and therefore covers the medial surface of the lobe.

The inferior surface, which is covered by skin, subcutaneous fat, platysma, and the deep fascia, is crossed by the facial vein and the cervical

Figure 1.10. The relationship of the superficial and deep lobes of the submandibular gland. Cross-sectional anatomy (a). The superficial lobe from outside (b). The relationship of the deep and superficial lobes to the mylo-hyoid muscle (c).

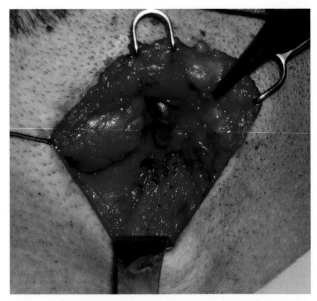

Figure 1.11. Superficial dissection of the left submandibular gland. The investing layer of the deep cervical fascia is elevated off of the submandibular gland and the facial vein is identified.

branch of the facial nerve, which loops down from the angle of the mandible and subsequently innervates the lower lip. The submandibular lymph nodes lie between the salivary gland and the mandible. Sometimes one or more lymph nodes may be embedded within the salivary gland.

The lateral surface of the superficial lobe is related to the submandibular fossa, a concavity on the medial surface of the mandible, and the attachment of the medial pterygoid muscle. The facial artery grooves its posterior part lying at first deep to the lobe and then emerging between its lateral surface and the mandibular attachment of the medial pterygoid muscle from which it reaches the lower border of the mandible.

The medial surface is related anteriorly to the mylohyoid from which it is separated by the mylohyoid nerve and submental vessels. Posteriorly, it is related to the styloglossus, the stylohyoid ligament, and the glossopharyngeal nerve separating it from the pharynx. Between these, the medial aspect of the lobe is related to hyoglossus muscle from which it is separated by styloglossus muscle, the lingual nerve, submandibular ganglion, hypoglossal nerve, and deep lingual vein. More inferiorly, the medial surface is related to the stylohyoid muscle and the posterior belly of the digastric.

The Deep Lobe

The deep lobe of the gland arises from the superficial lobe at the posterior free edge of the mylohyoid muscle and extends forward to the back of the sublingual gland (Figure 1.12). It lies between the mylohyoid muscle inferolaterally, the hyoglossus and styloglossus muscles medially, the lingual nerve superiorly and the hypoglossal nerve and deep lingual vein inferiorly.

The Submandibular Duct

The submandibular duct is about 5 cm long in the adult. The wall of the submandibular duct is thinner than that of the parotid duct. It arises from numerous tributaries in the superficial lobe and emerges from the medial surface of this lobe just behind the posterior border of the mylohyoid. It crosses the deep lobe, passing upward and slightly backward for 5 mm before running forward between the mylohyoid and hyoglossus muscles. As it passes forward, it runs between the sublingual gland and genioglossus to open into the floor of the mouth on

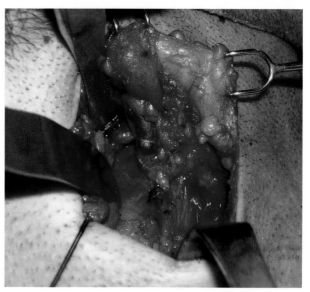

Figure 1.12. Deep dissection of the left submandibular gland. With the submandibular gland retracted, the facial artery is identified in proximity to the facial vein.

the summit of the sublingual papilla at the side of the lingual frenum just below the tip of the tongue. It lies between the lingual and hypoglossal nerves on the hyoglossus. At the anterior border of the hyoglossus muscle it is crossed by the lingual nerve. As the duct traverses the deep lobe of the gland it receives tributaries draining that lobe.

Blood Supply and Lymphatic Drainage

The arterial blood supply arises from multiple branches of the facial and lingual arteries. Venous blood drains predominantly into the deep lingual vein. The lymphatics drain into the deep cervical group of nodes, mostly into the jugulo-omohyoid node, via the submandibular nodes.

Nerve Supply to the Submandibular Gland
Parasympathetic Innervation

The secretomotor supply to the submandibular gland arises from the submandibular (sublingual) ganglion. This is a small ganglion lying on the upper part of the hyoglossus muscle. There are additional ganglion cells at the hilum of the gland. The submandibular ganglion is suspended from the lingual nerve by anterior and posterior filaments (Figure 1.13).

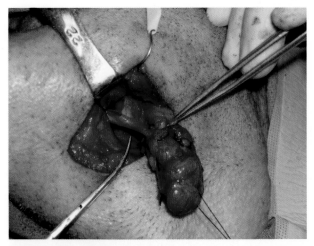

Figure 1.13. Clinical photograph showing the relationship of the lingual nerve to the submandibular gland.

The parasympathetic secretomotor fibers originate in the superior salivatory nucleus and the preganglionic fibers, then travel via the facial nerve, chorda tympani, and lingual nerve to the ganglion via the posterior filaments connecting the ganglion to the lingual nerve. They synapse within the ganglion, and the postganglionic fibers innervate the submandibular and sublingual glands (Figure 1.9). Some fibers are thought to reach the lower pole of the parotid gland.

Sympathetic Innervation

The sympathetic root is derived from the plexus on the facial artery. The postganglionic fibers arise from the superior cervical ganglion and pass through the submandibular ganglion without synapsing. They are vasomotor to the vessels supplying the submandibular and sublingual glands. Five or six branches from the ganglion supply the submandibular gland and its duct. Others pass back into the lingual nerve via the anterior filament to innervate the sublingual and other minor salivary glands in the region.

Sensory Innervation

Sensory fibers arising from the submandibular and sublingual glands pass through the ganglion without synapsing and join the lingual nerve, itself a branch of the trigeminal nerve.

The Sublingual Gland

EMBRYOLOGY

The sublingual gland arises in 20 mm embryos as a number of small epithelial thickenings in the linguogingival groove and on the outer side of the groove. Each thickening forms its own canal and so many of the sublingual ducts open directly onto the summit of the sublingual fold. Those that arise within the linguogingival groove end up draining into the submandibular duct.

ANATOMY

The sublingual gland is the smallest of the major salivary glands. It is almond shaped and weighs approximately 4 g. It is predominantly a mucous gland. The gland lies on the mylohyoid and is covered by the mucosa of the floor of the mouth, which is raised as it overlies the gland to form the sublingual fold. Posteriorly, the sublingual gland is in contact with the deep lobe of the submandibular gland. The sublingual fossa of the mandible is located laterally and the genioglossus muscle is located medially. The lingual nerve and the submandibular duct lie medial to the sublingual gland between it and the genioglossus.

Sublingual Ducts

The gland has a variable number of excretory ducts ranging from 8 to 20. The majority drain into the floor of the mouth at the crest of the sublingual fold. A few drain into the submandibular duct. Sometimes, a collection of draining ducts coalesce anteriorly to form a major duct (Bartholin's duct), which opens with the orifice of the submandibular duct at the sublingual papilla.

Blood Supply, Innervation, and Lymphatic Drainage

The arterial supply is from the sublingual branch of the lingual artery and also the submental branch of the facial artery. Innervation is via the sublingual ganglion as described above. The lymphatics drain to the submental nodes.

Minor Salivary Glands

Minor salivary glands are distributed widely in the oral cavity and oropharynx. They are grouped as labial, buccal, palatoglossal, palatal, and lingual glands. The labial and buccal glands contain both mucous and serous acini, whereas the palatoglossal glands are mucous secreting. The palatal glands, which are also mucous secreting, occur in both the hard and soft palates. The anterior and posterior lingual glands are mainly mucous. The anterior glands are embedded within the muscle ventrally and they drain via four or five ducts near the lingual frenum. The posterior lingual glands are located at the root of the tongue. The deep posterior lingual glands are predominantly serous. Additional serous glands (of von Ebner) occur around the circumvallate papillae on the dorsum of the tongue. Their watery secretion is thought to be important in spreading taste stimuli over the taste buds.

Histology of the Salivary Glands

The salivary glands are composed of large numbers of secretory acini, which may be tubular or globular in shape. Each acinus drains into a duct. These microscopic ducts coalesce to form lobular ducts. Each lobule has its own duct and these then merge to form the main ducts. The individual lobes and lobules are separated by dense connective tissue, which is continuous with the gland capsule. The ducts, blood vessels, lymphatics, and nerves run through and are supported by this connective tissue.

The acini are the primary secretory organs but the saliva is modified as it passes through the intercalated, striated, and excretory ducts before being discharged into the mouth and oropharynx (Figure 1.14). The lobules also contain significant amounts of adipose tissue particularly in the parotid gland. The proportion of adipose tissue relative to excretory acinar cells increases with age.

In the human parotid, the excretory acini are almost entirely serous. In the submandibular gland, again, the secretory units are mostly serous but there are additional mucous tubules and acini. In some areas the mucinous acini have crescentic "caps" of serous cells called serous demilunes. In the sublingual gland the acini are almost entirely mucinous, although there are occasional serous acini or demilunes.

The serous cells contain numerous proteinaceous secretory (zymogen) granules. These granules contain high levels of amylase. In addition, the secretory cells produce kallikrein, lactoferrin, and lysozyme. In mucous cells, the cytoplasm is packed with large pale secretory droplets.

Initially the secretory acini drain into intercalated ducts. These function mainly to conduct the saliva but they may also modify the electrolyte content and secrete immunoglobulin A. The intercalated ducts drain into striated ducts, which coalesce into intralobular and extralobular collecting ducts. The intercalated duct cells are very active metabolically and they transport potassium and bicarbonate into saliva. They reabsorb sodium and chloride ions so that the resulting saliva is hypotonic. They also secrete immunoglobulin A, lysozyme, and kallikrein. The immunoglobulin is produced by plasma cells adjacent to the striated duct cells and it is then transported through the epithelial lining into the saliva. The main collecting ducts are simple conduits for saliva and do not modify the composition of the saliva.

Myoepithelial cells are contractile cells closely related to the secretory acini and also much of the duct system. The myoepithelial cells lie between the basal lamina and the epithelial cells. Numerous cytoplasmic processes arise from them and surround the serous acini as basket cells. Those associated with the duct cells are more fusiform and are aligned along the length of the ducts. The cytoplasm of the myoepithelial cells contains actin myofilaments, which contract as a result of both parasympathetic and sympathetic activity. Thus the myoepithelial cells "squeeze" the saliva out of the secretory acini and ducts and add to the salivary secretory pressure.

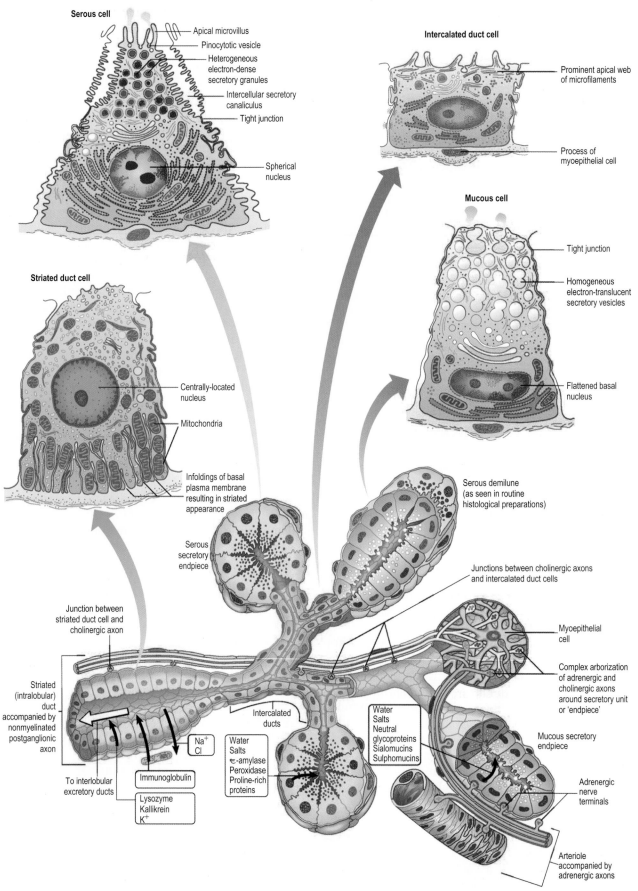

Serous cell

Apical microvillus
Pinocytotic vesicle
Heterogeneous electron-dense secretory granules
Intercellular secretory canaliculus
Tight junction
Spherical nucleus

Intercalated duct cell

Prominent apical web of microfilaments
Process of myoepithelial cell

Mucous cell

Tight junction
Homogeneous electron-translucent secretory vesicles
Flattened basal nucleus

Striated duct cell

Centrally-located nucleus
Mitochondria
Infoldings of basal plasma membrane resulting in striated appearance

Serous demilune (as seen in routine histological preparations)

Serous secretory endpiece

Junctions between cholinergic axons and intercalated duct cells

Myoepithelial cell

Complex arborization of adrenergic and cholinergic axons around secretory unit or 'endpiece'

Junction between striated duct cell and cholinergic axon

Striated (intralobular) duct accompanied by nonmyelinated postganglionic axon

To interlobular excretory ducts

Na⁺
Cl

Immunoglobulin

Lysozyme
Kallikrein
K⁺

Intercalated ducts

Water
Salts
∈-amylase
Peroxidase
Proline-rich proteins

Water
Salts
Neutral glycoproteins
Sialomucins
Sulphomucins

Mucous secretory endpiece

Adrenergic nerve terminals

Arteriole accompanied by adrenergic axons

Figure 1.14. Diagram showing the histology of the major components of the salivary glands. Published with permission, Elsevier Churchill Livingstone, Oxford, Standring S, Editor in Chief, Gray's Anatomy, 39th edition.

Control of Salivation

There is a continuous low background saliva production that is stimulated by drying of the oral and pharyngeal mucosa. A rapid increase in the resting levels occurs as a reflex in response to masticatory stimuli including the mechanoreceptors and taste fibers. Other sensory modalities such as smell are also involved. The afferent input is via the salivatory centers, which are themselves influenced by the higher centers. The higher centers may be facilitory or inhibitory depending on the circumstances. The efferent secretory drive to the salivary glands passes via the parasympathetic and sympathetic pathways. There are no peripheral inhibitory mechanisms.

Cholinergic nerves (parasympathetic) often accompany ducts and branch freely around the secretory endpieces (acini). Adrenergic nerves (sympathetic) usually enter the glands along the arteries and arterioles and ramify with them. Within the glands, the nerve fibers intermingle such that cholinergic and adrenergic axons frequently lie in adjacent invaginations of a single Schwann cell. Secretion and vasoconstriction are mediated by separate sympathetic axons, whereas a single parasympathetic axon may, through serial terminals, result in vasodilatation, secretion, and constriction of myoepithelial cells.

Secretory endpieces are the most densely innervated structures in the salivary glands. Individual acinar cells may have both cholinergic and adrenergic nerve endings. The secretion of water and electrolytes, which accounts for the volume of saliva produced, results from a complex set of stimuli that are largely parasympathetic. The active secretion of proteins into the saliva depends upon the relative levels of both sympathetic and parasympathetic stimulation.

Although the ducts are less densely innervated than secretory acini, they do influence the composition of the saliva. Adrenal aldosterone promotes resorption of sodium and secretion of potassium into the saliva by striated ductal cells. Myoepithelial cell contraction is stimulated predominantly by adrenergic fibers, although there may be an additional role for cholinergic axons.

Summary

- Although embryologically the parotid consists of a single lobe, anatomically the facial nerve lies in a distinct plane between the anatomical superficial and deep lobes.
- There are fixed anatomical landmarks indicating the origin of the extracranial facial nerve as it leaves the stylomastoid foramen.
- The lower pole of the parotid gland is separated from the posterior pole of the submandibular gland by only thin fascia. This can lead to diagnostic confusion in determining the origin of a swelling in this area.
- The relationship of the submandibular salivary duct to the lingual nerve is critical to the safe removal of stones within the duct.
- Great care must be taken to identify the lingual nerve when excising the submandibular gland. The lingual nerve is attached to the gland by the parasympathetic fibers synapsing in the submandibular (sublingual) ganglion.
- The sublingual gland may drain into the submandibular duct or it may drain directly into the floor of the mouth via multiple secretory ducts.

References

Berkovitz BKB, Langdon JD, Moxham BJ. 2003. The facial nerve and the parotid gland. In: Langdon JD, Berkovitz BKB, Moxham BJ (eds), Surgical Anatomy of the Infratemporal Fossa. London: Martin Dunitz, pp. 181–206.

Berkovitz BKB, Moxham BJ. 1988. A Textbook of Head and Neck Anatomy. London: Wolfe.

Bernstein L, Nelson RH. 1984. Surgical anatomy of the extraparotid distribution of the facial nerve. *Arch Otolaryngol* 110:177–183.

Davis RA, Anson BJ, Budinger JM, Kurth LE. 1956. Surgical anatomy of the facial nerve and parotid gland based on 350 cervicofacial halves. *Surg Gynecol Obstet* 102:385–412.

Ellis H. 1997. Clinical Anatomy (9th ed.). Oxford: Blackwell.

Flatau AT, Mills PR. 1995. Regional anatomy. In: Norman JE deB, McGurk M (eds.), Color Atlas and Text of the Salivary Glands. London: Mosby Wolfe, pp. 13–39.

Garetea-Crelgo J, Gay-Escoda C, Bermejo B, Buenechea-Imaz R. 1993. Morphological studies of the parotid lymph nodes. *J Cranio-Maxillo-Facial Surg* 21:207–209.

Gosain AK, Yousif NJ, Madiedo G et al. 1993. Surgical anatomy of the SMAS: A reinvestigation. *Plast Reconstr Surg* 92:1254–1263.

Hawthorn R, Flatau A. 1990. Temporomandibular joint anatomy. In: Norman JE deB, Bramley P (eds.), A Textbook and Colour Atlas of the Temporomandibular Joint. London: Mosby Wolfe, pp. 1–51.

Holt JJ. 1996. The stylomastoid area: Anatomic-histologic study and surgical approach. *Laryngoscope* 106:396–399.

Jost G, Levet Y. 1983. Parotid fascia and face lifting: A critical evaluation of the SMAS concept. *Plast Reconstr Surg* 74:42–51.

Langdon JD. 1998. Sublingual and submandibular gland excision. In: Langdon JD, Patel MF (eds.), Operative Maxillofacial Surgery. London: Chapman & Hall, pp. 376–380.

Langdon JD. 1998. Parotid surgery. In: Langdon JD, Patel MF (eds.), Operative Maxillofacial Surgery. London: Chapman & Hall, pp. 386–388.

Marks NJ. 1984. The anatomy of the lymph nodes of the parotid gland. *Clin Otolaryngol* 9:271–275.

McKean ME, Lee K, McGregor IA. 1985. The distribution of lymph nodes in and around the parotid gland: An anatomical study. *Br J Plast Surg* 38:1–5.

McMinn RMH, Hutchings RT, Logan BM. 1984. A Colour Atlas of Applied Anatomy. London: Wolfe.

Meningaud J-P, Bertolus C, Bertrand J-C. 2006. Parotidectomy: Assessment of a surgical technique including facelift incision and SMAS advancement. *J Cranio-Maxillofacial Surg* 34:34–37.

Mitz V, Peyronie M. 1976. The superficial musculo-aponeurotic system (SMAS) in the parotid and cheek area. *Plast Reconstr Surg* 58:80–88.

Thaller SR, Kim S, Patterson H et al. 1989. The submuscular aponeurotic system (SMAS): A histologic and comparative anatomy evaluation. *Plast Reconstr Surg* 86:691–696.

Wassef M. 1987. Superficial fascia and muscular layers in the face and neck: A histological study. *Aesthetic Plast Surg* 11:171–176.

Williams PL (ed.). 1995. Gray's Anatomy (38th ed.). Oxford: Blackwell.

Zigiotti GL, Liverani MB, Ghibellini D. 1991. The relationship between parotid and superficial fasciae. *Surg Radiol Anat* 13:293–300.

Chapter 2

Diagnostic Imaging of Salivary Gland Pathology

Pradeep K. Jacob, MD, MBA

Outline

Introduction

Anatomic and functional diagnostic imaging plays a central role in modern medicine. Virtually all specialties of medicine to varying degrees depend on diagnostic imaging for diagnosis, therapy, and follow-up of treatment. Because of the complexity of the anatomy, treatment of diseases of the head and neck, including those of the salivary glands, are particularly dependent on quality medical imaging and interpretation. Medical diagnostic imaging is divided primarily into two major categories, anatomic and functional. The *anatomic* imaging modalities include computed tomography (CT), magnetic resonance imaging (MRI), and ultrasonography (US). Although occasionally obtained, plain film radiography for the head and neck, including salivary gland disease, is mostly of historical interest. In a similar manner, the use of sialography has been significantly reduced, although both plain films and sialography are of some use in imaging sialoliths. *Functional* diagnostic imaging techniques include planar scintigraphy, single photon emission computed tomography (SPECT), positron emission tomography (PET), and magnetic resonance spectroscopy (MRS), all of which are promising technologies. Recently, the use of a combined anatomic and functional modality in the form of PET/CT has proved invaluable in head and neck imaging. Previously widely employed procedures including gallium radionuclide imaging are less important today than in the past.

Imaging Modalities

COMPUTED TOMOGRAPHY (CT)

Computed tomography has become indispensable in the diagnosis, treatment, and follow-up of diseases of the head and neck. The latest generation of multiple-row detector CT (MDCT) provides excellent soft tissue and osseous delineation. The rapid speed with which images can be obtained along with the high spatial resolution and tissue contrast make CT the imaging modality of choice in head and neck imaging. True volumetric data sets obtained from multidetector row scanners allow for excellent coronal, sagittal, or oblique reformation of images as well as a variety of 3-D renderings. This allows the radiologist and surgeon to characterize a lesion and assess involvement of adjacent structures or local spread from the orthogonal projections or three-dimensional rendering. The ability to manipulate images is critical when assessing pathology in complex anatomy, such as evaluation of parotid gland masses to determine deep lobe involvement, facial nerve involvement, or extension into the skull base. Images in the coronal plane are important in evaluating the submandibular gland in relation to the floor of the mouth. Lymphadenopathy and its relationship to the carotid sheath and its contents and other structures are also well delineated. CT is also superior to MRI in demonstrating bone detail and calcifications. CT is also the fastest method of imaging head and neck anatomy. Other advantages include

widespread availability of scanners, high-resolution images, and speed of image acquisition, which also reduces motion artifacts. Exposure to ionizing radiation and the administration of IV contrast are the only significant disadvantages to CT scanning.

CT Technique

The CT scanner contains a gantry, which holds an X-ray tube and a set of detectors. The X-ray tube is positioned opposite the detectors and is physically coupled. A "fan beam" of X-rays is produced and passes through the patient to the detectors as the tube and detector rotate around the patient. In the newer generation of scanners, the multiple rows of detectors are fixed around the gantry and only the tube rotates. A table carries the patient through the gantry. The detectors send signals, dependent on the degree of X-ray attenuation, to a computer, which uses this data to construct an image using complex algorithms.

For most CT studies (especially in the head and neck), intravenous contrast is administered. IV contrast is a solution consisting of organic compounds bonded with iodine molecules. Iodine is a dense atom with an atomic weight of 127, which is good at absorbing X-rays and is biocompatible. IV contrast readily attenuates the X-ray beam at concentrations optimal for vascular and soft tissue "enhancement," but short of causing attenuation-related artifacts. Streak artifacts, however, can occur if the concentration is too high, as seen occasionally at the thoracic inlet and supraclavicular region from dense opacification of the subclavian vein during rapid bolus injection of IV contrast.

CT of the neck should be performed with intravenous contrast whenever possible to optimize delineation of masses and inflammatory or infectious changes in the tissues and to enhance vascular structures. Imaging is obtained from the level of the orbits through the aortic arch in the axial plane with breath hold. The images are reconstructed using a computer algorithm to optimize soft tissue delineation, and displayed in soft tissue window and level settings (Figures 2.1 and 2.2). In a similar manner images are reconstructed using a computer algorithm to optimize bone details as more sharp and defined (Figure 2.3). The lung apex is often imaged in a complete neck evaluation and displayed using lung window settings

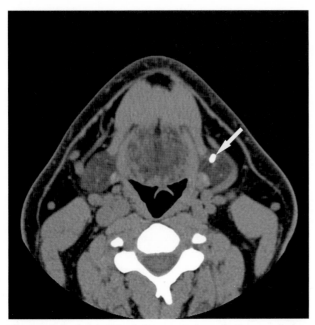

Figure 2.1. Axial CT of the neck in soft tissue window without contrast demonstrating poor definition between soft tissue structures. The blood vessels are unopacified and cannot be easily distinguished from lymph nodes. Note the sialolith (arrow) in the hilum of the left submandibular gland.

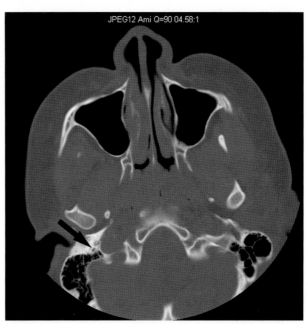

Figure 2.3. Axial CT of the skull base reconstructed in a sharp algorithm and in bone window and level display demonstrating sharp bone detail. Note the sharply defined normal right stylomastoid foramen (arrow).

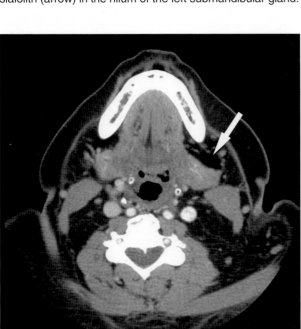

Figure 2.2. Axial CT of the neck in soft tissue window with IV contrast demonstrates improved visualization of structures with enhancement of tissues and vasculature. Note the small lipoma (arrow) anterior to the left submandibular gland, which distorts the anterior aspect of the gland with slight posterior displacement.

(Figure 2.4a). Dedicated CT scans of the chest are beneficial in the postoperative evaluation of patients with salivary gland malignancies, as lung nodules can be observed, possibly indicative of metastatic disease (Figure 2.4b). Multiplanar reformatted images of the neck are obtained typically in the coronal and sagittal planes (Figures 2.5 and 2.6), although they may be obtained in virtually any plane desired or in a 3-D rendering.

The Hounsfield unit (H) (named for Godfrey Hounsfield, inventor of the CT scanner) is the unit of density measurement for CT. These units are assigned based on the degree of attenuation of the X-ray beam by tissue in a given voxel (volume element) and are assigned relative to water (0 H) (Table 2.1). The scale ranges from −1024 H for air, to +4000 H for very dense bone. The images are created based on a grayscale from black (−1024 H) to white (+4000 H) and shades of gray. Despite the wide range of units, the majority of tissues in the human body are between −100 and +100 H. Soft tissues and parenchymal organs are in a range between 20 and 80 H, whereas fat is approximately −100 H. Simple fluid is 0 H, but proteinaceous fluid can be upward of 25 H. Unclotted and clotted

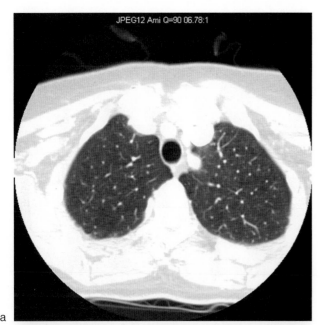

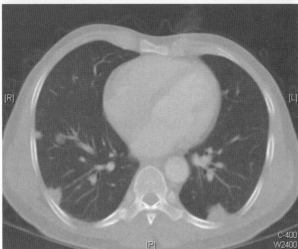

Figure 2.4. Axial CT of the neck at the thoracic inlet in lung windows demonstrating lung parenchyma (a). Axial image of dedicated CT of chest demonstrating cannon ball lesions in a patient previously treated for adenoid cystic carcinoma of the palate (b). These lesions are representative of diffuse metastatic disease of the lungs, but not pathognomonic of adenoid cystic carcinoma.

blood varies depending on the hemoglobin concentration and hematocrit, but average measurements are 50 H and 80 H, respectively. CT images are displayed using a combination of "window widths" (WW, range of CT numbers from black to white), and "window levels" (WL, position of the

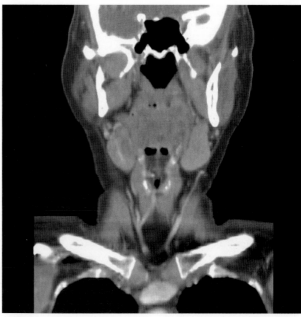

Figure 2.5. Coronal CT reformation of the neck in soft tissue window at the level of the submandibular glands. Orthogonal images with MDCT offer very good soft tissue detail in virtually any plane of interest in order to assess anatomic and pathologic relationships.

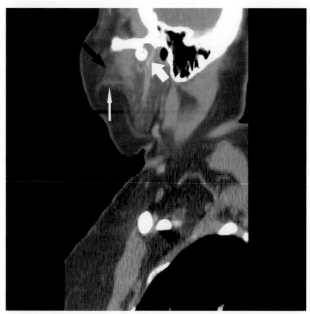

Figure 2.6. Sagittal CT reformation of the neck in soft tissue window at the level of the parotid gland. Note the accessory parotid gland (black arrow) sitting atop the parotid (Stenson's) duct (thin white arrow). Also note the retromandibular vein (large white arrow) and external auditory canal.

Table 2.1. CT density in Hounsfield units (H).

Tissue or Structure	Hounsfield Unit (H)
Water or CSF	0
Fat	−100
Soft tissue, muscle (a)	50–60
Unclotted blood (b)	35–50
Clotted blood (b)	50–75
Parotid gland (c)	−10 to +30
Submandibular gland (c)	+30–+60
Sublingual gland (d)	60–90
Bone	1000
Lung	−850
Air	−1024
Calcification	150–200
Grey matter	35–40
White matter	25–35

(a) Depends on degree of fat deposition.
(b) Depends on the hemoglobin concentration and hematocrit.
(c) Depends on age and fat deposition.
(d) Very limited evaluation secondary to partial volume effect.
CSF = cerebrospinal fluid.

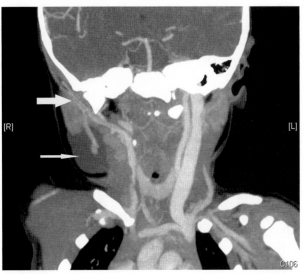

Figure 2.7. CT angiogram of the neck at the level of the parotid gland demonstrating the retromandibular vein and adjacent external carotid artery (large white arrow). Note the right cervical lymphangioma (thin white arrow) associated with the tail of the right parotid gland.

window on the scale), which are based on the attenuation characteristics of tissues. Typically, head and neck images are interpreted using "soft tissue windows" (WW 500 H, WL 30 H), "bone windows" (WW 2000, WL 500), or "lung windows" (WW 1500, WL −500). "Soft tissue windows" demonstrate the slight density differences of soft tissues, whereas "bone windows" demonstrate cortical and medullary features of bones with sharp detail. "Lung windows" demonstrate the sharp interface of air and the fine soft tissue components of lung parenchyma.

Although the density of the salivary glands is variable, the parotid glands tend to be slightly lower in density relative to muscle, secondary to a higher fat content, and become progressively more fat replaced over time. The CT density of parotid glands varies from −10 to +30 H. The submandibular glands are denser than parotid glands and are equivalent in density to muscle. The submandibular glands vary in density from +30 to +60 H.

CT angiography (CTA) is a powerful method that allows visualization of arterial vasculature, demonstrating the vascular anatomy of arteries and veins. CTA can be critical in preoperative evaluation to determine the degree of vascularity of lesions and to plan an appropriate surgical approach to minimize blood loss or perform preoperative embolization. CTA is obtained with fast image acquisition over a defined region of interest while administering a rapid IV contrast bolus timed to arrive in the region of interest during image acquisition. CTA images may be rendered in 3-D data sets and rotated in any plane (Figure 2.7). CTA is not only useful for preoperative planning; it can also be quite useful in diagnosis of salivary gland vascular pathology such as aneurysms or arteriovenous fistulae (AVFs) (Wong, Ahuja, and King et al. 2004).

CT scanning, as with all imaging modalities, is prone to artifacts. Artifacts can be caused by motion, very dense or metallic implants (dental amalgam), and volume averaging. Motion artifact is common and may result from breathing, swallowing, coughing, or sneezing during the image acquisition or from an unaware or uncooperative patient. Metallic implants cause complete attenuation of X-rays in the beam and result in focal loss of data and bright and dark streaks in the image. Because the image is created from a three-dimensional section of tissue averaged to form a two-dimensional image, the partial volume or volume averaging artifact results from partial inclusion of structures in adjacent images. Finally, the beam hardening artifact is produced by attenuation of low energy X-rays, by dense objects, from the energy spectrum of the X-ray beam, resulting in a residual average high energy beam (or hard X-rays), which results in loss of data and dark lines on the image. This phenomenon is often seen in the posterior fossa of head CT scans caused by the very dense petrous bones. A multidetector row CT scanner can help reduce metallic artifacts using advanced algorithms, and can reduce motion artifacts secondary to faster scanning speeds.

Advanced Computed Tomography

Newer CT techniques including CT perfusion and dynamic contrast enhanced multi-slice CT have been studied. Dynamic multi-slice contrast enhanced CT is obtained while scanning over a region of interest and simultaneously administering IV contrast. The characteristics of tissues can then be studied as the contrast bolus arrives at the lesion and "washes in" to the tumor, reaches a peak presence within the mass, and then decreases over time, that is, "washes out." This technique has demonstrated differences in various histologic types of tumors, for example, with early enhancement in Warthin's tumor with a time to peak at 30 seconds and subsequent fast washout. The malignant tumors show a time to peak at 90 seconds. The pleomorphic adenomas demonstrate a continued rise in enhancement in all four phases (Yerli, Aydin, and Coskum et al. 2007).

CT perfusion attempts to study physiologic parameters of blood volume, blood flow, mean transit time, and capillary permeability surface product. Statistically significant differences between malignant and benign tumors have been demonstrated with the mean transit time measurement. A rapid mean transit time of less then 3.5 seconds is seen with most malignant tumors, but with benign tumors or normal tissue the mean transit time is significantly longer (Rumboldt, Al-Okkaili, and Deveikis 2005).

MAGNETIC RESONANCE IMAGING (MRI)

Magnetic resonance imaging represents imaging technology with great promise in characterizing salivary gland pathology. The higher tissue contrast of MRI, when compared to CT, enables subtle differences in soft tissues to be demonstrated. Gadolinium contrast enhanced MRI further and accentuates the soft tissue contrast. Subtle pathologic states such as perineural spread of disease are better delineated when compared with CT. This along with excellent resolution and exquisite details make MRI a very powerful technique in head and neck imaging, particularly at the skull base. However, its susceptibility to motion artifacts and long imaging time as well as contraindication due to claustrophobia, pacemakers, aneurysm clips, and deep brain and vagal nerve stimulators limit its usefulness in the general population as a *routine* initial diagnostic and follow-up imaging modality. Many of the safety considerations are well defined and detailed on the popular Web site www.mrisafety.com.

MRI Technique

Although the physics and instrumentation of MRI are beyond the scope of this text, a fundamental understanding of the variety of different imaging sequences and techniques should be understood by clinicians in order to facilitate reciprocal communication of the clinical problem and understanding of imaging reports.

In contrast to CT, which is based on the use of ionizing radiation, MRI utilizes a high magnetic field and pulsed radiofrequency waves in order to create an image or obtain spectroscopic data. MRI is based on the proton (hydrogen ion) distribution throughout the body. The basic concept is that protons are normally oriented in a random state. However, once placed in the imaging magnet, a high magnetic field, a large proportion of protons align with the magnetic field. The protons remain aligned and precess (spin) in the magnetic field until an external force acts upon them and forces them out of alignment. This force is an applied radiofrequency pulse, used for a specified time and specified frequency by an antenna called a transmit coil. As the protons return to the aligned state, they give off energy in the form of their own radiofrequency pulse, determined by their local chemical state and tissue structure. The radiofrequency pulse given off is captured by an antenna, called a receive coil. The energy of the pulse and location is recorded and the process repeated multiple times and averaged, as the signal is weak. The recorded signal is used to form the image. Several different types of applied pulse sequences of radio waves result in different types of images.

The impact of MRI is in the soft tissue contrast that can be obtained, non-invasively. The relaxation times of tissues can be manipulated to bring out soft tissue detail. The routine sequences used in clinical scanning are spin-echo (SE), gradient echo (GRE), and echo-planar (EPI). Typical pulse sequences for head and neck and brain imaging include spin-echo T1, spin-echo T2, proton density (PD), FLAIR, dwi, post-contrast T1, and STIR. A variant of the spin-echo, the fast spin-echo sequence (FSE), allows for a more rapid acquisition of spin-echo images. Any one of these can be obtained in the three standard orientations of axial, coronal, and sagittal planes. Oblique planes may be obtained in special circumstances.

Spin-Echo T1

On T1 weighted images a short repetition time (tr) and short echo time (te) are applied, resulting in an image commonly used for anatomic depiction. Water signal is very low and is displayed as dark gray to black pixels on the grayscale. Fat is very bright, allowing tissue planes to be delineated. Fast flowing blood is devoid of signal and is therefore very black. Muscle tissue is an intermediate gray. Bone that has few free protons is also largely devoid of signal. Bone marrow, however, will vary depending on the relative percentage of red versus yellow marrow. Red marrow will have a signal similar to but slightly lower than muscle, whereas yellow marrow (fat replaced) will be bright. In the brain, cerebrospinal fluid (CSF) is dark, and flowing blood is black. Grey matter is dark relative to white matter (contains fatty myelin), but both are higher than CSF but less than fat. Cysts (simple) are dark in signal unless they are complicated by hemorrhage or infection or have elevated protein concentration, which results in an increased signal and slightly brighter display (Figure 2.8, Table 2.2).

Spin-Echo T2

The T2 images are obtained with a long tr and te. The T2 image is sensitive to the presence of water in tissues and depicts edema as a very bright signal. Therefore, CSF or fluid-containing structures such as cysts are very bright. Complicated cysts can vary in T2 images. If hemorrhagic, they can have a heterogenous or even uniformly dark signal caused by a susceptibility artifact. These

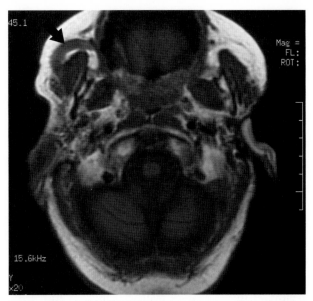

Figure 2.8. Axial MRI T1 weighted image at level of the skull base and brainstem without contrast demonstrating high signal in the subcutaneous fat, intermediate signal of the brain, and low signal of the CSF and mucosa. Note dilated right parotid duct (arrow).

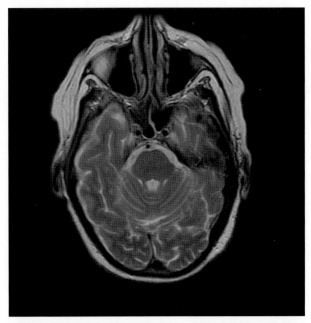

Figure 2.9. Axial MRI FSE T2 weighted image demonstrating the high signal of CSF and subcutaneous fat, intermediate signal of the brain and mucosa, and the low signal in the arteries.

artifacts can be caused by metals, melanin, forms of calcium, and the iron in hemoglobin. Increased tissue water from edema stands out as bright relative to the isointense soft tissue. The fast spin-echo T2 is a common sequence that is many times faster than the conventional spin-echo T2 but does alter the image. Fat stays brighter on the fast spin-echo (FSE) sequence relative to the conventional (Figure 2.9, Table 2.2).

Proton Density Images (PD)
Proton density images are obtained with a long tr but short te, resulting in an image with less tissue contrast but high signal to noise ratio. These are uncommonly used in the head and neck.

Gradient Recalled Echo Imaging (GRE)
Gradient recalled echo imaging is the second most common type of imaging sequence after the spin-

Table 2.2. Tissue characteristics on T1 and T2 MRI.*

	T1	T2
Increased signal	– Fat – Calcium (a) – Proteinaceous fluid (high) (b) – Slow-flowing blood – Melanin – Hyperacute hemorrhage (#) (oxyhemoglobin) – Subacute hemorrhage (intracellular and extracellular methemoglobin) – Gadolinium contrast – Manganese – Cholesterol	– Water (CSF) or edema – Proteinaceous fluid – Hyperacute hemorrhage (oxyhemoglobin – Subacute hemorrhage (extracellular methemoglobin) – Slow-flowing blood – Fat (FSE T2 scans)
Intermediate signal	– Hyperacute hemorrhage (oxyhemoglobin) – Acute hemorrhage (deoxyhemoglobin) – Calcium (a) – Grey matter – White matter (brighter than grey matter) – Soft tissue (muscle) – Proteinaceous fluid (b)	– Grey matter (brighter than white matter) – White matter – Proteinaceous fluid (b) – Calcium (a)
Decreased signal	– Water (CSF) or edema – Fast-flowing blood – Calcium (a) – Soft tissue – Acute hemorrhage (deoxyhemoglobin) – Chronic hemorrhage (hemosiderin) – Calcification – Air – Simple cyst (low protein)	– Calcium (a) – Melanin – Hemosiderin – Flowing blood – Hemorrhagic cyst – Iron deposition – Acute hemorrhage (deoxyhemoglobin) – Early subacute hemorrhage (intracellular methemoglobin) – Chronic hemorrhage (hemosiderin) – Air – Fast flow – Fat (conventional or non-FSE T2 scan)

(*) MRI signal on T1 and T2 predominantly from intracranial exam at 1.5T (Tesla).

(#) MRI signal of intracranial hemorrhage is quite complex and dependent on multiple factors with degrees of variability.

(a) Signal from calcium deposition is complex. Calcium concentration of under 30% by weight has high T1 signal and intermediate T2 signal, but over 40% has decreasing signal on T1 and T2. The surface area of the calcium particle also has an effect, with large surface area resulting in increased T1 signal (Henkelman, Watts, and Kucharczyk 1991).

(b) Depends on the protein concentration (complex cysts, abscess).

CSF = cerebrospinal fluid.

echo. This sequence is very susceptible (more than spin-echo T2) to magnetic field inhomogeneity and is commonly used in the brain to identify blood products and metal deposition such as iron, manganese, and non-metals such as calcium. This sequence is very sensitive but not specific. The "flip angle" used in obtaining GRE can be altered resulting in either T1 weighted (long flip angle) or T2 weighted (short flip angle) images (Figure 2.10).

Short Tau Inversion Recovery (STIR)

Short tau inversion recovery is commonly acquired because of its very high sensitivity to fluid and ready detection of subtle edema in tissues. When acquired in the conventional method, STIR also results in nulling the fat signal, thereby further increasing the signal of tissue fluid relative to background. This is the best sequence for edema, particularly when trying to determine bone invasion by tumors. It can also be useful in assessing skull base foramina (Figures 2.11 and 2.12).

Gadolinium (Gd) Contrast

Intravenous contrast with gadolinium, a paramagnetic element, alters (shortens) T1 and T2 relaxation times, which results in a brighter signal. Its

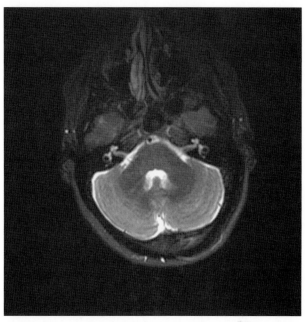

Figure 2.11. Axial MRI STIR image at the skull base demonstrating the high signal of CSF but suppression of subcutaneous fat signal.

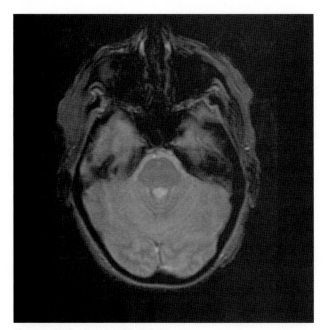

Figure 2.10. Axial MRI GRE image.

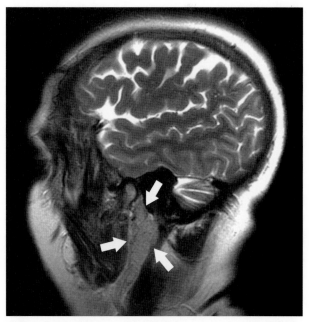

Figure 2.12. Sagittal MRI STIR image at the level of the parotid gland demonstrating the deep lobe seen through the stylomandibular tunnel (arrows). Note the parotid gland extending superiorly to the skull base.

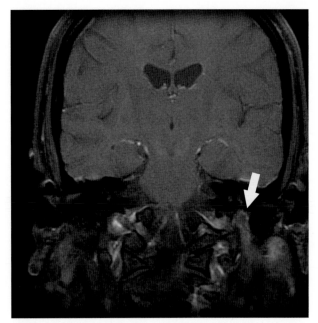

Figure 2.13. Coronal MRI T1 post-contrast fat saturated image of the skull base demonstrating a mass in the left parotid gland extending to the stylomastoid foramen (arrow). Note the mild vascular enhancement and suppression of fat high signal on T1 weighted image.

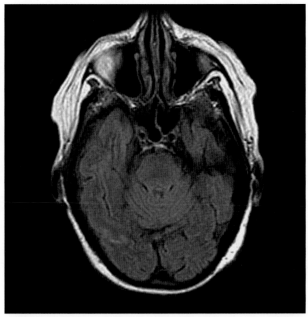

Figure 2.14. Axial MRI FLAIR image at the skull base demonstrating CSF flow-related artifactual increased signal in the right prepontine cistern.

effect is greater on T1 than on T2 weighted images. Areas of tissue that accumulate Gd will have a higher or brighter signal and "enhance." In the head and neck, post-contrast T1 images should be performed with fat saturation to null the fat signal and therefore increase the signal of Gd accumulation (Figure 2.13).

Fluid Attenuation Inversion Recovery (FLAIR)

Fluid attenuation inversion recovery is not as commonly used in the neck but is a necessity in brain imaging. By nulling the CSF signal, brain tissue edema from a variety of causes stands out and is easily identified. It is, however, not specific. FLAIR can be useful for assessing skull base or foraminal invasion by tumors. However, artifacts can result from CSF pulsation or high FiO_2 administration and can mimic pathologic processes such as subarachnoid hemorrhage or meningitis (bacterial, carcinomatous, viral, or aseptic) (Figure 2.14).

Diffusion Weighted Images (DWI)

Diffusion weighted images are not routinely clinically used in the neck or head but are indispens-

able in the brain. Typical intracranial application is for assessing acute stroke, but can be applied for the assessment of active multiple sclerosis (MS) plaques, and abscesses (Figure 2.15). The concept of DWI is based on the molecular motion of water and the sensitivity of certain MRI sequences to detect the diffusion or movement of water in tissues at the cellular level.

The use of DWI and specifically apparent diffusion coefficient (ADC) values and maps for salivary gland imaging are under investigation and show promise in differentiating benign from malignant tissues (Abdel Razek, Kandeel, and Soliman et al. 2007; Eida, Sumi, and Sakihama et al. 2007; Habermann, Gossrau, and Kooijman et al. 2007; Shah et al. 2003). The ADC values are affected by technical factors (b-value setting, image resolution, choice of region-of-interest, susceptibility artifacts, and adequate shimming) as well as physiologic factors (biochemical composition of tumors, hemorrhage, perfusion, and salivary flow) (Eida, Sumi, and Sakihama et al. 2007). The ADC values of salivary glands change with gustatory stimulation. Although there are mixed results reported, there is generally an increase in the ADC value from pre-stimulation to post-stimulation measurements (Habermann, Gossrau, and Kooijman et al.

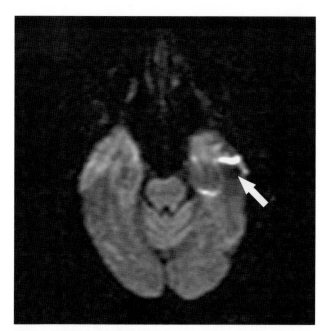

Figure 2.15. Axial MRI DWI image at the skull base demonstrating susceptibility artifact adjacent to the left temporal bone (arrow).

2007). The normal parotid, submandibular, and sublingual glands have measured ADC values of $0.63 \pm 0.11 \times 10^{-3}$ mm^2/s, $0.97 \pm 0.09 \times 10^{-3}$ mm^2/s, and $0.87 \pm 0.05 \times 10^{-3}$ mm^2/s (Eida, Sumi, and Sakihama et al. 2007). In pleomorphic adenomas the ADC maps demonstrate areas of cellular proliferation to have intermediate ADC levels and areas of myxomatous changes to have high ADC values (Eida, Sumi, and Sakihama et al. 2007). Warthin's tumor showed lymphoid tissue to have a very low ADC, necrosis with intermediate ADC, and low ADC in cysts among the lymphoid tissue (Eida, Sumi, and Sakihama et al. 2007). Among the malignant lesions, mucoepidermoid carcinoma shows low ADC in a more homogenous pattern, whereas the adenoid cystic carcinomas demonstrated a more speckled pattern with areas of low and high ADC likely from multiple areas of cystic or necrotic change (Eida, Sumi, and Sakihama et al. 2007). Lymphoma in salivary glands has been demonstrated to have a diffuse extremely low ADC likely from the diffuse uniform cellularity of lymphoma (Eida, Sumi, and Sakihama et al. 2007). In general, cystic, necrotic, or myxomatous changes tend to have higher ADC, and regions of cellularity, low ADC. Malignant tumors tend to show very low to intermediate ADC, whereas benign lesions have higher ADC, but with a heterogenous pattern. Overlaps do occur, for example, with Warthin's tumor demonstrating very low ADC regions and adenoid cystic carcinoma with areas of high ADC (Eida, Sumi, and Sakihama et al. 2007).

Evaluating postoperative changes for residual or recurrent tumors is also an area where DWI and ADC may have a significant impact. In general (with overlap of data), residual or recurrent lesions have been shown to have ADC values lower than post-treatment changes (Abdel Razek, Kandeel, and Soliman et al. 2007). The lower ADC may be a result of smaller diffusion spaces for water in intracellular and extracellular tissues in hypercellular tumors. The benign post-treatment tissue with edema and inflammatory changes has fewer barriers to diffusion and increased extracellular space resulting in a higher ADC (Abdel Razek, Kandeel, and Soliman et al. 2007).

Evaluation of connective tissue disorders with DWI has demonstrated early changes with an increase in ADC prior to changes on other MRI sequences. This may be a result of early edema and/or early lymphocellular infiltration (Patel et al. 2004). Therefore, DWI and ADC may play an important role in early assessment of connective tissue disorders and preoperative evaluation of salivary tumors, as well as surveillance for recurrent disease.

MR Spectroscopy (MRS)

Magnetic resonance spectroscopy falls under the category of functional MRI (fMRI), which contains a variety of different exams created to elucidate physiologic functions of the body. DWI, spectroscopy, perfusion weighted imaging (PWI), and activation studies are examples of fMRI. Of these, MRS of brain lesions is the most commonly performed functional study in clinical imaging. Spectroscopy is, after all, the basis for MRI. MRS attempts to elicit the chemical processes in tissues. Although a variety of nuclei may be interrogated, protons, demonstrating the highest concentration in tissues, are the most practical to evaluate. The majority of MRS studies are performed for the brain, but several recent studies have evaluated head and neck tumors. The need for a very homogenous magnetic field and patient cooperation (prevention of motion) are the keys to successful MRS. Susceptibility artifact and vascular pulsation artifact add to the challenge of MRS. With higher field strength magnets MRS shows promise in determining the biochemical nature of tissues (King, Yeung, and Ahuja et al. 2005).

As in brain tumors, the most reliable markers for tumors are choline and creatine. Choline is considered to be an important constituent of cell membranes. Increased levels of choline are thought to be related to increased biosynthesis of cell membranes, which is seen in tumors, particularly those demonstrating rapid proliferation. The choline signal is comprised of signals from choline, phosphocholine, phosphatidylcholine, and glycerophosphocholine. Elevation of the choline peak in the MR spectra is associated with tumors relative to normal tissue. This unfortunately can be seen in malignant lesions, inflammatory processes, and hypercellular benign lesions (King, Yeung, and Ahuja et al. 2005). Another important constituent is creatine, a marker for energy metabolism. Its peak is comprised of creatine and phosphocreatine. The reduction of the creatine peak in neoplasms may represent the higher energy demands of neoplasms. The elevation of choline and more importantly the elevation of the ratio of choline to creatine has been associated with neoplasms relative to normal tissue. The elevation of choline is not tumor specific and may be seen with squamous cell carcinomas as well as a variety of salivary gland tumors, including benign tumors. It has been described in Warthin's tumor, pleomorphic adenomas, glomus tumors, schwannomas, inflammatory polyps, and inverting papillomas (Shah et al. 2003). In fact, Warthin's tumor and pleomorphic adenoma demonstrate higher choline to creatine ratios than other tumors (King, Yeung, and Ahuja et al. 2005). King, Yeung, and Ahuja et al. also evaluated choline to water ratios and suggest that this may be an alternative method. Although the role of MRS in distinguishing between benign and malignant tumors may be limited, it nevertheless remains an important biomarker for neoplasms and plays a complementary role to other functional parameters and imaging characteristics (Shah et al. 2003). An area where MRS may play a more significant role is in a tumor's response to therapy and assessment of recurrence. Elevation of the choline to creatine ratio is seen in recurrent tumors, whereas the ratio remains low in post-treatment changes. Progressive reduction of choline is seen with a positive response to therapy and persistent elevation is seen in failure of therapy (Shah et al. 2003). Use of artificial intel-

ligence and neural network analysis of MR spectroscopy has demonstrated improved diagnostic accuracy of MRS using neural network analysis over linear discriminate analysis (Gerstle et al. 2000). Currently MRS of salivary gland tumors is under study and not employed clinically.

Dynamic Contrast Enhanced Magnetic Resonance Imaging

Dynamic contrast enhanced MRI has demonstrated improved diagnostic capability of tumor masses in the salivary glands and elsewhere in the body. Distinct enhancement curves can be generated based on the time points of acquisition resulting in improved differentiation of tumors (Alibek et al. 2007; Shah et al. 2003; Yabuuchi, Fukuya, and Tajima et al. 2002). However, data demonstrates similar characteristics in Warthin's tumor and malignant tumors, with a rapid increase in the signal intensity post-contrast. Pleomorphic adenoma demonstrates a more gradual increase in intensity (Alibek et al. 2007; Yabuuchi, Fukuya, and Tajima et al. 2002). Primary salivary duct carcinomas have also demonstrated the rapid enhancement as well as low ADC values as are seen with the more common primary malignancies of the salivary glands (Motoori, Iida, and Nagai et al. 2005).

Other Magnetic Resonance Imaging Techniques

In order to replace the invasive technique of digital subtraction sialography, attempts have been made to develop MR sialography. The techniques are based on acquiring heavily T2 weighted images in order to depict the ducts and branches. The lower spatial resolution and other technical factors have not allowed MR sialography to become a standard of care. This may change with newer single shot MR sequences and higher field strength magnets (Kalinowski et al. 2002; Shah et al. 2003; Takagi et al. 2005b). Dynamic MR sialography has also been used to assess function of parotid and submandibular glands at rest and under stimulation (Tanaka, Ono, and Habu et al. 2007).

An extension of this concept is MR virtual endoscopy. MR virtual endoscopy can provide high-resolution images of the lumen of salivary ducts comparable to sialoendoscopy (Su et al. 2006). Although this initial experience was a preoperative assessment of the technology, it appears to be a promising method of non-invasive assessment of the ducts. In a similar manner, MR microscopy is a high-resolution imaging technique employing tiny coils enabling highly detailed images of the glands (Takagi, Sumi, and Sumi et al. 2005a). This technique was used to demonstrate morphologic changes in Sjogren's syndrome.

Use of supraparamagnetic iron oxide particle MR contrast agents has been under investigation for several years. The particles used for evaluation of lymph nodes are 20 nm or less. These are intravenously injected and are taken up by the cells in the reticuloendothelial system (RES). Since normal lymph nodes have a RES that is intact they readily take up the iron oxide agents. MR imaging using T2 and T2* weighted images demonstrate susceptibility to the iron oxide and result in signal loss at sites of iron accumulation. Therefore, normal lymph nodes lose signal, whereas metastatic lymph nodes whose RES has been replaced by metastases do not take up the particles and do not lose signal (Shah et al. 2003). Although not a direct imaging technique for the salivary glands, it may prove to be useful in the evaluation of nodal metastases.

ULTRASONOGRAPHY (US)

Ultrasound is performed infrequently for head and neck imaging relative to CT and MRI. Although US is able to depict normal anatomy and pathology in the major salivary glands, it is limited in evaluation of the deep lobe of the parotid and submandibular glands (Figures 2.16 and 2.17). US is operator dependent and takes significantly longer to perform on bilateral individual salivary glands

when compared to contrast enhanced CT of the entire neck. US is quite effective at delineating cystic from solid masses and determining degree of vascularity. US can be used to image calculi and observe the resulting ductal dilatation. Normal lymph nodes and lymphadenopathy can also be reliably distinguished. US can be used to initially stage disease. It is not, however, optimal for post-therapy follow-up, be it radiation or surgery. When compared with CT or MRI, US significantly lacks in soft tissue resolution and contrast. Because of its real-time imaging capability and ease of hand-held imaging, US is quite good at image guided fine needle aspiration and biopsy. The application of color Doppler or power Doppler US can distinguish arteries from veins, which is critical for image guided biopsy (Figures 2.18 and 2.19). Eigh-

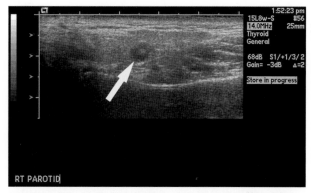

Figure 2.17. Ultrasound of the parotid gland demonstrating a normal intraparotid lymph node on a hyperechoic background. The lymph node is round and has a hypoechoic rim but demonstrates a fatty hyperechoic hilum (arrow).

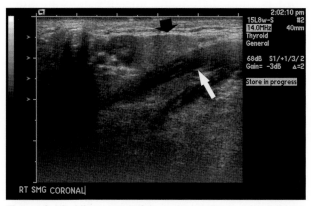

Figure 2.16. Ultrasound of the submandibular gland (black arrow) adjacent to the mylohyoid muscle (white arrow).

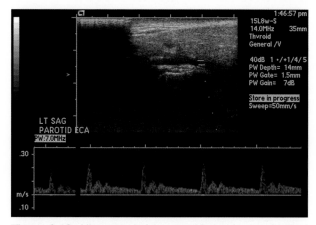

Figure 2.18. Ultrasound of the parotid gland in longitudinal orientation demonstrating the Doppler signal of the external carotid artery.

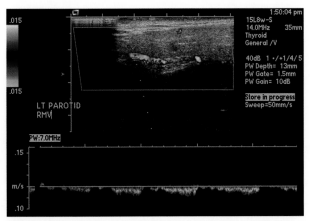

Figure 2.19. Ultrasound of the parotid gland in longitudinal orientation demonstrating the Doppler signal of the retro-mandibular vein.

teen gauge core biopsies of the parotid may be safely performed under US guidance (Wan, Chan, and Chen 2004).

US Technique

High-frequency transducers such as 5, 7.5, or 10 MHz are typically applied to image superficial small parts. Real-time imaging and image acquisition is performed by a technologist or physician. Doppler US may be applied to observe the vascularity of the glands (increased in inflammatory conditions) or tumors within the glands. Doppler US can easily determine arterial from venous channels.

RADIONUCLIDE IMAGING (RNI)

Radionuclide imaging has, throughout its history, been a functional imaging modality without the quality of anatomic depiction when compared with CT, MRI, or even US. The majority of radionuclide imaging has been performed with planar imaging systems that produce single view images of functional processes. All RNI exams employ a radioactive tracer either bound to a ligand (radiopharmaceutical) or injected directly (radionuclide). As the radionuclide undergoes radioactive decay it emits either a gamma ray (photon) and/or a particle such as an alpha particle (helium nucleus), beta particle (electron), or a positron (a positively charged electron). Gamma rays differ from X-rays in that gamma rays (for medical imaging) are an inherent nuclear event and are emitted from the nucleus of an unstable atom in order to achieve stability. X-rays (in the conventional sense) are produced in the electron cloud surrounding the nucleus. In medical imaging X-rays are artificially or intentionally produced on demand, whereas gamma rays (and other particles) are part of an on-going nuclear decay enabling unstable radioactive atoms to reach a stable state. The length of time it takes for one-half of the unstable atoms to reach their stable state is called their half-life. Radionuclide imaging involves the emission of a photon, which is imaged using a crystal or solid state detector. The detector may be static and produces images of the event in a single plane or the detector may be rotated about the patient in order to gather three-dimensional data and reconstruct a tomographic image in the same manner as a CT scanner. This is the basis for SPECT. Examples of planar images used in salivary gland diseases include Gallium (^{67}Ga) for evaluation of inflammation, infection, and neoplasms (lymphoma). SPECT, which produces tomographic cross-sectional images, is less commonly used in oncologic imaging, although novel radionuclides and ligands are under investigation. The recent introduction of SPECT/CT, a combined functional and anatomic imaging machine, may breathe new life into SPECT imaging.

POSITRON EMISSION TOMOGRAPHY (PET)

Positron emission tomography is a unique imaging modality that records a series of radioactive decay events. Positron emission is a form of radioactive decay in which a positron (positively charged electron) is emitted from the unstable atom in order to achieve a more stable state. The positron almost immediately collides with an electron (negatively charged) and undergoes an annihilation event in which both particles are destroyed and converted into pure energy. The annihilation event produces two gamma rays, each with 511 Kev (kilo electron volt) of energy, and traveling in 180-degree opposition. By using sophisticated solid state detectors and coincidence circuitry, the PET system is able to record the source of the event, thereby localizing the event in three-dimensional space. Using a complex algorithm similar to SPECT and CT, a three-dimensional block of data is produced and can be "sliced" in any plane, but most commonly in axial, coronal, and sagittal planes, as well as a maximum intensity projection (MIP) rendering.

PET radionuclides are produced in a cyclotron and are relatively short lived. Typical radionuclides include ^{18}F, ^{11}C, ^{15}O, ^{82}Rb, and ^{13}N. A variety of ligands have been labeled and studied for the evaluation of perfusion, metabolism, and cell surface receptors. The most commonly available is ^{18}F-deoxyglucose (FDG), which is used to study glucose metabolism of cells. Most common uses of FDG include oncology, cardiac viability, and brain metabolism. PET has a higher spatial resolution than SPECT. Both systems are prone to multiple artifacts, especially motion. Acquisition times for both are quite long, limiting the exam to patients who can lie still for prolonged periods of time. Both systems, but PET in particular, are very costly to install and maintain. Radiopharmaceuticals are now widely available to most institutions through a network of nuclear pharmacies.

The oncologic principle behind FDG PET is that neoplastic tissues can have a much higher metabolism than normal tissues and utilize glucose at a higher rate (Warburg 1925). Glucose metabolism in the brain was extensively studied using autoradiography by Sokoloff and colleagues at the National Institutes of Health (NIH) (Sokoloff 1961). The deoxyglucose metabolism is unique in that it mimics glucose and is taken up by cells using the same transporter proteins. Both glucose and deoxyglucose undergo phosphorylation by hexokinase to form glucose-6-phosphate. This is where the similarities end. Glucose-6-phosphate continues to be metabolized, eventually to form CO_2 and H_2O. Deoxyglucose-6-phosphate cannot be further metabolized and becomes trapped in the cell, as it cannot diffuse out through the cell membrane. Therefore, the accumulation of FDG reflects the relative metabolism of tissues (Sokoloff 1986). The characteristic increased rate of glucose metabolism by malignant tumors was initially described by Warburg and is the basis of FDG PET imaging of neoplasms (Warburg 1925).

FDG PET takes advantage of the higher utilization of glucose by neoplastic tissues to produce a map of glucose metabolism. Although the FDG PET system is sensitive, it is not specific. Several processes can elevate glucose metabolism, including neoplastic tissue, inflammatory or infected tissue, and normal tissue in a high metabolic state. An example of the latter includes uptake of FDG in skeletal muscle that was actively contracting during the uptake phase of the study. (Figure 2.20a–d). Another peculiar hypermetabolic phenomenon is brown adipose tissue (BAT) FDG uptake (Figure 2.21a–d). BAT is distributed in multiple sites in the body including interscapular, paravertebral, around large blood vessels, deep cervical, axillary, mediastinal, and intercostal fat, but is concentrated in the supraclavicular regions (Cohade et al. 2003; Tatsumi, Engles, and Ishimori et al. 2004). BAT functions as a thermogenic organ producing heat in mammals, and most commonly demonstrates uptake in the winter (Tatsumi, Engles, and Ishimori et al. 2004). BAT is innervated by the sympathetic nervous system, has higher concentration of mitochondria, and is stimulated by cold temperatures (Cohade, Mourtziks, and Wahl 2003; Tatsumi, Engles, and Ishimori et al. 2004). Administration of ketamine anesthesia in rats markedly increased FDG uptake presumably from sympathetic stimulation (Tatsumi, Engles, and Ishimori et al. 2004). Although typically described on FDG PET/CT exams, it can be demonstrated with ^{18}F-Fluorodopamine PET/CT, ^{99m}Tc-Tetrofosmin, and ^{123}I-MIBG SPECT as well as ^{201}TlCl and ^{3}H-l-methionine (Baba, Engles, and Huso et al. 2007; Hadi, Chen, and Millie et al. 2007). Propranolol and Reserpine administration appears to decrease the degree of FDG uptake, whereas diazepam does not appear to have as significant an effect (Tatsumi, Engles, and Ishimori et al. 2004). Exposure to nicotine and ephedrine also resulted in increased BAT uptake; therefore, avoiding these substances prior to PET scanning can prevent or reduce BAT uptake (Baba, Engles, and Huso et al. 2007). Preventing BAT uptake of FDG can be accomplished by having the patient stay in a warm ambient temperature for 48 hours before the study and by keeping the patient warm during the uptake phase of FDG PET (Cohade, Mourtzikos, and Wahl 2003; Delbeke, Coleman, and Guiberteau et al. 2006). Although somewhat controversial, diazepam or lorazepam and propranolol can reduce BAT uptake by blocking sympathetic activity as well as reducing skeletal muscle uptake from reduced anxiety and improved relaxation (Delbeke, Coleman, and Guiberteau et al. 2006). Understanding the distribution of BAT and the physiology that activates BAT, as well as recognizing the uptake of FDG in BAT in clinical studies, is critical in preventing a false positive diagnosis of supraclavicular, paravertebral, and cervical masses or lymphadenopathy.

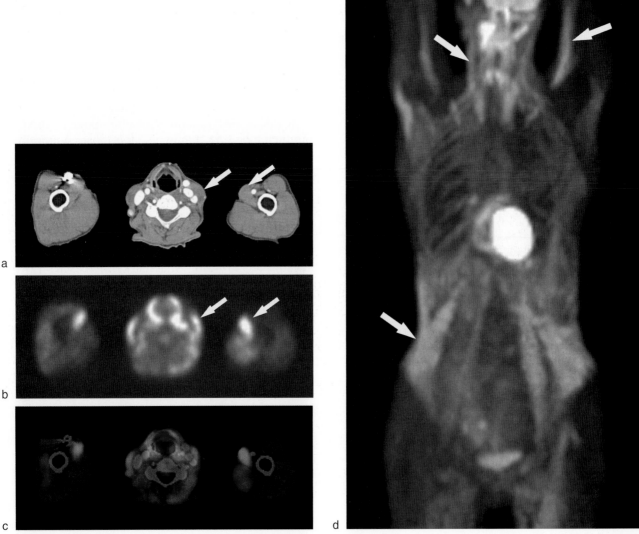

Figure 2.20. CT (a), PET (b), and fused PET/CT (c) images in axial plane, and an anterior MIP image (d) demonstrating skeletal muscle uptake in the sternocleidomastoid muscle and biceps muscle (arrows). Also note the intense uptake in the abdominal, psoas, and intercostal muscles on the MIP image. The very high focal uptake in the middle of the image is myocardial activity.

FDG uptake in all salivary glands in the normal state is usually mild and homogenous (Burrell and Van den Abbeele 2005; Wang et al. 2007) (Figures 2.22a and b and 2.23a and b). After therapy, radiation, or chemotherapy, the uptake can be very high (Burrell and Van den Abbeele 2005). Standardized uptake value (SUV), a semi-quantitative measurement of the degree of uptake of a radiotracer (FDG), may be calculated on PET scans. There are many factors that impact the

measurement of SUVs, including the method of attenuation correction and reconstruction, size of lesion, size of region of interest, motion of lesion, recovery coefficient, plasma glucose concentration, body habitus, and time from injection to imaging (Wang et al. 2007, Schoder, Erdi, and Chao et al. 2004 and Beaulieu, Kinaha, and Tseng et al. 2003).

A range of SUVs can be calculated in normal volunteers for each salivary gland. Wang et al.

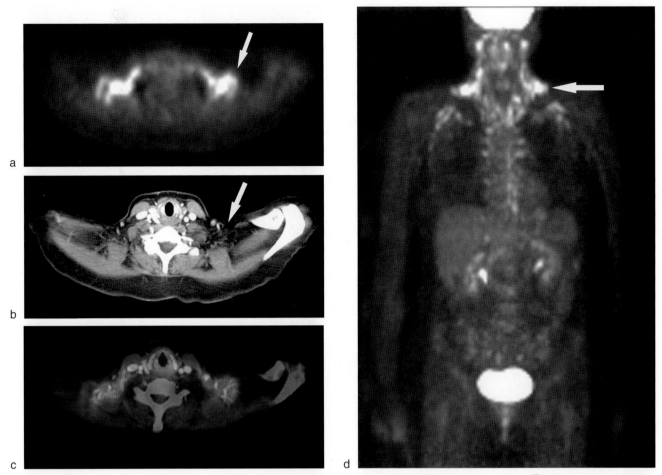

Figure 2.21. PET image (a), corresponding CT image (b), and a fused PET/CT image (c) in the axial plane demonstrating BAT uptake in the supraclavicular regions bilaterally, which could mimic lymphadenopathy (see arrows on Figures 2.21a and 2.21b). Direct correlation enabled by the PET/CT prevents a false positive finding. Note the similar uptake on the MIP image (arrow) (d) including paraspinal BAT uptake.

measured SUVs in normal tissues to determine the maximum SUV and mean SUV as well as assignment of an uptake grade ranging from none (mean SUV less than aortic blood pool), mild (mean SUV greater than mean SUV of aortic blood pool but less then 2.5), moderate (mean SUV between 2.5 and 5.0), and intense (mean SUV greater than 5.0). SUV greater than 2.5 was considered significant (Wang et al. 2007). Parotid glands (n = 97) had a range of SUVmax of 0.78–20.45 and an SUVmean range of 1.75 ± 0.79. Fifty-three percent of the SUV measurements fell into the "none" category, 33% into the "mild" category, and 14% into the "moderate" category. No SUV measurement fell into the "intense" category. Submandibular glands (n = 99) had an SUVmax range of 0.56–5.14 and an SUVmean of

2.22 ± 0.77. The uptake grades consisted of the following: 25% were in the "none" category, 44% in the "mild," and 31% were "moderate." The sublingual gland (n = 102) had an SUVmax range of 0.93–5.91 and an SUVmean of 4.06 ± 1.76. Four percent of these fell into the "none" category, 19% in the "mild," 54% in the "moderate," and 23% in the "intense" group (Wang et al. 2007). Similar work by Nakamoto et al. demonstrated a SUVmean of 1.9 ± 0.68 for the parotid gland, 2.11 ± 0.57 for the submandibular gland, and 2.93 ± 1.39 for the sublingual gland (Nakamoto, Tatsumi, and Hammoud et al. 2005). This demonstrates the wide range of normal uptake values (Table 2.3).

Although FDG does accumulate in the saliva, the concentration varies from 0.2 to 0.4 SUV but

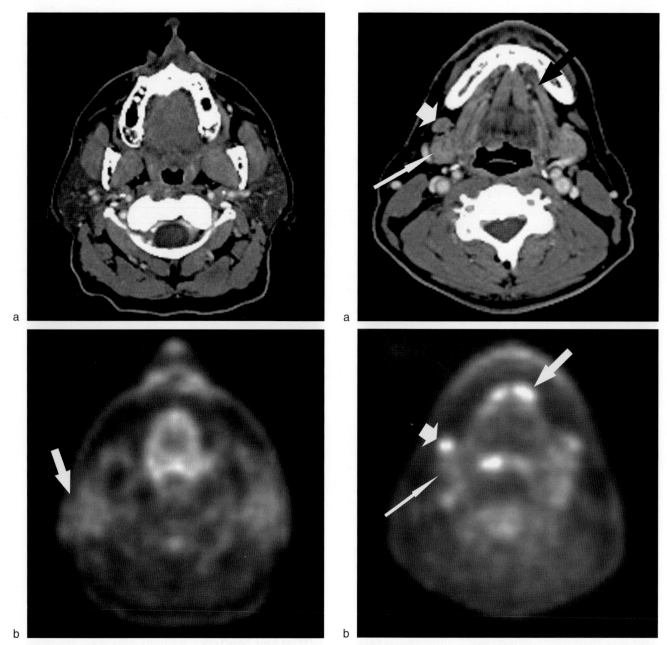

Figure 2.22. CT (a) and PET (b) images in axial plane demonstrating normal parotid gland activity (arrow).

Figure 2.23. CT (a) and PET (b) images in axial plane demonstrating normal submandibular (long thin arrow) and sublingual gland (medium arrow) activity. Note the abnormal uptake higher than and anterior to the submandibular glands (short fat arrow). Metastatic lymphadenopathy was diagnosed at the time of surgery.

does not influence FDG imaging (Stahl et al. 2002). SUV of greater then 2.5 has become a threshold for abnormal or neoplastic uptake (originally described by Patz et al.) (Patz, Lowe, and Hoffman et al. 1993; Wang et al. 2007). However, careful analysis must be undertaken when evaluating lesions based on SUVs, as there is a significant overlap of SUVs for malignant and benign tumors and inflammatory conditions. One cannot depend on SUV measurements alone and must take into consideration clinical data as well as radiologic imaging findings.

Table 2.3. SUV of salivary glands.

Gland	SUV Max (Range) (a)	SUV Mean ± SD (a)	SUV Mean ± SD (b)
Parotid gland	0.78–20.45	1.75 ± 0.79	1.90 ± 0.68
Submandibular gland	0.56–5.14	2.22 ± 0.77	2.11 ± 0.57
Sublingual gland	0.93–5.91	4.06 ± 1.76	2.93 ± 1.39

(a) Wang et al. 2007.
(b) Nakamoto, Tatsumi, and Hammoud et al. 2005.
SD = standard deviation.

POSITRON EMISSION TOMOGRAPHY/ COMPUTED TOMOGRAPHY (PET/CT)

Head and neck imaging has greatly benefited from the use of FDG PET imaging for the staging, restaging, and follow-up of neoplasms. The recent introduction of PET/CT has dramatically changed the imaging of diseases of the head and neck by directly combining anatomic and functional imaging.

The evaluation of the head and neck with FDG PET/CT has been significantly and positively affected with detection and demonstration of the extent of primary disease, lymphadenopathy, and scar versus recurrent or residual disease, pre-surgical staging, pre-radiosurgery planning, and follow-up post-therapy.

The role of FDG PET or PET/CT and that of conventional CT and MRI on the diagnosis, staging, restaging, and follow-up post-therapy of salivary gland tumors have been studied (Bui, Ching, and Carlos et al. 2003; de Ru, Van Leeuwen, and Van Benthem et al. 2007; Keyes, Harkness, and Greven et al. 1994; Otsuka et al. 2005; Roh, Ryu, and Choi et al. 2007). Although both CT and MRI are relatively equal in anatomic localization of disease and the effect of the tumors on local invasion and cervical nodal metastases, FDG PET/CT significantly improved sensitivity and specificity for salivary malignancies including nodal metastases (de Ru, Van Leeuwen, and Van Benthem et al. 2007; Jeong, Chung, and Son et al. 2007; Otsuka et al. 2005; Roh, Ryu, and Choi et al. 2007; Uchida, Minoshima, and Kawata et al. 2005).

Early studies have demonstrated FDG PET's relative inability to distinguish benign from malignant salivary neoplasms (Keyes, Harkness, and Greven et al. 1994). The variable uptake of FDG by pleomorphic adenomas and the increased uptake and SUVs by Warthin's tumor result in significant false positives (Jeong, Chung, and Son et al. 2007; Roh, Ryu, and Choi et al. 2007). In a similar manner, adenoid cystic carcinomas, which are relatively slower growing, may not accumulate significant concentrations of FDG and demonstrate low SUVs and therefore contribute to the false negatives (Jeong, Chung, and Son et al. 2007; Keyes, Harkness, and Greven et al. 1994). False negatives may also be caused by the relatively lower mean SUV of salivary tumors (SUV 3.8 ± 2.1) relative to squamous cell carcinoma (SUV 7.5 ± 3.4)(Roh, Ryu, and Choi et al. 2007). The low SUV of salivary neoplasms may also be obscured by the normal uptake of FDG by salivary glands (Roh, Ryu, and Choi et al. 2007). In general, FDG PET has demonstrated that lower grade malignancies tend to have lower SUV and vice versa for higher grade malignancies (Jeong, Chung, and Son et al. 2007; Roh, Ryu, and Choi et al. 2007). FDG PET has been shown to be more sensitive and specific compared to conventional CT or MRI (Cermik, Mavi, and Acikgoz et al. 2007; Otsuka et al. 2005; Roh, Ryu, and Choi et al. 2007). Small tumor size can contribute to false negative results and inflammatory changes contribute to false positive results (Roh, Ryu, and Choi et al. 2007). The use of concurrent salivary scintigraphy with [99]mTc-pertechnetate imaging can improve the false positive rate by identifying Warthin's tumors and oncocytomas, which tend to accumulate pertechnetate (and retain it after induced salivary gland washout) and have increased uptake of FDG (Uchida, Minoshima, and Kawata et al. 2005).

Diagnostic Imaging Anatomy

PAROTID GLAND

The average adult parotid gland measures 3.4 cm in AP, 3.7 cm in LR, and 5.8 cm in SI dimensions and is the largest salivary gland. The parotid gland is positioned high in the suprahyoid neck directly inferior to the external auditory canal (EAC) and wedged between the posterior border of the mandible and anterior border of the styloid process, sternocleidomastoid muscle, and posterior belly of the digastric muscle (Figures 2.24 through 2.30; also see figures 2.17 through 2.19). This position, as well as the seventh cranial nerve, which traverses the gland, divides the gland functionally

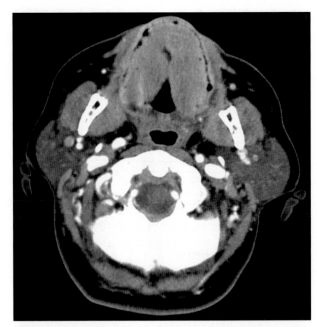

Figure 2.24. Axial CT of the neck demonstrates the intermediate to low density of the parotid gland.

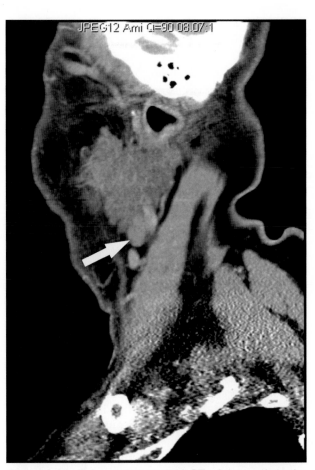

Figure 2.26. Reformatted sagittal CT of the neck at the level of the parotid gland demonstrating its relationship to adjacent structures including the external auditory canal. Note the slightly denser soft tissue density in the parotid tail, the so-called "earring lesion" of the parotid gland. Cervical lymphadenopathy (arrow) was diagnosed at surgery.

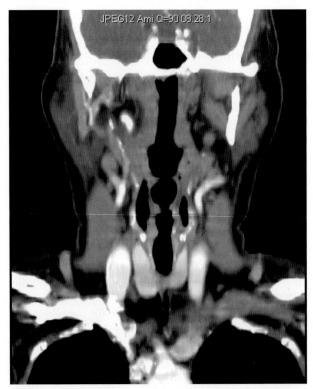

Figure 2.25. Reformatted coronal CT of the neck at the level of the parotid gland demonstrating its relationship to adjacent structures. Note the distinct soft tissue anatomy below the skull base.

(not anatomically) into superficial and deep "lobes." Its inferior extent is to the level of the angle of the mandible, where its "tail" is interposed between the platysma superficially and the sternocleidomastoid muscle (SCM) deep to the tail of the parotid. The parotid gland is surrounded by the superficial layer of the deep cervical fascia. The parotid space is bordered medially by the parapharyngeal space (PPS), the carotid space (CS), and the posterior belly of the digastric muscle. The anterior border is made up of the angle and ramus of the mandible along with the masticator space (MS). The posterior border is made up of the styloid and mastoid processes and the SCM. The gland traverses the stylomandibular tunnel, which

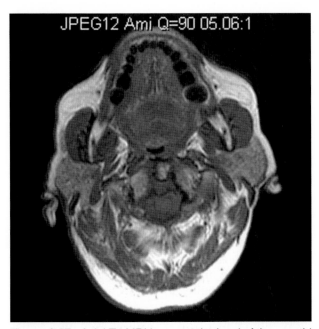

Figure 2.27. Axial T1 MRI image at the level of the parotid gland demonstrating the slightly higher signal as compared to skeletal muscle but less than subcutaneous fat.

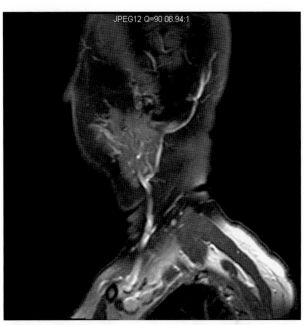

Figure 2.29. Sagittal fat suppressed T1 MRI image of the parotid gland demonstrating mild enhancement and lack of subcutaneous fat signal in the upper neck but incomplete fat suppression at the base of the neck.

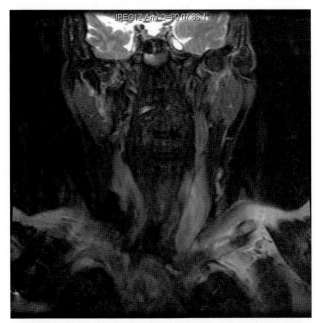

Figure 2.28. Coronal STIR MRI image at the level of the parotid gland demonstrating the nulling of the subcutaneous fat signal on STIR images and low signal from the partially fatty parotid gland.

is formed by the posterior border of the mandibular ramus, the anterior border of the sternocleidomastoid muscle, the anterior border of the stylomandibular ligament, and the anterior border of the posterior belly of the digastric muscle and the skull base on its superior aspect (Beale and Madani 2006; Som and Curtin 1996). The external carotid artery (ECA) and retromandibular vein (RMV) traverse the gland in a craniocaudal direction, posterior to the posterior border of the mandibular ramus. The seventh cranial nerve (CN 7) traverses the gland in the slightly oblique anteroposterior direction from the stylomastoid foramen to the anterior border of the gland passing just lateral to the RMV. The seventh cranial nerve divides into five branches (temporal, zygomatic, buccal, mandibular, and cervical) within the substance of the gland. Prior to entering the substance of the parotid gland, the facial nerve gives off small branches, the posterior auricular, posterior digastric, and the stylohyoid nerves. The intraparotid facial nerve and duct can be demonstrated by MRI using surface coils and high-resolution acquisition (Takahashi et al. 2005). Because the parotid gland encapsulates later in development than other salivary glands, lymph nodes become incorporated

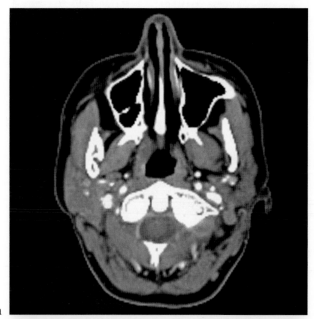

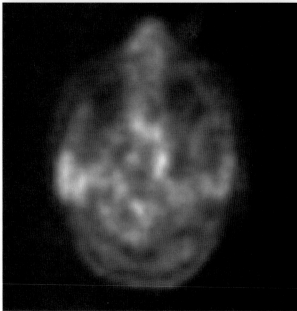

Figure 2.30. Axial CT scan (a) and corresponding PET scan (b) at the level of the parotid gland. Note the asymmetric slightly higher uptake on the right corresponding to partially resected parotid gland on the left, confirmed by CT.

into the substance of the gland. The parotid duct emanates from the superficial anterior part of the gland and is positioned along the superficial surface of the masseter muscle. Along the anterior aspect of the masseter muscle the duct turns medially, posterior to the zygomaticus major and minor muscle, to penetrate the buccinator muscle and

terminate in the oral mucosa lateral to the maxillary second molar. Fifteen to 20% of the general population also has an accessory parotid gland that lies along the surface of the masseter muscle in the path of the parotid duct.

In the pediatric population, the parotid gland is isodense to skeletal muscle by CT and becomes progressively but variably fatty replaced with aging. Therefore the CT density will progressively decrease over time (Drumond 1995). By MRI the parotid gland is isointense to skeletal muscle on T1 and T2 weighted images, but with progressive fatty replacement demonstrates progressive increase in signal (brighter) similar to but remaining less than subcutaneous fat. Administration of iodinated contrast for CT results in slight enhancement (increase in density and therefore brightness). Administration of intravenous gadolinium (Gd) contrast results in an increase in signal (T1 shortening) and therefore brightness on MRI scans. By US the acoustic signature is isoechoic to muscle, but with fatty replacement becomes hyperechoic (more heterogenous grey). Therefore, masses tend to stand out as less echogenic foci. Normal uptake on FDG PET varies but is mild to moderate relative to muscle and decreases over age.

SUBMANDIBULAR GLAND (SMG)

The submandibular gland is located in the upper neck in the submandibular space (SMS) and the posterior oral cavity in the sublingual space (SLS). The SMG is more difficult to measure, but the average adult superficial SMG measures 3.5 cm in oblique AP, 1.4 cm in oblique LR, and 3.3 cm in SI dimensions. The gland "wraps" around the posterior border of the mylohyoid muscle and traverses the two spaces. The superficial portion is in the SMS adjacent to level one lymph nodes (level 1b). The deep portion of the submandibular gland is located in the SLS. The SMS is bordered inferiorly by the hyoid bone and platysma and superiorly by the mylohyoid muscle. It is bordered laterally by the mandible and it is surrounded by the superficial layer of deep cervical fascia. Its medial border is a combination of the mylohyoid sling and anterior belly of the digastric muscle (Beale and Madani 2006) (Figures 2.31 through 2.37).

The submandibular duct emanates from the anterior-superior aspect of the gland and turns anteriorly and lies along the superior surface of the mylohyoid muscle between the genioglossus muscle medially and the sublingual gland laterally. The

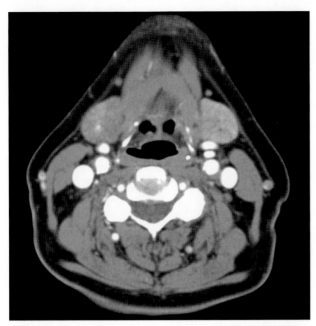

Figure 2.31. Axial CT at the level of the submandibular gland demonstrating density higher than skeletal muscle.

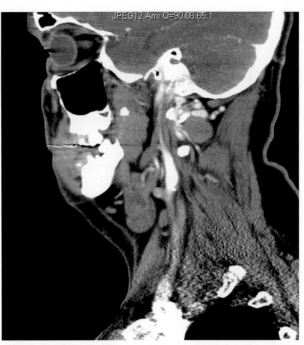

Figure 2.33. Reformatted sagittal CT at the level of the submandibular gland demonstrating its relationship to the floor of the mouth. Note the slight notch at the hilum of the gland. Majority of the gland "hangs" below the mylohyoid muscle.

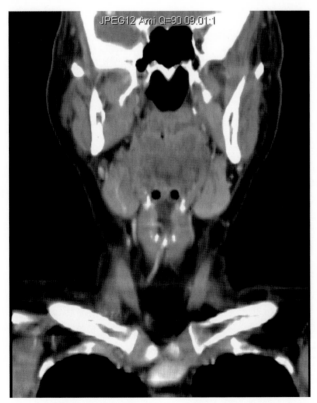

Figure 2.32. Reformatted coronal CT at the level of the submandibular gland demonstrating its relationship to the mylohyoid muscle and floor of the mouth.

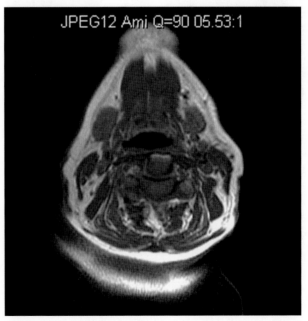

Figure 2.34. Axial T1 MRI of the submandibular gland demonstrating slight hyperintensity to muscle. Note the bright subcutaneous fat.

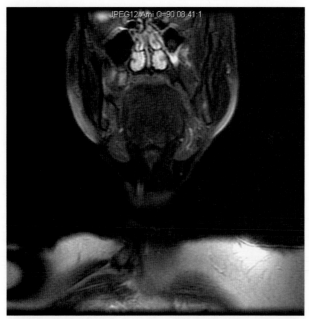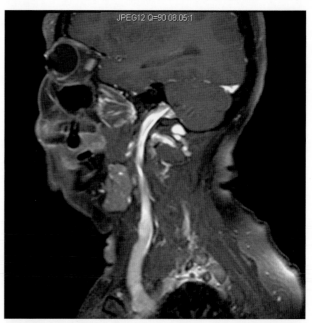

Figure 2.35. Coronal fat saturated T2 MRI of the submandibular gland. Note the slightly incomplete fat suppression and the engorged and edematous mucosa of the nasal cavity and turbinates.

Figure 2.36. Sagittal T1 fat saturated MRI of the submandibular gland demonstrating the well-defined appearance on a fat suppressed background. Note the slight notch at the hilum. Also note the entire internal jugular vein is visualized.

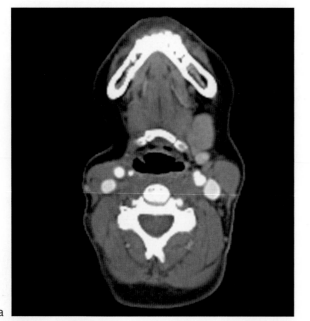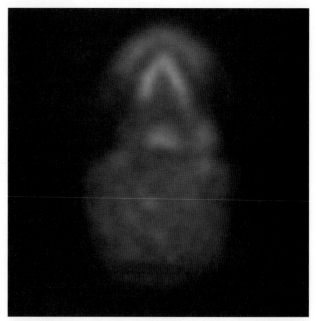

a   b

Figure 2.37. Axial CT (a) and corresponding PET (b) of the submandibular gland demonstrating slight normal uptake. Note the strong asymmetry of uptake on the PET corresponds to the absent submandibular gland on the right confirmed by the CT.

ducts open into the anterior medial (paramidline) floor of the mouth at the sublingual papillae.

On CT scans the submandibular gland has a density that is isodense to slightly hyperdense relative to skeletal muscle. The gland does not become as fatty replaced as the parotid gland. The SMG demonstrates a signal characteristic similar to that of skeletal muscle on T1 and T2 weighted images and is less intense when compared to the parotid gland secondary to less fatty replacement. The FDG uptake is moderate but higher than that of the parotid gland. The SMG undergoes contrast enhancement by CT and MRI (Kaneda 1996).

SUBLINGUAL GLAND (SLG)

The sublingual gland is the smallest of the major salivary glands and is the least likely to be involved with pathology. The SLG measures approximately 3.5 cm in oblique AP, 1.0 cm in oblique LR, and 1.5 cm in SI dimensions. Anatomically, the SLGs are located in the floor of the mouth and lie on the superior surface of the mylohyoid muscle, bordered anteriorly and laterally by the mandible, and medially by the submandibular duct, genioglossus muscle, and geniohyoid muscle. The submandibular gland serves as its posterior border (Figures 2.38 through 2.40). The sublingual gland commu-

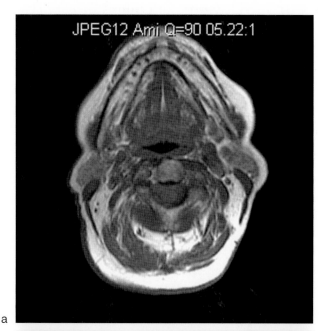

a

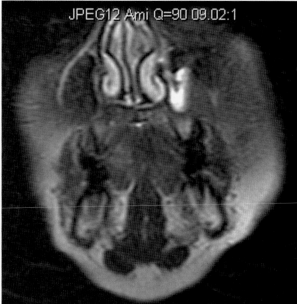

b

Figure 2.39. Axial contrast enhanced T1 MRI of the sublingual gland demonstrating enhancement (a). Note the deep lobe of the submandibular glands seen at the posterior margin of the sublingual glands. Coronal T2 weighted image demonstrating the sublingual gland "cradled" between the mandible laterally, the genioglossus muscle medially, the geniohyoid muscle inferomedially, and the combined mylohyoid and digastric muscles inferiorly (b).

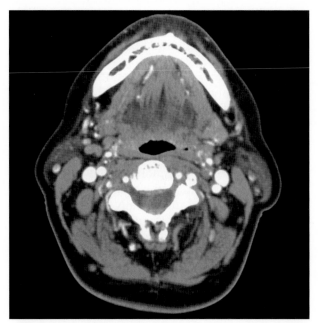

Figure 2.38. Axial CT of the neck at the level of the sublingual gland demonstrating mild normal enhancement along the lateral floor of the mouth.

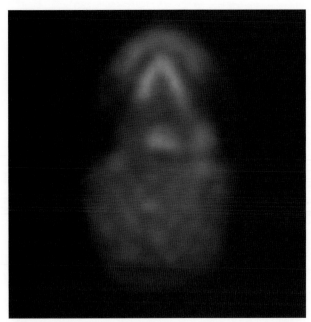

Figure 2.40. Axial PET of the sublingual gland demonstrating the intense uptake seen in the sublingual glands bilaterally medial to the mandible (photopenic linear regions).

nicates with the oral cavity via multiple small ducts (ducts of Rivinus) that open into the floor of the mouth adjacent to the sublingual papilla. These small ducts may be fused and form a larger single duct (duct of Bartholin) and empty into the submandibular duct (Beale and Madani 2006).

The SLG can be seen by CT and MRI and is similar in appearance to the SMG, although smaller (Sumi et al. 1999a). FDG uptake is less well defined since it is small and closely approximated to adjacent skeletal muscle, but the uptake is moderate.

Occasionally accessory salivary tissue is found in the SMS along the anterior aspect (anterior to the normal submandibular gland). This is caused by herniation of SLG through defects in the mylohyoid muscle, called a mylohyoid boutonniere, which typically occurs between the anterior and posterior parts of the mylohyoid muscle. The accessory gland may be accompanied by sublingual branches of the facial artery and vein. Although the accessory tissue may mimic a tumor, this should be readily identified as normal since the accessory tissue has the same characteristics on CT and MRI as normal sublingual or submandibular gland (Hopp, Mortensen, and Kolbenstvedt

2004; White, Davidson, and Harnsberger et al. 2001).

MINOR SALIVARY GLANDS

The minor salivary glands are unevenly distributed throughout the upper aerodigestive tract and are submucosal in location. They are more concentrated in the oral mucosa, where they inhabit the mucosa of the hard and soft palate, buccal mucosa, and floor of the mouth, as well as the mucosa of the lips, gingiva, and tongue. They are also found in the pharynx (nasal and oral), sinonasal spaces, larynx, trachea, and bronchi. Functionally they are either mucinous (predominantly in the palatal mucosa) or mixed seromucinous glands. The serous minor salivary glands are found only on the tongue at the circumvallate papilla. The minor salivary glands do not have large defined ducts but do contain multiple small excretory ducts. MRI of minor salivary glands has been achieved with high-resolution surface coils of the upper and lower lips. Patients with Sjogren's disease had a smaller gland area relative to normal, best demonstrated in the upper lip (Sumi et al. 2007).

Pathology of the Salivary Glands

Pathologic states of the salivary glands include tumors (epithelial and non-epithelial), infections and inflammation, autoimmune diseases, vascular lesion, and non-salivary tumors.

Of all salivary gland tumors, the vast majority (80%) are found in the parotid gland. The submandibular gland contains approximately 10%, with the remainder in the sublingual and minor salivary glands. Of all parotid gland tumors, 80% are benign and 20% malignant. About 50% of submandibular gland tumors are benign and the vast majority of sublingual gland tumors are malignant. About 50% of minor salivary gland tumors are benign. The smaller the gland, the more likely that a mass within it is malignant. The pleomorphic adenoma and papillary cystadenoma lymphomatosum (Warthin's) account for the vast majority of benign salivary tumors, with the former being the more common at about 80% of benign and the latter less common at about 15% of benign masses. Most of the malignant salivary gland tumors are represented by mucoepidermoid and adenoid cystic carcinomas.

Malignancies of the parotid gland may result in metastatic involvement of intraparotid and adjacent level II and III jugular chain lymph nodes. The SMG drains primarily into adjacent level Ib lymph nodes and then into the jugular chain and deep cervical nodes. The SLG drains into both level IA and IB nodes and then subsequently into the jugular chain and deep cervical nodes.

VASCULAR LESIONS

Lymphangioma (Cystic Hygroma)

The cystic hygroma is included in this discussion because of its transpatial location and the fact that it may mimic other cystic masses. It is typically multilocular and has an epicenter in the posterior triangle, but it may be found in the submandibular space and less commonly in the sublingual space. The imaging characteristics are those of cysts and follow fluid density on CT and signal intensity on MRI, although they do typically demonstrate internal architecture from septation with varying thickness. CT typically demonstrates isodensity to simple fluid or slight hyperdensity if infected or if it contains products of hemorrhage (Koeller et al. 1999; Makariou, Pikis, and Harley 2003) (Figure 2.41). US demonstrates anechoic spaces consistent with simple fluid with septa of variable thickness. Like cystic lesions (and a few solid lesions), there is increased through-transmission. Infection and hemorrhage cause variable degrees of echogenicity and thicker septations (Koeller et al. 1999; Makariou, Pikis, and Harley 2003). MRI, however, can be variable on both T1 and T2 sequences based on the fluid characteristics. With simple fluid, T1 and T2 are isointense to simple fluid (CSF), but with infection or hemorrhage products, the increased protein concentration as well as cellular debris and iron from hemoglobin can result in varying degrees of T1 hyperintensity and variable hypo- or hyperintensity on T2 (Figure 2.42). Any of these modalities may demonstrate fluid-fluid or fluid-debris layers. Both CT and MRI will demonstrate enhancement in the setting of infection (Macdonald, Salzman, and Hansberger 2003). These lesions are more common in the pediatric age group, although small lesions may persist into adulthood. When found in the submandibular or sublingual space, they may be mistaken for a ranula (especially giant or plunging ranulae) and less likely hemangioma or thyroglossal duct cyst if midline (Kurabayashi, Ida, and Yasumoto et al.

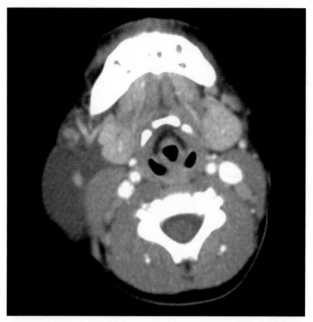

Figure 2.41. Axial contrast enhanced CT of the neck at the level of the submandibular glands demonstrating a low-density structure on the right of approximately fluid density (compare to the CSF in the spinal canal), which is intermediate in density relative to the muscles and subcutaneous fat. A large lymphangioma associated with the right submandibular gland was diagnosed.

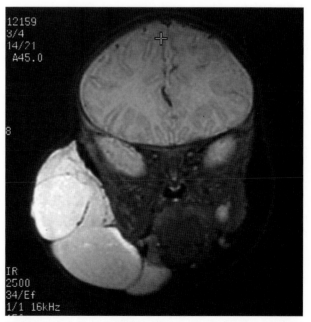

Figure 2.42. Coronal STIR MRI of the face of a different patient with a very large lymphangioma with large septations. Note the lymphangioma fluid is brighter than the CSF and there is fat suppression of the subcutaneous fat.

2000; Macdonald, Salzman, and Hansberger 2003). Although dermoids are in the differential diagnosis, they are usually identified by their imaging characteristics secondary to their contents of fat and dermal elements. Epidermoid cysts may be more difficult to differentiate from cystic hygromas and ranulae because of similar imaging characteristics (Koeller et al. 1999). Because the lymphangiomas have a vasculolymphatic origin, they may be associated with venous anomalies and rarely saccular venous aneurysms (Makariou, Pikis, and Harley 2003). Vascular flow signals may be seen with Doppler US. The venous anomalies or aneurysms may be difficult to differentiate from other vascular malformations; however, their association with typical findings of lymphangiomas may assist in diagnosis.

Hemangioma

Hemangiomas are typically found in the pediatric age group. The majority are of the cavernous type and less likely the capillary type. They are best demonstrated by MRI and show marked enhancement. They are also very bright on T2 MRI. Foci of signal void may be vascular channels or phleboliths (Figures 2.43 through 2.45). They are typically slow flow lesions and may not be angiographically evident. US can vary from hypoechoic to heterogenous (Wong, Ahuja, and King et al. 2004).

Other rare vascular lesions within salivary glands, most commonly the parotid gland, include aneurysms, pseudoaneurysms, and arteriovenous fistulae (AVFs). The aneurysms or pseudoaneurysms are most commonly associated with trauma or infection (mycotic). MRI in high flow lesions demonstrates "flow voids" or an absence of signal, but slow flow lesions or turbulent flow can demonstrate a heterogenous signal mimicking a mass. Contrast enhancement and magnetic resonance angiography (MRA) can help delineate vascular lesions from masses. CT without contrast, however, demonstrates a mass or masses isodense to skeletal muscle or normal blood vessels. With contrast the often large vascular channels become more obvious, although smaller lesions may still mimic a mass. US (especially Doppler US) can reveal characteristic flow patterns of arterial waveforms in the venous channels for AVFs. US can also delineate aneurysms with their turbulent flow patterns. Angiography is typically reserved for endovascular treatment. CTA or MRA is useful for non-invasive assessment of arterial feeders and

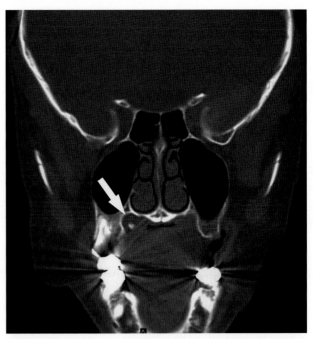

Figure 2.43. Direct coronal CT displayed in bone window demonstrating smooth erosion of the hard palate on the right lateral aspect, along with a dense calcification consistent with a phlebolith (arrow). A hemangioma is presumed based on this CT scan.

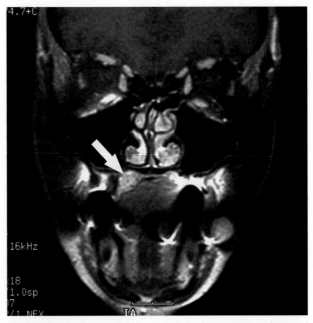

Figure 2.44. Coronal fat suppressed contrast enhanced T1 MRI image corresponding to the same level as Figure 2.43, demonstrating a sharply marginated homogenously enhancing mass (arrow).

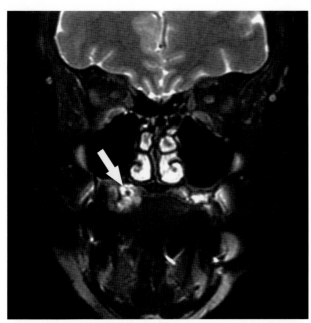

Figure 2.45. Coronal fat saturated T2 MRI image demonstrating a well-demarcated hyperintense mass with a focal signal void centrally. A hemangioma containing a phlebolith (arrow) was presumed based on this MRI.

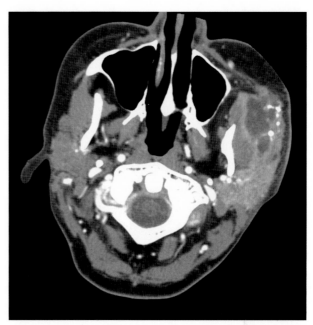

Figure 2.46. Axial CT with contrast at the level of the masseter muscles demonstrating a left accessory parotid gland abscess.

venous anatomy in AVFs and in defining aneurysms (Wong, Ahuja, and King et al. 2004).

ACUTE SIALADENITIS

Acute sialadenitis may be bacterial or viral in nature and may be a result of obstruction from a calculus, stricture, or mass (see chapters 3 and 5). Viral parotitis or mumps may be caused by a variety of viruses but most commonly the paromyxovirus is the culprit. The patient presents with an enlarged, tender, and painful gland. Acute suppurative parotitis (sialadenitis) presents in a similar manner as viral parotitis with the additional sign of purulent exudate. Oral bacterial pathogens are the causative agents, with staphylococcal and streptococcal species being the most common. CT scan demonstrates an enlarged gland with ill-defined margins and infiltration of the surrounding fat by edema fluid. The gland, especially the parotid, is increased in density because of the edema fluid, which is of higher density than fat. CT contrast demonstrates heterogenous enhancement and may show an abscess. On T1 MRI scan the overall gland signal may be decreased slightly from the edema but does enhance heterogenously with contrast. T2 MRI scan shows increased signal secondary to edema. Both CT and MRI may demonstrate enhancement and enlargement of the parotid (or sublingual) duct. US shows slight decrease in echogenicity relative to normal. These patterns are not unique to bacterial or viral infection or inflammation and may be seen with autoimmune diseases such as Sjogren's syndrome or a diffusely infiltrating mass. The surrounding subcutaneous fat also demonstrates heterogenous increased density from edema resulting in a "dirty fat" appearance. There is also thickening of fascia and the platysma muscle (Bialek, Jakubowski, and Zajkowski et al. 2006; Madani and Beale 2006a; Shah 2002).

With acute submandibular sialadenitis the gland becomes enlarged and may be associated with a dilated duct if a sialolith is present. By CT the calculus may be readily identified but not as easily seen by MRI. There may be varying degrees of cellulitis or frank abscess formation. The inflamed gland undergoes greater contrast enhancement. MRI demonstrates an enlarged heterogenous gland with a dilated fluid-filled duct and gland, which on T2 images is of high signal. On ultrasound the acutely inflamed gland demonstrates enlargement with focal hypoechoic foci (Bialek, Jakubowski, and Zajkowski et al. 2006; Madani and Beale 2006a; Shah 2002) (Figures 2.46 through 2.48).

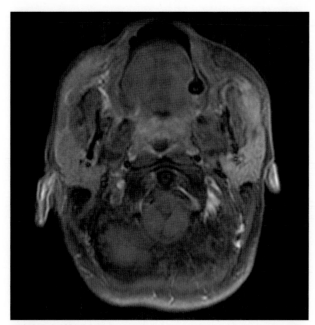

Figure 2.47. Axial contrast enhanced fat saturated T1 MRI demonstrating heterogenous enhancement consistent with abscess of the left accessory parotid gland.

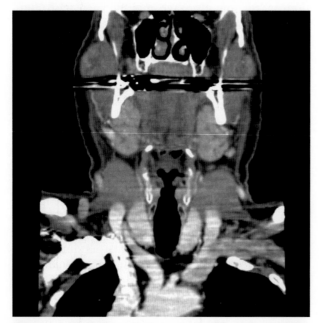

Figure 2.48. Reformatted coronal CT demonstrating enlargement and enhancement of the submandibular glands consistent with viral sialadenitis.

CHRONIC SIALADENITIS

The etiology of chronic inflammatory states of the salivary glands varies by the particular gland in question. Chronic inflammatory changes in the parotid gland tend to be related to autoimmune disease (Sjogren's syndrome), recurrent suppurative parotitis, or radiation injury. Other etiologies include granulomatous infections such as tuberculosis or sarcoidosis. Chronic inflammation of the submandibular gland and to a lesser degree the sublingual gland is more commonly due to obstructive disease, particularly sialolithiasis. In the chronically inflamed state the glands are enlarged but over longer periods of time progressively reduced in size, and heterogenous density may be seen on CT with extensive fibrosis and small focal (punctate) calcification. The density on CT is often increased due to cellular infiltration and edema during acute phases of exacerbation. The surrounding subcutaneous fat may not show signs of edema as is seen with acute sialadenitis. MRI demonstrates similar changes with heterogenous signal on both T1 and T2. The duct or ducts may be dilated, strictured, or both. Both may be visible by contrast CT and MRI (Bialek, Jakubowski, and Zajkowski et al. 2006; Madani and Beale 2006a; Shah 2002; Sumi et al. 1999b). Chronic sclerosing sialadenitis (aka Kuttner tumor) can mimic a mass of the salivary (most commonly submandibular) glands (Huang et al. 2002). It presents with a firm, enlarged gland mimicking a tumor. The most common etiology is sialolithiasis (50–83%), but other etiologies include chronic inflammation from autoimmune disease (Sjogren's syndrome), congenital ductal dilatation and stasis, and disorders of secretion (Huang et al. 2002). It is best diagnosed by gland removal and pathologic examination as fine needle aspiration biopsy may be misleading (Huang et al. 2002). Chronic sialadenitis can also be caused by chronic radiation injury. US studies have demonstrated a difference in imaging characteristics between submandibular sialadenitis caused by acalculus versus calculus disease. The acalculus sialadenitis submandibular gland US demonstrates multiple hypoechoic lesions, mimicking cysts, with diffuse distribution throughout a heterogenous hypoechoic gland. They do not, however, demonstrate increased through-transmission, which is typically seen with cysts and some soft tissue tumors. Sialadenitis caused by calculus disease demonstrates hyperechoic glands relative to the adjacent digastric muscle, but some are iso- or hypoechoic relative to the contralateral gland (Ching, Ahuja, and King et al. 2001).

HIV-LYMPHOEPITHELIAL LESIONS

These lesions are comprised of mixed cystic and solid masses within the parotid (much less in the SMG and SLG). CT shows multiple cystic and solid masses with associated parotid enlargement. IV contrast shows mild peripheral enhancement in the cysts and more heterogenous enhancement in the solid lesions (Figure 2.49). MRI of the cysts is typical with low signal on T1 and high on T2. The more solid lesions are of heterogenous soft tissue signal on T1 and increase on T2. Contrast MRI images follow the same pattern as CT (Holliday 1998). The US images show heterogenous cystic lesions with internal architecture of septation and vascularity and a slightly hypoechoic signal of the solid masses. Mural nodules may be seen in a predominantly cystic lesion. Associated cervical lymphadenopathy is commonly seen, as well as hypertrophy of tonsillar tissues. Differential diagnosis of these findings includes Sjogren's syndrome, lymphoma, sarcoidosis, other granulomatous diseases, metastases, and Warthin's tumor (Kirshenbaum and Nadimpalli et al. 1991; Madani and Beale 2006a; Martinoli, Pretolesi, and Del Bono et al. 1995; Shah 2002; Som, Brandwein, and Silver 1995).

MUCOUS ESCAPE PHENOMENA

The mucous escape phenomenon most commonly results from obstruction in the sublingual gland resulting in a back-up of salivary secretions (see chapter 4). Ductal obstruction may be caused by calculi, stricture from prior infection, or trauma. The chronic dilatation of the duct and accumulation of fluid produces a cystic mass by CT, MRI, and US. The simple ranula remains in the sublingual space and typically presents with a unilocular, well-demarcated, and homogenous structure unless complicated by hemorrhage or infection. The walls may enhance slightly if a ranula remains contained above the mylohyoid muscle. However, it may rupture into the surrounding tissues and extravasate along a path of least resistance and extend inferiorly into the submandibular space or posteriorly into the parapharyngeal space, under which circumstances it is termed a "plunging ranula" (see chapter 4). The non-plunging ranula has a dilated ovoid configuration on axial images, but when it herniates into the submandibular space the dilated space shrinks into a tail-like configuration in the sublingual space. The tail sign is pathognomonic for ranulae and may be seen in both simple and plunging types. The ranula can usually be differentiated from a hemangioma and lymphangioma by its lack of internal architecture (unless complicated). The ranulae are typically homogenous internally with well-defined margins, unless infected or hemorrhagic, and follow fluid density on CT (isodense to simple fluid) and intensity on MRI (low on T1 and high on T2). Both simple and plunging ranulae have these characteristics. The plunging component may be in the parapharyngeal space if the lesion plunges posterior to the mylohyoid muscle or in the anterior submandibular space if it plunges through the anterior and posterior portions of the mylohyoid muscle or through a defect in the muscle. Involvement of the parapharyngeal space and the submandibular space results in a large cystic mass termed "giant ranula" and may mimic a cystic hygroma

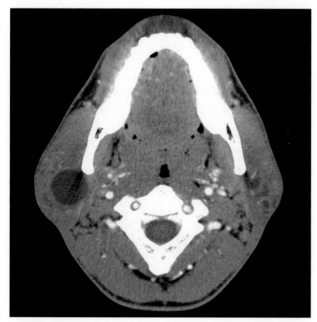

Figure 2.49. Axial CT demonstrating a large cystic lesion in the right parotid gland and multiple small lesions in the left parotid diagnosed as lymphoepithelial cysts.

(Kurabayashi, Ida, and Yasumoto et al. 2000; Macdonald, Salzman, and Hansberger 2003; Makariou, Pikis, and Harley 2003; Cholankeril and Scioscia 1993).

SIALADENOSIS (SIALOSIS)

Sialadenosis, also known as sialosis, is a painless bilateral enlargement of the parotid glands and less commonly the submandibular and sublingual glands (see chapter 6). It is typically bilateral and without inflammatory changes. No underlying mass is present. It has been associated with mal-nutrition, alcoholism, medications, and a variety of endocrine abnormalities, the most common of which is diabetes mellitus. In the early stages there is gland enlargement, but it may progress to fatty replacement and reduction in size by late stages. By CT there is a slight increase in density of the entire gland in the early setting, but the density decreases in the late stage when the gland is pre-dominantly fatty. On T1 weighted MRI images in the early stage, the gland demonstrates a slight decrease in signal corresponding to the lower fat content and increased cellular component. T2 images show a slight increase in signal (Bialek, Jakubowski, and Zajkowski et al. 2006; Madani and Beale 2006a; Som and Curtin 1996).

SIALOLITHIASIS

Approximately 80–90% of salivary calculi form in the submandibular gland due to the chemistry of the secretions as well as the orientation and size of the duct in the floor of the mouth. Eighty percent of submandibular calculi are radio-opaque, while approximately 40% of parotid sialoliths are radio-opaque (see chapter 5). CT without contrast is the imaging modality of choice as it easily depicts the dense calculi (Figures 2.50 through 2.52). MRI is less sensitive and may miss calculi. Vascular flow voids can be false positives on MRI. MR sialogra-phy as previously discussed may become more important in the assessment of calculi not readily visible by CT or for evaluation of strictures, and it is more important as part of therapeutic maneu-vers. US can demonstrate stones over 2 mm with distal shadowing (Bialek, Jakubowski, and Zajkowski et al. 2006; Madani and Beale 2006a; Shah 2002).

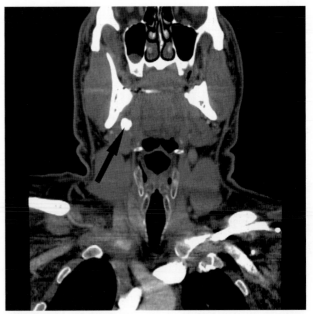

Figure 2.50. Reformatted coronal contrast enhanced CT of the submandibular gland demonstrating a sialolith in the hilum of the right submandibular gland.

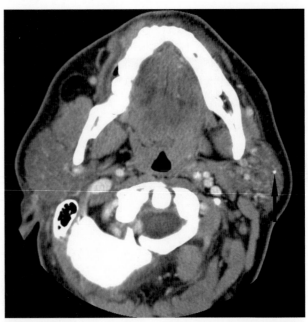

Figure 2.51. Axial contrast enhanced CT of the parotid gland demonstrating a small left parotid sialolith (arrow).

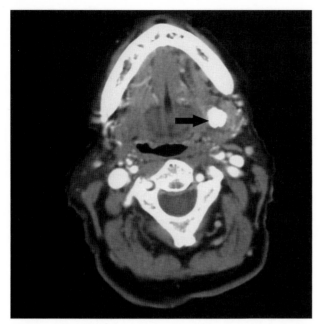

Figure 2.52. Axial contrast enhanced CT at the level of the submandibular glands with a very large left hilum sialolith (arrow).

SJOGREN'S SYNDROME

This autoimmune disease affects the salivary glands and lacrimal glands and is called "primary Sjogren's" if no systemic connective tissue disease is present, but it is considered secondary Sjogren's if the salivary disease is associated with systemic connective tissue disease (Madani and Beale 2006a). The presentations vary radiographically according to stage. Typically early in the disease the gland may appear normal on CT and MRI. Early in the course of the disease there may be premature fat deposition, which may be demonstrated radiographically and may be correlated with abnormal salivary flow (Izumi, Eguchi, and Hideki et al. 1997). Also in the early course of the disease tiny cysts may form consistent with dilated acinar ducts and either enlarge or coalesce as the disease progresses. These can give a mixed density appearance of the gland with focal areas of increased and decreased density by CT and areas of increased and decreased signal on T1 and T2 MRI giving a "salt and pepper" appearance (Takashima, Takeuchi, and Morimoto et al. 1991; Takashima, Tomofumi, and Noguchi et al. 1992). There may be diffuse glandular swelling from the inflammatory reaction, or this may present as a focal area of swelling. The diffuse swelling may mimic viral or bacterial sialadenitis. The focal swelling may mimic a tumor, benign or malignant, including lymphoma. Pseudotumors may be cystic lesions from coalescence or formation of cysts or dilatation of ducts, or they may be solid from lymphocytic infiltrates (Takashima, Takeuchi, and Morimoto et al. 1991; Takashima, Tomofumi, and Noguchi et al. 1992). As glandular enlargement and cellular infiltration replace the fatty elements, the gland appears denser on CT and lower in signal on T1 and T2 MRI. But when chronic inflammatory changes have progressed, tiny or coarse calcifications may develop. The cysts are variable in size, and the larger cysts may represent confluent small cysts or abscesses. The CT and MRI appearance can be similar to that of lymphoepithial lesions seen with HIV but does include calcifications. Typically there is no diffuse cervical lymphadenopathy. The development of cervical adenopathy may indicate development of lymphoma (Takashima, Tomofumi, and Noguchi et al. 1992). Solid nodules or masses can also represent underlying lymphoma (non-Hodgkin's type) to which these patients are prone. The latter stages of the disease produce a smaller and more fibrotic gland (Bialek, Jakubowski, and Zajkowski et al. 2006; Madani and Beale 2006a; Shah 2002).

SARCOIDOSIS

Sarcoidosis is a granulomatous disease of unknown etiology (see chapter 6). It typically presents with bilateral parotid enlargement. It may be an asymptomatic enlargement or may mimic a neoplasm with facial nerve palsy. The parotid gland usually demonstrates multiple masses bilaterally, which is a nonspecific finding and can also be seen with lymphoma, tuberculosis (TB), or other granulomatous infections, including cat-scratch disease. There is usually associated cervical lymphadenopathy. The CT characteristics of the masses are slightly hypodense to muscle but hyperdense to the more fatty parotid gland. MRI also demonstrates nonspecific findings. Doppler US demonstrates hypervascularity, which may be seen with any inflammatory process. The classically described "panda sign" seen with uptake of ^{67}Ga-citrate in sarcoidosis is also not pathognomonic for this disease and may be seen with Sjogren's syndrome, mycobacterial diseases, and lymphoma.

CONGENITAL ANOMALIES OF THE SALIVARY GLANDS

First Branchial Cleft Cyst

This congenital lesion is in the differential diagnosis of cystic masses in and around the parotid gland along with lymphoepithelial lesions, abscesses, infected or necrotic lymph nodes, cystic hygromas, and Sjogren's syndrome. Pathologically the first branchial cleft cyst is a remnant of the first branchial apparatus. Radiographically it has typical characteristics of a benign cyst if uncomplicated by infection or hemorrhage, with water density by CT and signal intensity by MRI. It may demonstrate slightly increased signal on T1 and T2 images if the protein concentration is elevated and may be heterogenous if infected or hemorrhagic. Contrast enhancement by either modality is seen if infection is present. Ultrasound demonstrates hypoechoic or anechoic signal if uncomplicated and hyperechoic if infected or hemorrhagic. There is no increase in FDG uptake unless complicated. Anatomically it may be intimately associated with the facial nerve or branches. They are classified as type I (Figure 2.53) if found in the external auditory canal (the less common of the two types) and type II if found in the parotid gland or adjacent to the angle of the mandible (Figure 2.54) and may extend into the

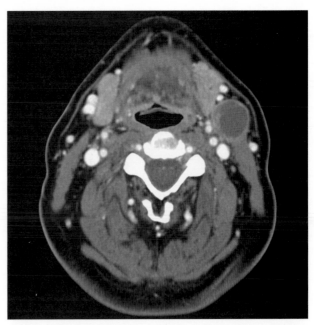

Figure 2.54. Axial contrast enhanced CT of the maxillofacial soft tissues with a cystic mass interposed between the left submandibular gland and sternocleidomastoid muscle, consistent with a type II branchial cleft cyst.

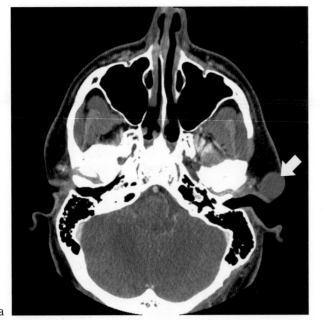

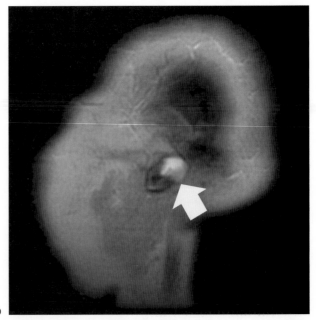

a   b

Figure 2.53. Axial contrast enhanced CT (a) of the head with a cystic mass at the level of the left external auditory canal and sagittal T2 MRI of a different patient (b) consistent with a type I branchial cleft cyst.

parapharyngeal space. It may have a fistulous connection to the external auditory canal or the skin surface. Infected or previously infected cysts may mimic a malignant tumor. Although not typically associated with either the parotid or submandibular glands, the second branchial cleft cyst, which is found associated with the sternocleidomastoid muscle and carotid sheath, may extend superiorly to the tail of the parotid or antero-inferiorly to the posterior border of the submandibular gland. It has imaging characteristics similar to the first branchial cleft cyst. Therefore this must be differentiated from cervical chain lymphadenopathy or exophytic salivary masses. The third and fourth branchial cleft cysts are rare, are not associated with the salivary glands, and are found in the posterior triangle and adjacent to the thyroid gland, respectively (Koeller et al. 1999).

NEOPLASMS—SALIVARY, EPITHELIAL

Benign

Pleomorphic Adenoma

Pleomorphic adenoma (PA) is the most common tumor of the salivary glands and is comprised of epithelial, myoepithelial, and stromal components. It is also the most common benign tumor of the minor salivary glands (Jansisyanont, Blanchaert, and Ord 2002). Typically unilateral, lobulated, and most commonly sharply marginated, the PA can vary in size, be up to 8 cm in long dimension, and involve superficial and deep parotid lobes. The lobulated regions are sometimes referred to as a "cluster of grapes" (Shah 2002). The majority (80%) are located in the superficial lobe of the parotid gland. Small lesions are better circumscribed, have homogenous enhancement, and are of uniform soft tissue density (skeletal muscle). There can be mild to moderate enhancement and the lesion is relatively homogenous. The larger lesions have a heterogenous density, enhancement pattern, and low attenuation foci from necrosis and cyst formation as well as calcification. The T1 signal can be as variable as the density on CT but tends to follow muscle or soft tissue signal against a background of fat of the normal parotid gland (Figure 2.55). The masses may be hypointense when small, and then become heterogenous with the cystic and calcific changes, and can be hyperintense secondary to areas of hemorrhage and calcifications. The T2 imaging characteristic is that of

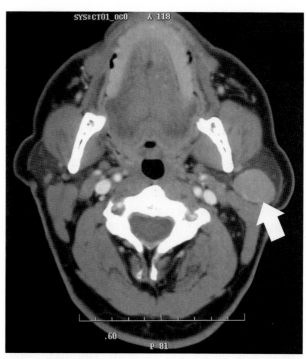

Figure 2.55. Axial contrast enhanced CT of the parotid gland with a heterogenous mass with cystic changes. A pleomorphic adenoma (arrow) was diagnosed at surgery.

high signal intensity, with a thin low signal rim, except when hemorrhage may cause the signal to be heterogenous. The cystic or necrotic regions will tend to be low to intermediate signal on T1 and high on T2. There is mild homogenous enhancement when small and heterogenous when large. US usually demonstrates a homogenous hypoechoic mass but may also have heterogenous hypoechoic features with slight increase in through-transmission (Madani and Beale 2006b). These features may be shared with other benign and malignant lesions, but only tumors that have both lobulation of the contour and a well-defined pseudocapsule are benign (Ikeda, Tsutomu, and Ha-Kawa et al. 1996). The tumor's components, cellular or myxoid, determine the MRI signal. The hypercellular regions have lower signal on T2 and STIR sequences as well as reduced ADC values on DWI and earlier time vs. signal intensity curves (TIC) peak on dynamic MRI (Motoori, Yamamoto, and Ueda et al. 2004). The high cellular components may be seen with other tumor types including malignant types. The myxoid components, which are more diagnostic of PAs, result in high T2 and STIR signal, high ADC values on DWI, and progressive enhancement on dynamic MRI (Motoori, Yamamoto, and Ueda et al. 2004). In fact, of the three types of PAs, myxoid, cellular, and classic, the myxoid is the most common and the most common to recur (Moonis, Patel, and Koshkareva et al. 2007). MRI with T2 and STIR sequences has been shown to be quite sensitive in detecting recurrent PA of the myxoid type by demonstrating the focal, diffuse, or multifocal high signal of the myxoid material (Kinoshita and Okitsu 2004; Moonis, Patel, and Koshkareva et al. 2007). While most PAs demonstrate the benign and non-aggressive features of smooth margins and homogenous enhancement, the more aggressive and invasive features may be seen with carcinoma-ex pleomorphic adenoma, which is seen in areas of previously or concurrently benign PAs. Carcinoma-ex pleomorphic adenomas can result in distance metastatic foci, including the brain (Sheedy et al. 2006). Heterogenous signal within PAs can indicate a concurrent high-grade malignancy, which can be low on T1 and T2 (Kinoshita and Okitsu 2004). FDG PET can be variable but tends to have increased uptake (Figure 2.56). Benignancy cannot be determined by imaging and therefore the differential includes primary parotid malignancy, metastases, and lymphoma as well as benign Warthin's tumors (Madani and Beale 2006b; Shah 2002; Thoeny 2007).

Warthin's Tumor

Papillary cystadenoma lymphomatosum, or Warthin's tumor, is the second most common benign lesion of the salivary glands. These tumors are typically well marginated but inhomogenous and found in the parotid tail of the superficial lobe. Fifteen percent present as bilateral or multicentric disease (Madani and Beale 2006b). There is by CT a heterogenous density and very mild enhancement (Figure 2.57). They typically have small cysts but do not demonstrate calcifications; therefore differential includes lymphoepithelial cysts, primary neoplasms, metastatic disease, and lymphoma. MRI signal on T1 is generally low but may be heterogenous, and T2 is either high signal based on its more cystic features or heterogenous. If the tumor is primarily solid, the imaging characteristics may mimic a PA with relatively homogenous hypoechoic architecture. Contrast with Gd follows CT characteristics. FDG uptake can be high on PET imaging. Warthin's tumors contain oncocytes and

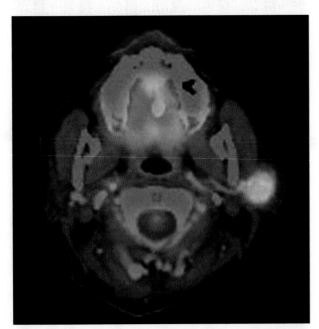

Figure 2.56. Axial PET/CT fused image demonstrating intense FDG uptake in a parotid mass. Pleomorphic adenoma was diagnosed at surgery.

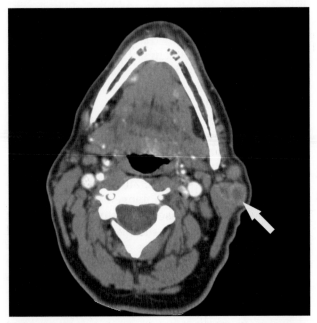

Figure 2.57. Axial contrast enhanced CT of a heterogenous parotid mass at the tail of the gland, with multiplicity and cystic or necrotic changes, diagnosed as a Warthin's tumor (arrow).

are thought to be the mechanism by which they tend to accumulate ^{99}mTc-pertechnetate. The ^{99}mTc-pertechnetate uptake and retention after lemon juice stimulated washout by the normal tissue is a good indicator of the diagnosis of Warthin's tumor (Miyake, Matsumoto, and Hori et al. 2001). This pattern is much less commonly seen by other lesions such as lymphoepithelial cysts, PAs, and oncocytomas. This technique allows visualization of Warthin's tumors as small as 9 mm (Miyake, Matsumoto, and Hori et al. 2001). By its peripheral location and cystic components, it can be mistaken for a necrotic lymph node or second branchial cleft cyst. The tail of the parotid region can be difficult to differentiate from adjacent cervical lymphadenopathy. However, coronal images can aid in determining the site of origin. If the lesion is medial to the parotid tail it is more likely cervical jugular chain lymphadenopathy and if it is more laterally located, it is more likely an exophytic tumor from the parotid gland (Hamilton et al. 2003).

Oncocytoma

These relatively rare tumors exist primarily in the parotid gland. Their imaging characteristics are that of PAs except that they do accumulate ^{99}mTc-pertechnetate. They are also reported to have high ^{18}F-FDG uptake. They are considered benign but may have some invasive features.

Malignant Tumors
Mucoepidermoid Carcinoma

Mucoepidermoid carcinoma is the most common malignant lesion of the salivary glands. It is also the most common salivary malignancy in the pediatric population. One-half occur in the parotid gland and the other half in minor salivary glands (Jansisyanont, Blanchaert, and Ord 2002; Shah 2002). The imaging characteristics of mucoepidermoid carcinoma are based on histologic grade. The low-grade lesions are sharply marginated and inhomogenous, mimicking PA and Warthin's tumor. These well-differentiated lesions can have increased signal on T2 weighted sequences. The low-grade lesions are more commonly cystic (Madani and Beale 2006b). The high-grade, invasive lesions mimic adenoid cystic carcinoma and lymphoma or large heterogenous PAs or carcinoma ex-pleomorphic adenoma. They tend to have a lower signal of T2. Contrast enhanced studies

demonstrate enhancement in the more solid components (Bialek, Jakubowski, and Zajkowski et al. 2006; Lowe, Stokes, and Johnson et al. 2001; Madani and Beale 2006b; Sigal, Monnet, and De Baere et al. 1992) (Figures 2.58 through 2.60). Therefore standard imaging cannot exclude a malignant neoplasm. Defining the tumor's extent is critical. Contrast MRI, especially in the coronal

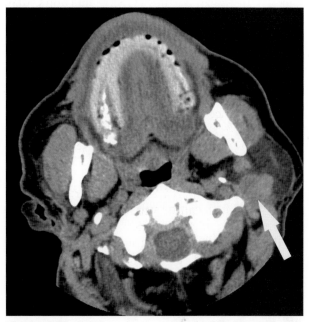

Figure 2.58. Axial contrast enhanced CT demonstrating an ill-defined mass diagnosed as a mucoepidermoid carcinoma (arrow).

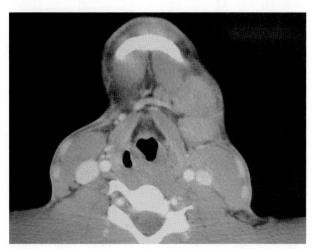

Figure 2.59. Axial contrast enhanced CT demonstrating large bulky cervical lymphadenopathy with ill-defined borders diagnosed as a mucoepidermoid carcinoma.

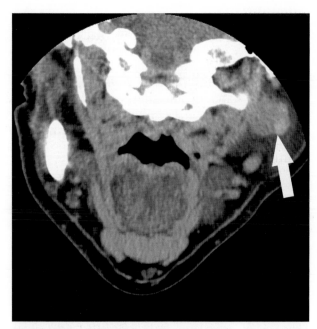

Figure 2.60. Reformatted coronal contrast enhanced CT demonstrating an ill-defined heterogenous density mass diagnosed as a mucoepidermoid carcinoma (arrow).

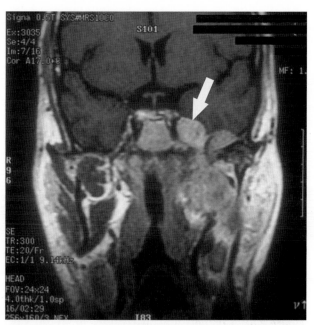

Figure 2.61. Coronal contrast enhanced MRI of the skull base demonstrating a mass extending through the skull base via the left foramen ovale (arrow) diagnosed as an adenoid cystic carcinoma originating from a minor salivary gland of the pharyngeal mucosa.

or sagittal plane, is essential to identify perineural invasion into the skull base.

Adenoid Cystic Carcinoma

Adenoid cystic carcinoma has similar characteristics to mucoepidermoid carcinoma in that their imaging findings are based on histologic grade. Adenoid cystic carcinoma is the most common malignant neoplasm of the submandibular and sublingual glands, as well as the minor salivary glands in the palate. These tumors have a high rate of local recurrence, higher rate of distance metastases as opposed to nodal disease, and may recur after a long latency period (Madani and Beale 2006b). MRI is the imaging method of choice demonstrating high signal due to increased water content. Contrast enhanced fat saturated images are critical to evaluate for perineural spread, which is demonstrated by nerve thickening and enhancement (Madani and Beale 2006b; Shah 2002). CT can be helpful to evaluate bone destruction or foraminal widening. It is important to define the tumor's extent and identify perineural invasion into the skull base (Figures 2.61 through 2.65).

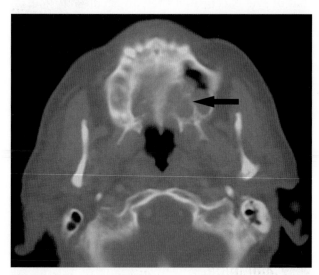

Figure 2.62. Axial CT in bone window demonstrating a mass eroding through the left side of the hard palate and extending into the maxillary sinus (arrow) diagnosed as adenoid cystic carcinoma.

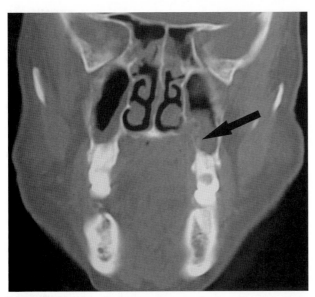

Figure 2.63. Coronal CT corresponding to the case illustrated in Figure 2.62 with a mass eroding the hard palate and extending into the left maxillary sinus (arrow).

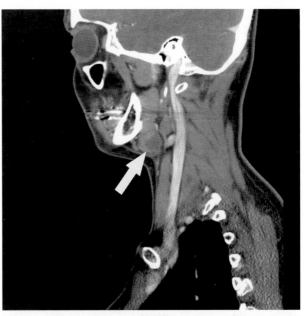

Figure 2.65. Reformatted sagittal contrast enhanced CT corresponding to the case illustrated in Figure 2.64.

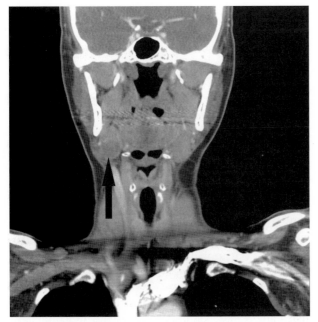

Figure 2.64. Reformatted contrast enhanced coronal CT with a mass in the right submandibular gland (arrow) diagnosed as an adenoid cystic carcinoma.

NEOPLASMS—NON-SALIVARY

Benign
Lipoma
In the cervical soft tissues, lipomas are slightly more commonly seen within the parotid gland rather than peri-parotid. Lipomas of the salivary glands are uncommon (Shah 2002). The CT and MRI characteristics are those of subcutaneous fat with CT density very low (−100 H) and hyperintense on both T1 and T2. Lipomas tend to be echogenic on US. They may be uniform on imaging but may have areas of fibrosis. The heterogenous density from fibrosis, or hemorrhage, carries the additional differential diagnosis of liposarcoma or other neoplasms (Som, Brandwein, and Silver 1995) (Figures 2.66 and 2.67).

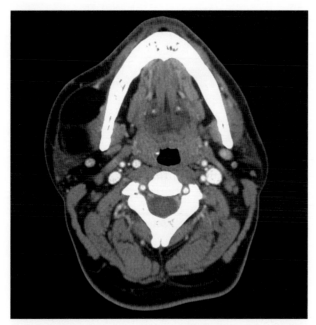

Figure 2.66. Axial contrasted enhanced CT of the head with a fat density mass at the level of the parotid gland and extending to the submandibular gland, diagnosed as a lipoma.

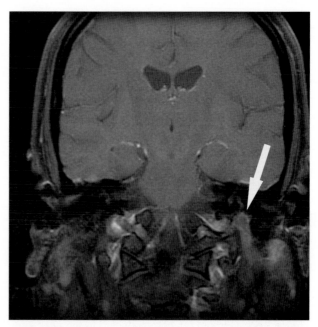

Figure 2.68. Coronal T1 contrast enhanced MRI demonstrating a mass in the left parotid gland with smooth margins. The mass extends superiorly into the skull base at the stylomastoid foramen (arrow). A benign schwannoma was diagnosed.

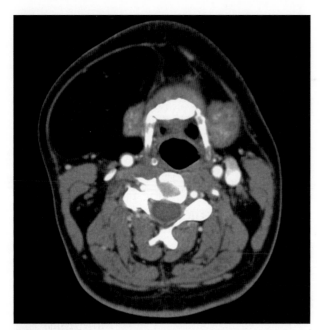

Figure 2.67. Axial contrast enhanced CT through the submandibular gland with fat density mass partially surrounding the gland. A lipoma was diagnosed.

Neurogenic Tumors

Neurogenic tumors are uncommon in the salivary glands but when encountered are most commonly found in the parotid gland. The majority of the

facial nerve schwannomas are on the intratemporal facial nerve with only 9% extra-temporal and in the parotid gland (Shimizu, Iwai, and Ikeda et al. 2005) (Figures 2.68 through 2.70). These are difficult to preoperatively diagnose as they do not typically present with facial nerve dysfunction. As seen in other parts of the body, they tend to be sharply marginated and have an ovoid shape along the axis of the involved nerve, such as the facial nerve. The CT density is that of soft tissue but post-contrast both enhance (schwannoma slightly greater then neurofibroma). Both are seen as low signal on T1 and high on T2. MRI enhancement pattern follows that of CT. They may demonstrate a target sign appearance with peripheral hyperintensity relative to a central hypointensity (Martin et al. 1992; Shimizu, Iwai, and Ikeda et al. 2005; Suh, Abenoza, and Galloway et al. 1992). However, this sign is not pathognomonic and may be seen in schwannomas or neurofibromas. Increased uptake is seen on FDG PET in both diseases. The neurofibroma may be associated with Von Recklinghausen's disease. Although the vast majority of schwannomas and neurofibromas are benign, they are reported as demonstrating increased uptake (hypermetabolism of glucose) of ^{18}F-FDG

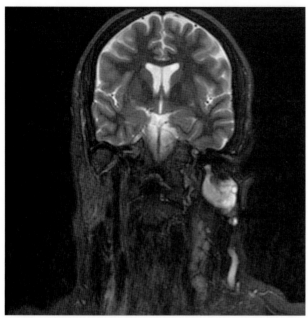

Figure 2.69. Coronal T2 MRI corresponding to the case illustrated in Figure 2.68.

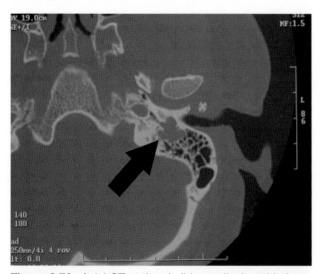

Figure 2.70. Axial CT at the skull base displayed in bone window showing dilatation of the stylomastoid foramen with soft tissue mass (arrow). A benign schwannoma was diagnosed.

on PET imaging (Hsu et al. 2003). Although the calculated SUV can be helpful in differentiating benign from malignant lesions, there is a significant overlap (Ioannidis and Lau 2003). There is difficulty in separating low-grade malignant lesions from benign lesions (Ioannidis and Lau 2003) (Figures 2.71 and 2.72). Plexiform neurofibromas are also slow-growing and rare. They present with

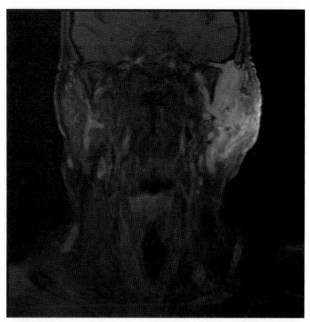

Figure 2.71. Coronal T1 contrast image showing a very ill-defined mass with heterogenous enhancement in the parotid gland with skull base extension via the stylomastoid foramen. A malignant schwannoma was diagnosed.

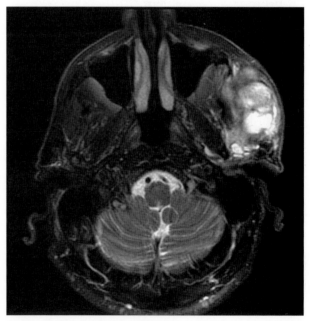

Figure 2.72. Axial T2 MRI image corresponding to the case illustrated in Figure 2.71.

multiple cord-like masses and are also far more common in the parotid gland relative to other salivary glands. By CT and MRI they are sometimes described as a "branching" pattern or "bag of worms" secondary to the multiple lesions growing along nerve branches. They have CT and MRI signal characteristics similar to the neurofibromas and schwannomas including the "target sign" (Aribandi et al. 2006; Lin and Martel 2001). The target sign may also be seen by US as a hypoechoic periphery surrounding a subtle slightly hyperechoic center. There may also be slight increased through-transmission (Lin and Martel 2001).

Malignant

Lymphoma

Both primary and secondary lymphomas of the salivary glands are rare. Primary lymphoma of the salivary glands is the mucosa-associated lymphoid tissue subtype (MALT). MALT lymphomas constitute about 5% of non-Hodgkin's lymphomas (Jhanvar and Straus 2006). These lymphomas are seen in the gastrointestinal tract and are associated with chronic inflammatory or autoimmune diseases. The salivary glands do not typically contain MALT but may in the setting of chronic inflammation (Ando, Matsuzaki, and Murofushi 2005). The MALT lymphomas found in the gastrointestinal tract are not typically associated with Sjogren's syndrome. The MALT lymphoma, a low-grade B-cell type, tends to be a slow-growing neoplasm. Metastases tend to be to other mucosal sites, a demonstration of tissue tropism. The MALT lymphomas are amenable to radiotherapy but can relapse in the contralateral gland, demonstrating tropism for the glandular tissue (MacManus et al. 2007). In Sjogren's syndrome, there is an approximately forty-fold increased incidence of developing lymphoma compared to age-controlled populations. Of the various subtypes of lymphoma that are seen associated with Sjogren's syndrome (follicular, diffuse large B-cell, large cell, and immunoblastic), the MALT subtype is the most common at around 50% (Tonami, Munetaka, and Yokota et al. 2002). The parotid gland is the most commonly affected (80%). Less commonly the submandibular and rarely the sublingual gland may be involved. Clinically, it may present with a focal mass or diffuse unilateral or bilateral glandular swelling.

[67]Ga-citrate scintigraphy had been the standard imaging modality used to assess staging and post-therapy follow-up for lymphomas (Hodgkin's and non-Hodgkin's) for many decades. PET/CT with FDG is quickly becoming the standard for staging and follow-up for many lymphoma subtypes (Jhanvar and Straus 2006).

The imaging findings in salivary lymphomas, however, are not specific. CT may demonstrate focal or diffuse low to intermediate density mass with cystic areas and calcifications. MRI shows the soft tissue areas to be isointense to skeletal muscle on T1 images and hypointense relative to fat on T2 images along with diffuse enhancement post-contrast (Tonami, Munetaka, and Yokota et al. 2002). Although there may be cystic changes demonstrated by CT, MRI, or US, they are thought to be dilated ducts as a result of compression of terminal ducts (Ando, Matsuzaki, and Murofushi 2005). The US characteristics of MALT lymphoma may demonstrate multifocal hypoechoic intraparotid nodules and cysts (which may be dilated ducts), and calcification as well. Large B-cell intraparotid lymphoma has been described as a hypoechoic, homogenous, well-marginated mass exhibiting increased through-transmission (a characteristic of cysts) and hypervascularity (Eichhorn, Iakovos, and Ridder 2002). Although there are reports of hypermetabolism in MALT lymphomas, PET imaging findings are also not conclusive (Mac-Manus et al. 2007). Uptake in the tumor and a

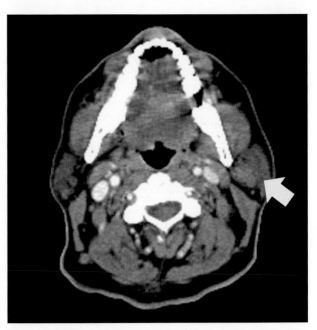

Figure 2.73. Axial CT scan with contrast at the level of the parotid tail demonstrating an ill-defined heterogeneously enhancing mass adjacent to or exophytic from the parotid tail medially (arrow). Lymphoma in cervical lymphadenopathy was diagnosed at surgery.

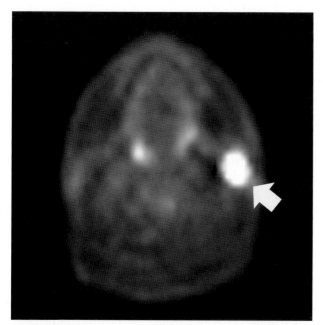

Figure 2.74. Axial PET scan image corresponding to the case in Figure 2.73. A large mass of the left parotid gland (arrow) is noted.

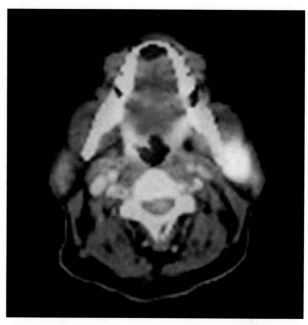

Figure 2.75. Fused axial PET/CT image corresponding to the case illustrated in Figure 2.73.

background of chronic inflammatory changes of chronic sialadenitis may result in variably elevated uptake of FDG.

Secondary lymphomas (Hodgkin's and non-Hodgkin's) are also quite rare, with the histology most commonly encountered being of the large cell type. There is typically extraglandular lymphadenopathy associated. The imaging features are also nonspecific, although there is usually no associated chronic sialadenitis (Figures 2.73 through 2.75).

Metastases

Intraglandular lymph nodes are found in the parotid gland due to its early encapsulation during development. The sublingual gland and submandibular gland do not contain lymph nodes. The parotid and periparotid lymph nodes are the first order nodal site for lesions that affect the scalp, skin of the upper face, and external ear (Ollila and Leland et al. 1999). The most common malignancy to metastasize to the parotid nodes is squamous cell carcinoma, followed by melanoma and less commonly Merkel cell carcinoma (Bron, Traynor, and McNeil et al. 2003) (Figures 2.76 through 2.78).

The imaging findings are not specific. CT in early stages demonstrates the nodes to have sharp

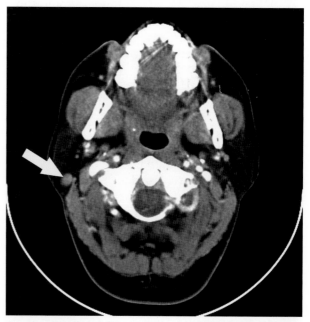

Figure 2.76. Axial CT of a mass in the right parotid gland with homogenous enhancement. The patient had a history of right facial melanoma. Metastatic melanoma was diagnosed at surgery.

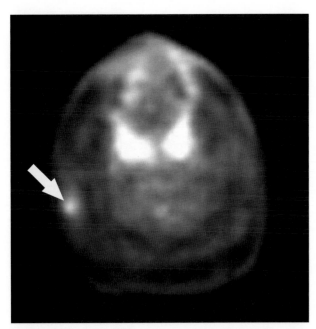

Figure 2.77. Axial PET scan corresponding to the case illustrated in Figure 2.76. The mass in the right parotid gland (arrow) is hypermetabolic. Also note two foci of intense uptake corresponding to inflammatory changes in the tonsils.

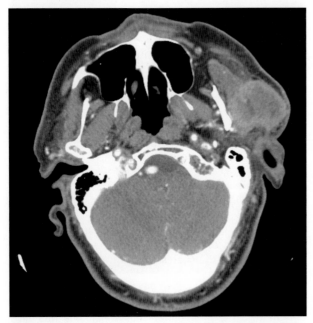

Figure 2.78. Axial contrast enhanced CT scan through the parotid glands demonstrating a large mass of heterogenous density and enhancement partially exophytic from the gland. Metastatic squamous cell carcinoma from the scalp was diagnosed.

margins and round or ovoid architecture but without a fatty hilum. Late in the disease, mass can mimic infected or inflammatory nodes with heterogenous borders, enhancement, and necrosis. Late in the disease with extranodal spread the margins blur and are ill-defined. Contrast enhancement is heterogenous. Similar findings are seen on MRI with T1 showing low to intermediate signal pre-contrast and homogenous to heterogenous signal post-contrast depending on intranodal versus extranodal disease. PET with FDG is abnormal in infectious, inflammatory, and neoplastic etiology and is not typically helpful within the parotid, but can aid in localizing the site of the primary lesion as well as other sites of metastases. This can be significant since the incidence of clinically occult neck disease is high in skin cancer metastatic to the parotid gland (Bron, Traynor, and McNeil et al. 2003). Local failure was highest with metastatic squamous cell carcinoma and distant metastases were higher in melanoma (Bron, Traynor, and McNeil et al. 2003).

With either squamous cell carcinoma or melanoma there is also a concern for perineural invasion and spread. Tumors commonly known to have perineural spread in addition to the above include adenoid cystic carcinoma, lymphoma, and schwannoma. The desmoplastic subtype of melanoma has a predilection for neurotropism (Chang, Fischbein, and McCalmont et al. 2004). The perineural spread along the facial nerve in the parotid gland and into the skull base at the stylomastoid foramen must be carefully assessed. MRI with contrast is the best means of evaluating the skull base foramina for perineural invasion. Gadolinium enhanced T1 MRI in the coronal plane provides optimal view of the skull base (Chang, Fischbein, and McCalmont et al. 2004). There may also be symptomatic facial nerve involvement with lymphadenopathy from severe infectious adenopathy or inflammatory diseases such as sarcoidosis.

Summary

- Among the choices for imaging of the salivary glands, CT with IV contrast is the most commonly performed procedure. Coronal and sagittal reformatted images provide excellent evaluation of soft tissues in orthogonal planes. The latest generation MDCT scanners provide rapid image acquisition reducing motion artifact and produce exquisite multi-planar reformatted images.

- US has the inherent limitation of being operator dependent and poor at assessing deep lobe of the parotid gland and surveying the neck for lymphadenopathy, as well as time consuming relative to the latest generation MDCT scanners.
- MRI should not be used as a primary imaging modality but reserved for special situations, such as assessment of the skull base for perineural spread of tumors. Although MRI provides similar information to CT, it is more susceptible to motion and has longer image acquisition time but has better soft tissue delineation.
- PET/CT can also be utilized for initial diagnosis and staging but excels in localizing recurrent disease in post-surgical or radiation fields. Its limitation is specificity, as inflammatory diseases and some benign lesions can mimic malignant neoplasms, and malignant lesions such as adenoid cystic carcinoma may not demonstrate significantly increased uptake of FDG. A major benefit is its ability to perform combined anatomic and functional evaluation of the head and neck as well as upper and lower torso in the same setting. The serial acquisitions are fused in order to provide a direct anatomic correlate to a focus of radiotracer uptake.
- Newer MRI techniques such as dynamic contrast enhancement, MR sialography, diffusion weighted imaging, MR spectroscopy, and MR microscopy are challenging PET/CT in functional evaluation of salivary gland disease and delineation of benign versus malignant tumors. However, PET/CT with novel tracers may repel this challenge.
- Conventional radionuclide scintigraphic imaging has largely been displaced. However, conventional scintigraphy with ^{99m}Tc-pertechnetate can be useful for the evaluation of masses suspected to be Warthin's tumor or oncocytoma, which accumulate the tracer and retain it after washout of the normal gland with acid stimulants. The advent of SPECT/CT in a similar manner to PET/CT may breathe new life into older scintigraphic exams.
- Radiology continues to provide a very significant contribution to clinicians and surgeons in the diagnosis, staging, and post-therapy follow-up of disease. Because of the complex anatomy of the head and neck, imaging is even more important in evaluation of diseases affecting this region. The anatomic and functional imaging, as well as the direct fusion of data from these methods, has had a beneficial effect on disease treatment and outcome. A close working relationship is important between radiologists and clinicians and surgeons in order to achieve these goals.

References

Abdel Razek A, Kandeel A, Soliman N et al. 2007. Role of diffusion-weighted echo-planar MR imaging in differentiation of residual or recurrent head and neck tumors and post-treatment changes. *Am J Neuroradiol* 28:1146–1152.

Alibek S, Zenk J, Bozzato A, Lell M et al. 2007. The value of dynamic MRI studies in parotid tumors. *Academic Radiology* 14:701–710.

Ando M, Matsuzaki M, Murofushi, T. 2005. Mucosa-associated lymphoid tissue lymphoma presents as diffuse swelling of the parotid gland. *Am J Otolaryngol* 26:285–288.

Aribandi M, Wood W, Elston D, Weiss, D. 2006. CT features of plexiform neurofibroma of the submandibular gland. *Am J Neuroradiol* 27:126–128.

Baba S, Engles J, Huso D et al. 2007. Comparison of uptake of multiple clinical radiotracers into brown adipose tissue under cold-stimulated and nonstimulated conditions. J Nucl Med 48:1715–1723.

Beale T, Madani G. 2006. Anatomy of the salivary glands. *Semin Ultrasound CT MRI* 27:436–439.

Beaulieu S, Kinaha P, Tseng J et al. 2003. SUV varies with time after injection in ^{18}F-FDG PET of breast cancer: Characterization and method to adjust for time differences. *J Nucl Med* 44:1044–1050.

Bialek E, Jakubowski W, Zajkowski P et al. 2006. US of the major salivary glands: Anatomy and spatial relationships, pathologic conditions and pitfalls. *Radiographics* 26:745–763.

Bron L, Traynor S, McNeil E et al. 2003. Primary and metastatic cancer of the parotid: Comparison of clinical behavior in 232 cases. *Laryngoscope* 113(6):1070–1075.

Bui C, Ching A, Carlos R et al. 2003. Diagnostic accuracy of 2-[fluorine-18]-fluro-2-deoxy-D-glucose positron emission tomography imaging in non-squamous tumors of the head and neck. *Invest Radiol* 38:593–601.

Burrell S, Van den Abbeele A. 2005. 2-deoxy-2-(F-18)-fluoro-D-glucose positron emission tomography of the head and neck: An atlas of normal uptake and variants. *Mol Imaging Biol* 7:244–256.

Cermik T, Mavi A, Acikgoz G et al. 2007. FDG PET in detecting primary and recurrent malignant salivary gland tumors. *Clin Nucl Med* 32(4):286–291.

Chang P, Fischbein N, McCalmont T et al. 2004. Perineural spread of malignant melanoma of the head and neck: Clinical and imaging features. *Am J Neuroradiol* 25:5–11.

Ching A, Ahuja A, King A et al. 2001. Comparison of the sonographic features of acalculous and calculous submandibular sialadenitis. *J Clin Ultrasound* 29(6): 332–338.

Cholankeril J, Scioscia P. 1993. Post-traumatic sialoceles and mucoceles of the salivary glands. *Clinical Imaging* 17(1):41–45.

Cohade C, Mourtzikos K, Wahl R. 2003. USA-Fat: Prevalence is related to ambient outdoor temperature—evaluation with ^{18}F-FDG PET/CT. *J Nucl Med* 44:1267–1270.

Cohade C, Osman M, Pannu H, Wahl R. 2003. Uptake in supraclavicular area fat (USA-Fat): Description on ^{18}F-FDG PET/CT. *J Nucl Med* 44:170–176.

de Ru JA, Van Leeuwen M, Van Benthem P et al. 2007. Do magnetic resonance imaging and ultrasound add anything to the workup of parotid gland tumors? *J Oral and Maxillofac Surg* 65:945–952.

Delbeke D, Coleman R, Guiberteau M et al. 2006. Procedure guidelines for tumor imaging with ^{18}F-FDG PET/CT. *J Nucl Med* 47:887–895.

Drumond J. 1995. Tomographic measurements of age changes in the human parotid gland. *Gerodontology* 12(1):26–30.

Eichhorn K, Iakovos A, Ridder G. 2002. Malignant non-Hodgkin's lymphoma mimicking a benign parotid tumor: Sonographic findings. *J Clin Ultrasound* 30(1):42–44.

Eida S, Sumi M, Sakihama N et al. 2007. Apparent diffusion coefficient mapping of salivary gland tumors: Prediction of the benignancy and malignancy. *Am J Neuroradiol* 28:116–121.

Gerstle R, Aylward S, Kromhout-Schiro S, Mukherji S et al. 2000. The role of neural networks in improving the accuracy of MR spectroscopy for the diagnosis of head and neck squamous cell carcinoma. *Am J Neuroradiol* 21:1133–1138.

Habermann C, Gossrau P, Kooijman H et al. 2007. Monitoring of gustatory stimulation of salivary glands by diffusion weighted MR imaging: Comparison of 1.5 T and 3 T. *Am J Neuroradiol* 28:1547–1551.

Hadi M, Chen C, Millie W et al. 2007. PET/CT, and ^{123}I-MIBG SPECT: A study of patients being evaluated for pheochromocytoma. *J Nucl Med* 48:1077–1083.

Hamilton B, Salzman K, Wiggins R, Harnsberger H. 2003. Earring Lesions of the Parotid Tail. *Am J Neuroradiol* 24:1757–1764.

Henkelman R, Watts J, Kucharczyk W. 1991. High signal intensity in MR images in calcified brain tissue. *Radiology* 179:199–206.

Holliday R. 1998. Benign lymphoepithelial parotid cysts and hyperplastic cervical adenopathy in AIDS-risk patients: A new CT appearance. *Radiology* 168:439–441.

Hopp E, Mortensen B, Kolbenstvedt A. 2004. Mylohyoid herniation of the sublingual gland diagnosed by magnetic resonance imaging. *Dentomaxillofacial Radiology* 33:351–353.

Hsu C, Lee C, Wang F, Fang C. 2003. Neurofibroma with increased uptake of F-18-fluoro-2-deoxy-D-glucose interpreted as a metastatic lesion. *Annals of Nuclear Medicine* 17:609–611.

Huang C, Damrose E, Bhuta S, Abemayor E. 2002. Kuttner tumor (chronic sclerosing sialadenitis). *Am J Otolaryngol* 23(6):394–397.

Ikeda M, Motoori K, Hanazawa T et al. 2004. Warthin tumor of the parotid gland: Diagnostic value of MR imaging with histopathologic correlation. *Am J Neuroradiol* 25:1256–1262.

Ikeda K, Tsutomu K, Ha-Kawa S et al. 1996. The usefulness of MR in establishing the diagnosis of parotid pleomorphic adenoma. *Am J Neuroradiol* 17:555–559.

Ioannidis J, Lau J. 2003. ^{18}F-FDG PET for the diagnosis and grading of soft-tissue sarcoma: A meta-analysis. *J Nucl Med* 44:717–724.

Izumi M, Eguchi K, Hideki N et al. 1997. Premature fat deposition in the salivary glands associated with Sjogren's syndrome: MR and CT evidence. *Am J Neuroradiol* 18(5):951–958.

Jansisyanont P, Blanchaert R, Ord R. 2002. Intraoral minor salivary gland neoplasm: A single institution experience of 80 cases. *Int J Oral Maxillofac Surg* 31(3):257–261.

Jeong H, Chung M, Son Y et al. 2007. Role of 18-F-FDG PET/CT in management of high-grade salivary gland malignancies. *J Nucl Med* 48:1237–1244.

Jhanvar Y, Straus D. 2006. The role of PET in lymphoma. *J Nucl Med* 47:1326–1334.

Kalinowski M, Heverhagen J, Rehberg E, Klose K et al. 2002. Comparative study of MR sialography and digital subtraction sialography for benign salivary gland disorders. *Am J Neuroradiol* 23:1485–1492.

Kaneda T. 1996. MR of the submandibular gland: Normal and pathologic states. *AJR* 17:1575–1581.

Keyes J, Harkness B, Greven K et al. 1994. Salivary gland tumors: Pretherapy evaluation with PET. *Radiology* 192:99–102.

King A, Yeung D, Ahuja A et al. 2005. Salivary gland tumors at in-vivo proton MR spectroscopy. *Radiology* 237:563–569.

Kinoshita T, Okitsu T. 2004. MR imaging findings of parotid tumors with pathologic diagnostic clues: A pictorial essay. *Clinical Imaging* 28:93–101.

Kirshenbaum K, Nadimpalli S et al. 1991. Benign lymphoepithelial parotid tumors in AIDS patients: CT and MR findings in nine cases. *Am J Neuroradiol* 12:271–274.

Koeller K, Alamo L, Adair C, Smirniotopoulos J. 1999. Congenital cystic masses of the neck: Radiologic-pathologic characteristics. *Radiographics* 19:121–146.

Kurabayashi T, Ida M, Yasumoto M et al. 2000. MRI of ranulas. *Neuroradiology* 42(12):917–922.

Lin J, Martel W. 2001. Cross-sectional imaging of peripheral nerve sheath tumors: Characteristic signs on CT, MR imaging and sonography. *AJR* 176:75–82.

Lowe L, Stokes L, Johnson J et al. 2001. Swelling at the angle of the mandible: Imaging of the pediatric parotid gland and periparotid region. *Radiographics* 21:1211–1227.

Macdonald A, Salzman K, Hansberger H. 2003. Giant ranula of the neck: Differentiation from cystic hygroma. *Am J Neuroradiol* 24:757–761.

MacManus M, Ryan G, Lau E, Wirth A, Hicks R. 2007. Positron emission tomography of stage IV mucosa-associated lymphoid tissue lymphoma confined to the four major salivary glands. *Australian Radiology* 51:68–70.

Madani G, Beale T. 2006a. Inflammatory conditions of the salivary glands. *Semin Ultrasound CT MRI* 27:440–451.

Madani G, Beale T. 2006b. Tumors of the salivary glands. *Semin Ultrasound CT MRI* 27:452–464.

Makariou E, Pikis A, Harley E. 2003. Cystic hygroma of the neck: Associated with a growing venous aneurysm. *Am J Neuroradiol* 24:2102–2104.

Martin N, Serkers O, Mompoint D, Nahum H. 1992. Facial nerve neuromas: MR imaging-report of four cases. *Neuroradiology* 34:62–67.

Martinoli C, Pretolesi F, Del Bono V et al. 1995. Benign lymphoepithelial parotid lesion in HIV-positive patients: Spectrum of findings at gray-scale and Doppler sonography. *AJR* 165:975–979.

Miyake H, Matsumoto A, Hori Y et al. 2001. Warthin's tumor of parotid gland on Tc-99m pertechnetate scintigraphy with lemon juice stimulation: Tc99m uptake, size, and pathologic correlation. *Eur Radiol* 11(12):2472–2478.

Moonis G, Patel P, Koshkareva Y et al. 2007. Imaging characteristics of recurrent pleomorphic adenoma of the parotid gland. *Am J Neuroradiol* 28:1532–1536.

Motoori K, Iida Y, Nagai Y et al. 2005. MR imaging of salivary duct carcinoma. *Am J Neuroradiol* 26:1201–1206.

Motoori K, Yamamoto S, Ueda T et al. 2004. Inter- and intratumoral variability in magnetic resonance imaging of pleomorphic adenoma. *J Comput Assist Tomogr* 28:233–246.

Nakamoto Y, Tatsumi M, Hammoud D et al. 2005. Normal FDG distribution patterns in the head and neck: PET/CT evaluation. *Radiology* 234:879–885.

Ollila DF, Leland ER et al. 1999. Parotid region lymphatic mapping and sentinel lymphadenopathy for cutaneous melanoma. *Ann of Surg Oncol* 6(2):150–154.

Otsuka H, Graham M, Kogame M, Nishitani H. 2005. The impact of FDG-PET in the management of patients with salivary gland malignancy. *Annals of Nuclear Medicine* 19(8):691–694.

Patel R, Carlos R, Midia M, Mukherji S. 2004. Apparent diffusion coefficient mapping of the normal parotid gland and parotid involvement in patients with systemic connective tissue disorders. *Am J Neuroradiol* 25:16–20.

Patz E, Lowe V, Hoffman J et al. 1993. Focal pulmonary abnormalities: Evaluation with F-18 fluorodeoxyglucose PET scanning. *Radiology* 188:487–490.

Roh J, Ryu C, Choi S et al. 2007. Clinical utility of ^{18}F-FDG PET for patients with salivary gland malignancies. *J Nucl Med* 48:240–246.

Rumboldt Z, Al-Okkaili R, Deveikis J. 2005. Perfusion CT for head and neck tumors: A pilot study. *Am J Neuroradiol* 26:1178–1185.

Schoder H, Erdi Y, Chao K et al. 2004. Clinical implications of different image reconstruction parameters for interpretation of whole-body PET studies in cancer patients. *J Nucl Med* 45:559–566.

Shah G. 2002. MR imaging of salivary glands. *Mag Reson Clin of N Am* 10:631–662.

Shah G, Fischbein N, Patel R, Mukherji S. 2003. Newer MR imaging techniques for head and neck. *Magn Reson Clin of N Am* 11:449–469.

Sheedy S, Welker K, Delone D, Gilbertson J. 2006. CNS metastases of carcinoma ex pleomorphic adenoma of the parotid gland. *Am J Neuroradiol* 27:1483–1485.

Shimizu K, Iwai H, Ikeda K et al. 2005. Intraparotid facial nerve schwannoma: A report of five cases and an analysis of MR imaging results. *Am J Neuroradiol* 26:1328–1330.

Sigal R, Monnet O, De Baere T et al. 1992. Adenoid cystic carcinoma of the head and neck: Evaluation with MR imaging and clinical-pathologic correlation in 27 patients. *Radiology* 184:95–101.

Sokoloff L. 1961. Local cerebral circulation at rest and during altered cerebral activity induced by anesthesia or visual stimulation. In Kety SS, Elkes J (eds.), The Regional Chemistry, Physiology and Pharmacology of the Nervous System. Oxford: Pergamon Press, pp 107–117.

Sokoloff L. 1986. Cerebral circulation, energy metabolism, and protein synthesis: General characteristics and principles of measurement. In Phelps M, Mazziotta J, Schelbert H (eds.), Positron Emission Tomography and Autoradiography: Principles and Applications for the Brain and Heart. New York: Raven Press, pp. 1–71.

Som P, Brandwein M, Silver A. 1995. Nodal inclusion cysts of the parotid gland and parapharyngeal space: A discussion of lymphoepithelial, AIDS-related parotid and branchial cysts, cystic Warthin's tumors, and cysts in Sjogren's syndrome. *Laryngoscope* 105(10):1122–1128.

Som P, Curtin H (eds.). 1996. Head and Neck Imaging (3rd ed.). St. Louis: Mosby, pp. 823–914.

Stahl A, Dzewas B, Schwaige W, Weber W. 2002. Excretion of FDG into saliva and its significance for PET imaging. *Nuklearmedizin* 41:214–216.

Su Y, Liao G, Kang Z, Zou Y. 2006. Application of magnetic resonance virtual endoscopy as a presurgical procedure before sialoendoscopy. *Laryngoscope* 116:1899–1906.

Sugai S. 2002. Mucosa-associated lymphoid tissue lymphoma in Sjogren's syndrome. *AJR* 179:485–489.

Suh J, Abenoza P, Galloway H et al. 1992. Peripheral (extracranial) nerve tumors: Correlation of MR imaging and histologic findings. *Radiology* 183:341–346.

Sumi M, Izumi M, Yonetsu K, Nakamura T. 1999a. Sublingual gland: MR features of normal and diseased states. *AJR* 172(3):717–722.

Sumi M, Izumi M, Yonetsu K, Nakamura T. 1999b. The MR imaging assessment of submandibular gland sialoadenitis secondary to sialolithiasis: Correlation with CT and histopathologic findings. *Am J Neuroradiol* 20:1737–1743.

Sumi M, Yamada T, Takagi Y, Nakamura T. 2007. MR imaging of labial glands. *Am J Neuroradiol* 28:1552–1556.

Takagi Y, Sumi M, Sumi T et al. 2005a. MR microscopy of the parotid glands in patients with Sjogren's syndrome: Quantitative MR diagnostic criteria. *Am J Neuroradiol* 26:1207–1214.

Takagi Y, Sumi M, Van Cauteren M, Nakamura T. 2005b. Fast and high resolution MR sialography using a small surface coil. *J Magn Reson Imaging* 22:29–37.

Takahashi N, Okamoto K, Ohkubo M, Kawana M. 2005. High-resolution magnetic resonance of the extracranial facial nerve and parotid duct: Demonstration of the branches of the intraparotid facial nerve and its relation to parotid tumours by MRI with a surface coil. *Clinical Radiology* 60:349–354.

Takashima S, Takeuchi N, Morimoto S et al. 1991. MR imaging of Sjogren's syndrome: Correlation with sialography and pathology. *J Comput Assist Tomogr* 15(3):393–400.

Takashima S, Tomofumi N, Noguchi Y et al. 1992. CT and MR appearances of parotid pseudotumors in Sjogren's syndrome. *J Comput Assist Tomogr* 16(3):376–383.

Tanaka T, Ono K, Habu M et al. 2007. Functional evaluation of the parotid and submandibular glands using dynamic magnetic resonance sialography. *Dentomaxillofacial radiology* 36:218–223.

Tatsumi M, Engles J, Ishimori T et al. 2004. Intense ^{18}F-FDG uptake in brown fat can be reduced pharmacologically. *J Nucl Med* 45:1189–1193.

Thoeny H. 2007. Imaging of salivary gland tumors. *Cancer Imaging* 7:52–62.

Tonami H, Matoba M, Yokota H et al. 2005. Diagnostic value of FDG PET and salivary gland scintigraphy for parotid tumors. *Clin Nucl Med* 30(3):170–176.

Tonami H, Munetaka M, Yokota H et al. 2002. Mucosa-associated lymphoid tissue lymphoma in Sjogren's syndrome: Initial and follow-up imaging features. *AJR* 179:485–489.

Uchida Y, Minoshima S, Kawata T et al. 2005. Diagnostic value of FDG PET and salivary gland scintigraphy for parotid tumors. *Clin Nucl Med* 30:170–176.

Wan Y, Chan S, Chen Y. 2004. Ultrasonography-guided core-needle biopsy of parotid gland masses. *Am J Neuroradiol* 25:1608–1612.

Wang Y, Chiu E, Rosenberg J, Gambhir S. 2007. Standardized uptake value atlas: Characterization of physiological 2-deoxy-2-[^{18}F]fluoro-D-glucose uptake in normal tissues. *Mol Imaging Biol* 9(2):83–90.

Warburg O. 1925. Uber den Stoffwechsel der Carcinom-Zelle. *Klinsche Wochenschrift* 4:534–536.

White D, Davidson H, Harnsberger H et al. 2001. Accessory salivary tissue in the mylohyoid boutonniere: A clinical and radiologic pseudolesion of the oral cavity. *Am J Neuroradiol* 22:406–412.

Wong K, Ahuja A, King A et al. 2004. Vascular lesion in the parotid gland in adult patients: Diagnosis with high-resolution ultrasound and MRI. *British J of Radiol* 77:600–606.

Yabuuchi H, Fukuya T, Tajima T et al. 2002. Salivary gland tumors: Diagnostic value of gadolinium enhanced dynamic MR imaging with histopathologic correlation. *Radiology* 226:345–354.

Yerli H, Aydin E, Coskum M et al. 2007. Dynamic multislice CT of parotid gland. *J Comput Assist Tomogr* 31(2):309–316.

Chapter 3
Infections of the Salivary Glands

Introduction

Most non-neoplastic swellings of the major salivary glands represent acute or chronic infections of these glands. Sialadenitis, a generic term to describe infection of the salivary glands, has a diverse range of signs and symptoms and predisposing factors. Although any of the major and minor salivary glands can become infected, these conditions most commonly occur in the parotid (Figure 3.1) and submandibular (Figure 3.2) glands, with minor salivary gland and sublingual gland infections being very rare. From an etiologic standpoint, these infections may be related to underlying bacterial, viral, fungal, mycobacterial, parasitic, or immunologically mediated infections (Miloro and Goldberg 2002). The most common of these diagnoses include acute bacterial parotitis and acute submandibular sialadenitis (see Table 3.1). A number of risk factors may predispose patients to sialadenitis. The classic risk factor is the hospitalized patient who recently underwent surgery with general anesthesia. Dehydration may exacerbate this condition. In general terms, stasis and decreased salivary flow predispose patients to sialadenitis, although medications and comorbid diagnoses may also contribute to this problem (see Table 3.2).

General Considerations

Evaluation and treatment of the patient with sialadenitis begins with a thorough history and physical examination. The setting in which the evaluation occurs, for example, a hospital ward vs. an office, may provide information as to the underlying cause of the infection. Many cases of acute bacterial parotitis (ABP) occur in elderly debilitated patients, some of whom are admitted to the hospital, who demonstrate inadequate fluid intake with resultant dehydration. This notwithstanding, many cases of acute bacterial parotitis and submandibular sialadenitis are evaluated initially in an outpatient setting. The formal history taking begins by obtaining the chief complaint. Sialadenitis commonly begins as swelling of the salivary gland with pain due to stretching of that gland's innervated capsule. Patients may or may not describe the perception of pus associated with salivary secretions, and the absence of pus may be confirmed on physical examination.

History taking is important so as to disclose the acute or chronic nature of the problem that will

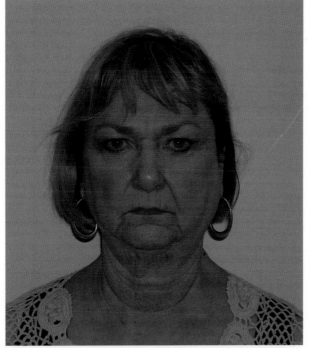

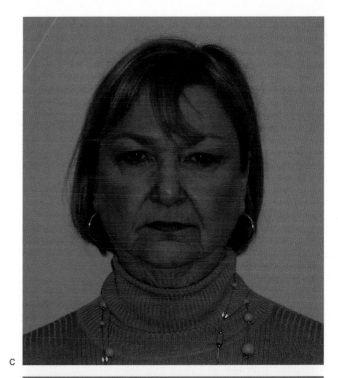

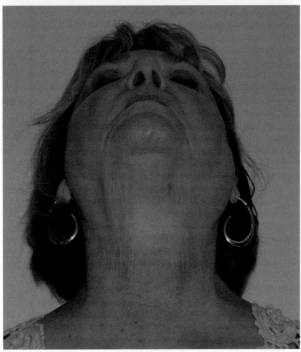

Figures 3.1a and 3.1b. A 55-year-old woman with a 1-week history of pain and swelling in the left parotid gland. No pus was present at Stenson's duct. The diagnosis was community acquired acute bacterial parotitis. Conservative measures were instituted, including the use of oral antibiotics, warm compresses to the left face, sialogogues, and digital massage.

Figures 3.1c and 3.1d. Two weeks later, she was asymptomatic, and physical examination revealed resolution of her swelling.

68

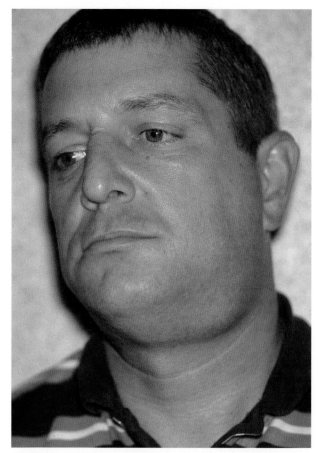

Figure 3.2a. A 45-year-old man with a 6-month history of left submandibular pain and swelling. A clinical diagnosis of chronic submandibular sialadenitis was made.

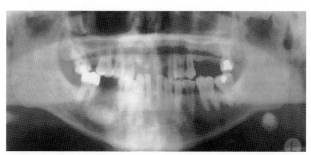

Figure 3.2b. A screening panoramic radiograph was obtained that revealed the presence of a large sialolith in the gland. As such, the obstruction of salivary outflow by the sialolith was responsible for the chronic sialadenitis. This case underscores the importance of obtaining a screening panoramic radiograph in a patient with a clinical diagnosis of sialadenitis, as it permitted expedient diagnosis of sialolithiasis.

Table 3.1. Classification of salivary gland infections.

Bacterial infections
  Acute bacterial parotitis
  Chronic bacterial parotitis
  Chronic recurrent juvenile parotitis
  Acute suppurative submandibular sialadenitis
  Chronic recurrent submandibular sialadenitis
  Acute allergic sialadenitis
Viral infections
  Mumps
  HIV/AIDS
  Cytomegalovirus
Fungal infections
Mycobacterial infections
  Tuberculosis
  Atypical mycobacteria
Parasitic infections
Autoimmune-related infections
  Systemic lupus erythematosus
  Sarcoidosis
  Sjogren's syndrome

Table 3.2. Risk factors associated with salivary gland infections.

Modifiable risk factors
  Dehydration
  Recent surgery and anesthesia
  Malnutrition
  Medications
    Antihistamines
    Diuretics
    Tricyclic antidepressants
    Phenothiazines
    Antihypertensives
    Barbiturates
    Antisialogogues
    Anticholinergics
    Chemotherapeutic agents
  Sialolithiasis
  Oral infection
Non-modifiable risk factors
  Advanced age
Relatively non-modifiable risk factors
  Radiation therapy where cytoprotective agents were
    not administered
  Renal failure
  Hepatic failure
  Congestive heart failure
  HIV/AIDS
  Diabetes mellitus
  Anorexia nervosa/bulimia
  Cystic fibrosis
  Cushing's disease

69

significantly impact on how the sialadenitis is ultimately managed. For the purpose of prognosis and the anticipation as to the possible need for future surgical intervention, an acute sialadenitis is somewhat arbitrarily classified as one where symptoms are less than 1 month in duration, while a chronic sialadenitis is defined as having been present for longer than 1 month. In addition, the history will permit the clinician to assess the risk factors associated with the condition. In so doing, the realization of modifiable vs. relatively non-modifiable vs. non-modifiable risk factors can be determined. For example, dehydration, recent surgery, oral infection, and some medications represent modifiable risk factors predisposing patients to sialadenitis. On the other hand, advanced age is a non-modifiable risk factor, and chronic medical illnesses and radiation therapy constitute relatively non-modifiable risk factors associated with these infections. The distinction between modifiable and relatively non-modifiable risk factors is not intuitive. For example, dehydration is obviously modifiable. The sialadenitis associated with diabetes mellitus may abate clinically as evidenced by decreased swelling and pain; however, the underlying medical condition is not reversible. The same is true for HIV/AIDS. While much medical comorbidity can be controlled and palliated, these conditions often are not curable such that patients may be fraught with recurrent sialadenitis at unpredictable time frames following the initial event. As such these and many other risk factors are considered relatively non-modifiable.

Other features of the history, such as the presence or absence of prandial pain, may direct the physical and radiographic examinations to the existence of an obstructive phenomenon. The presence of medical conditions and the use of medications to manage these conditions are very important elements of the history taking of a patient with a chief complaint suggestive of sialadenitis. They may be determined to be of etiologic significance when the physical examination confirms the diagnosis of sialadenitis. Musicians playing wind instruments who present for evaluation of bilateral parotid swelling and pain after a concert may have acute air insufflation of the parotid glands as part of the "trumpet blower's syndrome" (Miloro and Goldberg 2002). Recent dental work, specifically the application of orthodontic brackets, may result in traumatic introduction of bacteria into the ductal system with resultant retrograde sialadenitis. Deep facial lacerations proximal to an imaginary line connecting the lateral canthus of the eye to the oral commissure, and along an imaginary line connecting the tragus to the mid-philtrum of the lip, may violate the integrity of Stenson's duct. While a thorough exploration of these wounds with cannulation and repair of Stenson's duct is meticulously performed, it is possible for foreign bodies to result in obstruction of salivary flow with resultant parotid swelling. A number of autoimmune diseases with immune complex formation can also be responsible for sialadenitis, and confirmation of their diagnosis should be sought during the history and physical examination.

After the history has been completed, the physical examination should be performed. In the patient with suspected sialadenitis, the examination is focused on the head and neck and begins with the extraoral examination followed by the intraoral examination. In particular, the salivary glands should be assessed in a bimanual fashion for asymmetries, erythema, tenderness to palpation, swellings, and warmth. In so doing, one of the most important aspects of this examination is to rule out the presence of a tumor. A neoplastic process of the parotid gland presents as a *discrete* mass within the gland, with or without symptoms of pain. An infectious process presents as a *diffuse* enlargement of the parotid gland that is commonly symptomatic. It is possible for an indurated inflammatory lymph node within the parotid gland to simulate neoplastic disease. The distinction in the character of the parotid gland is important so as to not waste time treating a patient for an infectious process when they have a tumor in the parotid gland, particularly in the event of a malignancy. Evidence of facial trauma, including healing facial lacerations or ecchymoses, should be ascertained. The intraoral examination focuses on the observation of the quality and quantity of spontaneous and stimulated salivary flow. It is important to understand, however, that the anxiety and sympathomimetic response associated with the examination is likely to decrease salivary flow. Nonetheless, an advanced case of sialadenitis will often allow the clinician to appreciate the flow of pus from the salivary ducts (Figure 3.3). If pus is not observed, mucous plugs, small stones, or "salivary sludge" may be noted. As part of the examination, it may be appropriate to perform cannulation of the salivary duct with a series of lacrimal probes (Figure 3.4). This maneuver may dislodge obstructive material or diagnose an obstruction. The decision to perform this instrumentation, however, must not be made indiscriminately. This procedure

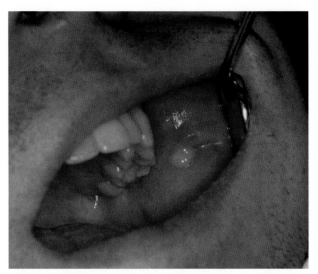

Figure 3.3. Pus expressed from Stenson's duct that reflects an acute bacterial parotitis.

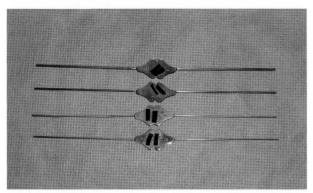

Figure 3.4. Lacrimal probes are utilized to probe the salivary ducts. The four shown in this figure incrementally increase in size. Cannulation of salivary ducts begins with the smallest probe and proceeds sequentially to the largest so as to properly dilate the duct. It is recommended that patients initiate a course of antibiotics prior to probing salivary ducts so as to not exacerbate the sialadenitis by introducing oral bacteria into the gland.

may introduce bacteria into the salivary duct that normally colonize around the ductal orifice, thereby permitting retrograde contamination of the gland. This procedure is probably contraindicated in acute bacterial parotitis. The head and neck examination concludes by palpating the regional lymph nodes, including those in the preauricular and cervical regions.

Radiographs of the salivary glands may be obtained after performing the history and physical examination. Since radiographic analysis of the salivary glands is the subject of chapter 2, they will not be discussed in detail in this chapter. Nonethe-

less, plain films and specialized imaging studies may be of value in evaluating patients with a clinical diagnosis of sialadenitis. Screening plain radiographs such as a panoramic radiograph and/or an occlusal radiograph is important data to obtain when a history exists that suggests an obstructive phenomenon. The presence of a sialolith on plain films, for example, represents very important information with which to direct therapy. It permits the clinician to identify the etiology of the sialadenitis and to remove the stone at an early time frame. Such expedience may permit the avoidance of chronicity such that gland function can be maintained.

Bacterial Salivary Gland Infections

ACUTE BACTERIAL PAROTITIS (ABP)

World history indicates that acute bacterial parotitis played a significant role in its chronicles, particularly in the United States. We are told that the first case of ABP occurred in Paris in 1829 in a 71-year-old man where the parotitis progressed to gangrene (McQuone 1999; Miloro and Goldberg 2002). As mumps plays a role in the differential diagnosis of infectious parotitis, Brodie's distinction between acute bacterial parotitis and viral mumps in 1834 represents a major inroad into the understanding of this pathologic process (Brodie 1834; Goldberg and Bevilacqua 1995). Prior to the modern surgical era, ABP was not uncommonly observed, and indeed represented a dreaded complication of major surgery, with a mortality rate as high as 50% (Goldberg and Bevilacqua 1995). Ineffective postoperative intravascular volume repletion with resultant diminished salivary flow and dry mouth were the norm rather than the exception. President James Garfield sustained a gunshot wound to the abdomen in July 1881 and developed chronic peritonitis and ultimately died several months later. The terminal event was described as suppurative parotitis that led to sepsis (Goldberg and Bevilacqua 1995). It has been pointed out that upper and lower aerodigestive tract surgeries require patients to be without oral nutritional intake or with limited oral intake postoperatively (McQuone 1999). The reduction of salivary stimulation predisposes these patients to acute bacterial parotitis, with an estimated incidence of 1 in 1,000 postoperative patients (Andrews, Abemayor, and Alessi et al. 1989). Other figures showed 3.68 cases per 10,000 operations in the preantibiotic era compared with 0.173 cases per 10,000 operations in the antibiotic era (Robinson

1955). The prophylactic use of antibiotics has probably contributed to the reduction of cases of acute bacterial parotitis. In addition, intraoperative and postoperative intravenous hydration became well accepted in the 1930s, particularly during World War II, therefore also contributing to the reduction in the incidence of ABP. In 1958 Petersdorf reported 7 cases of staphylococcal parotitis, and the 1960s ushered in several reports of ABP as a disease making a comeback (Goldberg and Bevilacqua 1995; Petersdorf, Forsyth, and Bernanke 1958). Of Petersdorf's 7 cases, 5 of the patients had undergone surgery, and 2 of the patients died in the hospital. Oral and maxillofacial surgeons began to report cases of ABP in the literature in the 1960s (Goldberg and Harrigan 1965; Guralnick, Donoff, and Galdabini 1968).

The parotid gland's relative propensity for infection results from physiologic and anatomic factors. Parotid saliva differs from that of the submandibular and sublingual glands. Parotid saliva is predominantly serous compared to the mucinous saliva from the submandibular and sublingual glands. Mucoid saliva contains lysosomes and IgA antibodies that protect against bacterial infection. Mucins also contain sialic acid, which agglutinates bacteria, thereby preventing its adherence to host tissues. Glycoproteins found in mucins bind epithelial cells, thereby inhibiting bacterial attachment to the epithelial cells of the salivary duct.

Variants of ABP and Their Etiology

Over the past several decades changes have occurred in the bacterial flora of the oral cavity that directly reflect the identification of organisms in ABP. In part, this change is evident due to the increased incidence of nosocomial and opportunistic infections in patients who are immunocompromised as well as those critically ill patients in hospital intensive care units whose mouths became colonized with micro-organisms that were previously only rarely found in the oral cavity. Moreover, improved culturing techniques have permitted the identification of anaerobes that were previously difficult to recover in the microbiology laboratory. Finally, the occasionally indiscriminate use of antibiotics has allowed for the occupation of other organisms in the oral cavity such as Gramnegative enteric organisms. Bacterial Darwinism has also occurred such that iatrogenically and genetically altered staphylococcal organisms have developed penicillin resistance.

Acute bacterial parotitis has two well-defined presentations, *community acquired* and *hospital acquired* variants. Numerous factors predispose the parotid gland to sialadenitis. Retrograde infection is recognized as the major cause of ABP. As a result of acute illness, sepsis, trauma, or surgery, depleted intravascular volume may result in diminished salivary flow that in turn diminishes the normal flushing action of saliva as it passes through Stenson's duct. Patients with salivary secretions of modest flow rates show bacteria at the duct papillae and in cannulated ducts, while patients with salivary secretions of high rates show bacteria at the duct papillae but not within the duct (Katz, Fisher, and Levine 1990). In a healthy state, fibronectin exists in high concentrations within parotid saliva, which promotes the adherence of *Streptococcus* species and *S. aureus* around the ductal orifice of Stenson's duct (Katz, Fisher, and Levine 1990). Low levels of fibronectin as occur in the unhealthy host are known to promote the adherence of Pseudomonas and E. coli. This observation explains the clinical situation whereby colonization as a result of dehydration leads to a Gram-positive sialadenitis in ABP compared to the development of Gram-negative sialadenitis of the parotid gland in immunocompromised patients (Miloro and Goldberg 2002). Depending on the health of the host, therefore, specific colonized bacteria are able to infect the parotid gland in a retrograde fashion. Hospital acquired ABP still shows cultures of *Staphylococcus aureus* in over 50% of cases (Goldberg and Bevilacqua 1995). Methicillin resistant *Staphylococcus aureus* should be ruled out in this population of inpatients. Critically ill and immunocompromised inpatients may also show *Pseudomonas*, *Klebsiella*, *Escherichia coli*, *Proteus*, *Eikenella corrodens*, *Haemophilus influenzae*, *Prevotella*, and *Fusobacterium* species. Postoperative parotitis has been reported from 1 to 15 weeks following surgery, but most commonly occurs within 2 weeks after surgery (McQuone 1999). The peak incidence of this disease seems to be between postoperative days 5 and 7.

Community acquired ABP is diagnosed five times more commonly than hospital acquired ABP and is diagnosed in emergency departments, offices, and outpatient clinics. This variant of ABP is most commonly associated with staphylococcal and streptococcal species. As community acquired methicillin resistant *Staphylococcus aureus* becomes more common in society, this organism will become more prevalent in community acquired

ABP. Etiologic factors in community acquired ABP include medications that decrease salivary flow, trauma to Stenson's duct, cheek biting, toothbrush trauma, trumpet blower's syndrome, and medical conditions such as diabetes, malnutrition, and dehydration from acute or chronic gastrointestinal disorders with loss of intravascular volume. Sialoliths present in Stenson's duct with retrograde infection are less common than in Wharton's duct, but this possibility should also be considered in the patient with community acquired ABP.

Diagnosis of ABP

Diagnosis of ABP requires a thorough history and physical examination followed by laboratory and radiographic corroboration of the clinical diagnosis. Whether occurring in out-patient or in-patient arenas, a history of use of antisialogogue medications, dehydration, malnutrition, diabetes mellitus, immunosuppression, surgery, or systemic disease supports this diagnosis. A predilection for males exists for ABP, and the average age at presentation is 60 years (Miloro and Goldberg 2002). A systemic disorder will result in both glands being affected, but when one gland is affected, the right gland seems to be involved more commonly than the left gland (Miloro and Goldberg 2002). The declaration of acute requires that the parotitis has been present for one month or shorter.

The classic symptoms include an abrupt history of painful swelling of the parotid region, typically when eating. The physical findings are commonly dramatic, with parotid enlargement, often displacing the ear lobe, and tenderness to palpation. If Stenson's duct is patent, milking the gland may produce pus (Figure 3.3). A comparison of salivary flow should be performed by also examining the contralateral parotid gland as well as the bilateral submandibular glands. The identification of pus should alert the clinician to the need to obtain a sterile culture and sensitivity. Constitutional symptoms may be present, including fever and chills, and temperature elevation may exist as long as the gland is infected. If glandular obstruction is present without infection, temperature elevation may not be present. Laboratory values will show a leukocytosis with a bandemia in the presence of true bacterial infection, with elevated hematocrit, blood urea nitrogen, and urine specific gravity if the patient is dehydrated. Electrolyte determinations should be performed in this patient population, particularly in in-patients and out-

patients who are malnourished. Probing of Stenson's duct is considered contraindicated in ABP. The concern is for pushing purulent material proximally in the gland, although an argument exists that probing may relieve duct strictures and mucous plugging.

The radiographic assessment of ABP is discussed in detail in chapter 2. Briefly, plain films are of importance so as to rule out sialoliths, and special imaging studies are indicated to further image the parotid gland. The presence of an intraparotid abscess on special imaging studies, for example, may direct the clinician to the need for expedient incision and drainage.

Treatment of ABP

The treatment of ABP is a function of the setting in which ABP is diagnosed, as well as the severity of the disease within the parotid gland and the presence of medical comorbidities (Figure 3.5). In the outpatient setting, the presence or absence of pus will assist in directing specific therapy. The presence of pus should result in culture and sensitivity. Early species-specific antibiotic therapy is the sine qua non of treatment of ABP. Empiric antibiotic therapy should be based on a Gram stain of ductal exudates. In general terms, an anti-staphylococcal penicillin or a first-generation cephalosporin is a proper choice. Antibiotics should be changed if cultures and sensitivities show methicillin resistant staphylococcal species, in which case clindamycin is indicated in community acquired ABP. In the absence of pus, empiric antibiotic therapy should be instituted as described above. Antibiotic compliance is often difficult for patients such that once- or twice-daily antibiotics are always preferable. In all patients with community acquired ABP, other general measures should be followed including the stimulation of salivary flow with digital massage, the use of dry heat, and the use of sour ball candies. Sugarless sour ball candies should be recommended for diabetics or those with impaired glucose tolerance. Some elderly and debilitated out-patients may require admission to the hospital, in which case intravenous antibiotic therapy will be instituted and incision and drainage may be required. Alteration of anti-sialogogue medications should be accomplished as soon as possible. In the out-patient setting, these commonly include urinary incontinence medications, loop diuretics, beta blockers, and antihistamines. Glycemic control in diabetics is beneficial in the control of ABP. Finally, effective

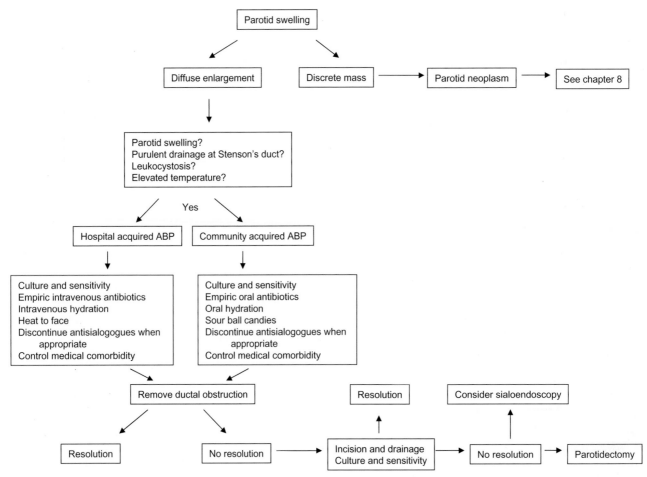

Figure 3.5. Algorithm for treatment of acute bacterial parotitis.

control of viral load in HIV infected patients is of utmost importance.

Imaging of out-patients with community acquired ABP is based on the severity of the clinical disease, its chronicity, and the clinician's suspicion for intra-parotid abscess. Obtaining routine plain films, such as panoramic and occlusal radiographs, is certainly indicated. The main purpose of obtaining these films is to investigate for the presence of a sialolith. It may be acceptable, however, to defer special imaging studies in these patients until refractory infection develops. Patients with severe symptoms, fever, and concern for abscess formation within the parotid gland should be imaged with CT scans in an expedient fashion. Except in the presence of severe immunosuppression or other medical comorbidity, refractory infections are uncommonly seen in ABP.

The general principles of the management of hospital acquired ABP are identical to those of the community acquired ABP. As previously described,

however, the risk factors differ. In these in-patients, rehydration should be performed with caution to avoid cardiac overload. Empiric intravenous antibiotics should be instituted in these patients, and confirmed as to their efficacy with culture and sensitivity of purulent parotid exudates whenever possible. The use of heat to the affected gland is appropriate in this setting, as well. The in-patient should be monitored closely for clinical improvement. Despite the institution of conservative measures, if the patient's course deteriorates within 48–72 hours as evident by increased swelling and pain, or an increase in white blood cell count, an incision and drainage procedure is indicated (Figure 3.6). Such a procedure must be guided by CT scans so as to explore all loculations of pus. A needle aspiration of a parotid abscess is unlikely to represent a definitive drainage procedure, although it will permit the procurement of a sample of pus prior to instituting antibiotic therapy in preparation for incision and drainage.

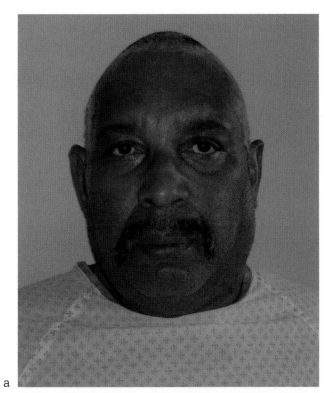
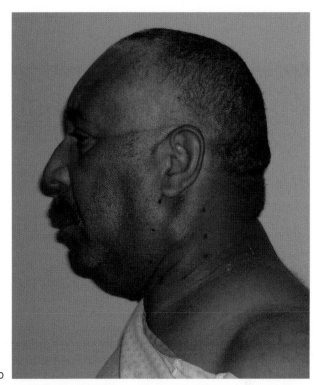

a
b

Figures 3.6a and 3.6b. A 65-year-old man with a 2-week history of left parotid/neck swelling and pain.

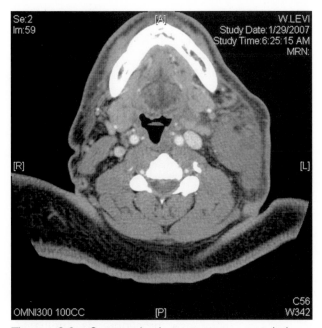

Figure 3.6c. Computerized tomograms revealed an abscess within the left parotid gland.

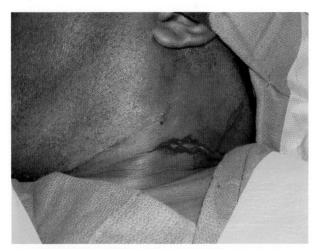

Figure 3.6d. The patient underwent incision and drainage in the operating room for a diagnosis of community acquired acute bacterial parotitis with abscess formation. Methicillin resistant *Staph aureus* species were cultured.

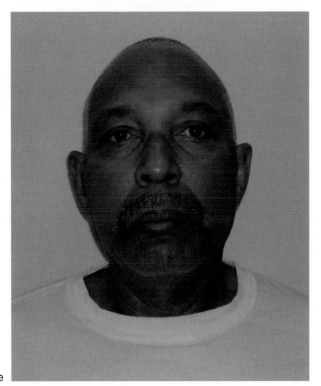
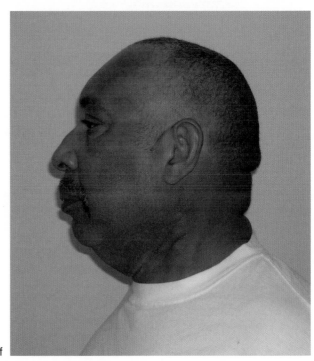

e

f

Figures 3.6e and 3.6f. At 2 months postoperatively he showed resolution of the disease.

CHRONIC (RECURRENT OR REFRACTORY) BACTERIAL PAROTITIS

Chronic bacterial parotitis occurs in at least three clinical settings. The first is one in which the patient defers evaluation such that the condition has persisted for at least 1 month. The second includes the setting in which acute bacterial parotitis was managed conservatively but without resolution (refractory sialadenitis). Finally, it is possible for an untreated parotitis to become recurrent such that periods of remission separate recurrent episodes of ABP. The parotid gland may demonstrate evidence of latent infection despite clinical resolution of the disease. The result is scarring in the gland such that function is impaired. Histology will show dilation of glandular ducts, abscess formation, and atrophy (Patey 1965). Pus is rarely observed in chronic bacterial parotitis (Baurmash 2004). Rather, there is a marked reduction of salivary flow, and the parotid secretions are viscous and milky in appearance. The microbiologic etiology of chronic bacterial parotitis is most commonly streptococci and staphylococci, but other organisms may be found as a function of the patient's immune status, the setting in which the parotitis originally occurred, and medical comor-

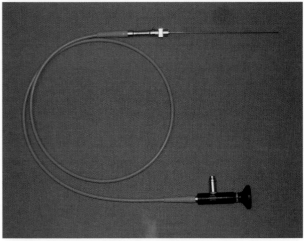

Figure 3.7a. The miniature endoscope for diagnostic and interventional sialoendoscopic procedures (Karl Storz Endoscopy-America, Inc., Culver City California). The instrumentation seen here is utilized for diagnostic procedures only. The endoscope may be connected to an operating sheath for interventional procedures (see chapter 5).

bidity. It has been suggested that the accumulation of a semisolid material that obstructs the parotid duct is the culprit in chronic bacterial parotitis (Baurmash 2004). The clinical course of the disease shows pain and swelling waxing and waning.

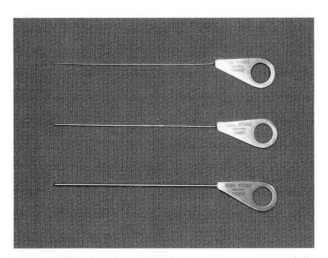

Figure 3.7b. A series of duct dilators are sequentially inserted into Stenson's duct prior to placing the sialoendoscope.

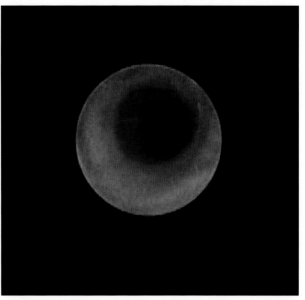

Figure 3.7d. A representative image is noted that demonstrates normal findings in a patient with chronic parotid pain. The sialoendoscopy procedure, including dilatation and irrigation of the duct, resulted in resolution of symptoms.

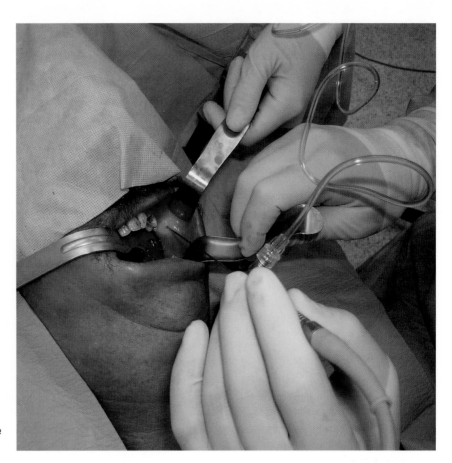

Figure 3.7c. The sialoendoscope placed into Stenson's duct.

Treatment of Chronic Bacterial Parotitis

Treatment of chronic bacterial parotitis centers on palliative therapy with parotidectomy reserved as a last resort. Effective treatment is centered on the gland inflammation as well as the precipitated intraductal material. Patients should be treated with culture specific systemic antibiotics, ductal antibiotic irrigations during periods of remission, analgesics, and avoidance of dehydration and anti-sialogogue medications (Goldberg and Bevilacqua 1995). Sialoendoscopy represents a technique that may obviate the need for aggressive surgical intervention (Hasson 2007; Nahlieli et al. 2006). Sialoendoscopic findings of patients with chronic obstructive parotitis include ductal stricture, mucous plugs, and desquamative epithelial cells

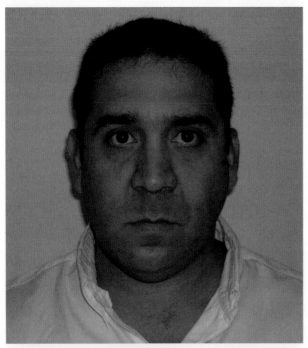

a

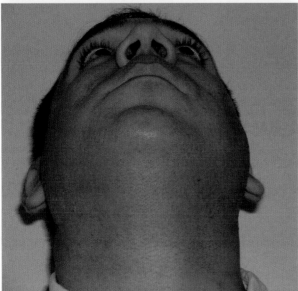

b

Figures 3.8a and 3.8b. A 35-year-old man with a 2-year history of left parotid pain and swelling.

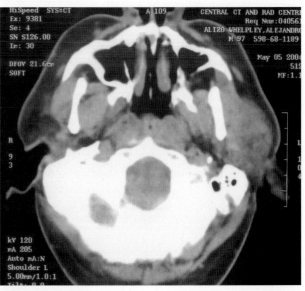

Figure 3.8c. Computerized tomograms showed sclerosis of the parotid parenchyma as well as a suspected abscess. The patient underwent left superficial parotidectomy with a clinical and radiographic diagnosis of chronic bacterial parotitis with abscess formation.

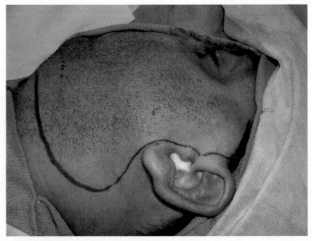

Figure 3.8d. The superficial parotidectomy was accessed with a standard incision.

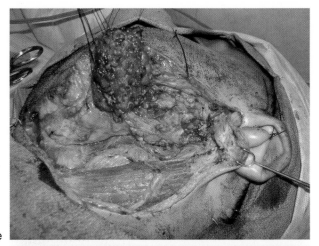

e

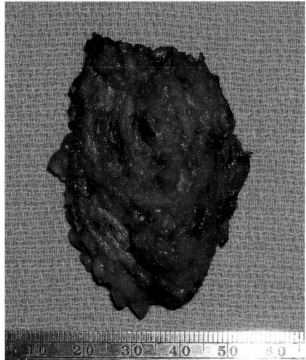

f

Figures 3.8e and 3.8f. A nerve-sparing approach was followed (e) that allowed for delivery of the specimen (f).

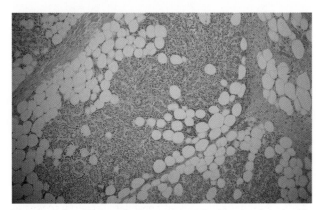

Figure 3.8g. Histopathology showed chronic sialadenitis with abscess formation.

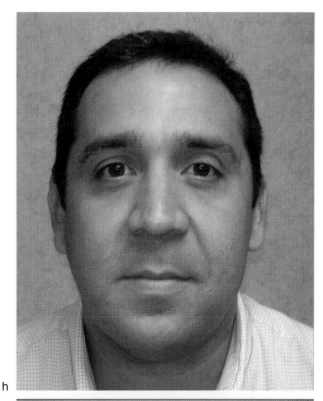

h

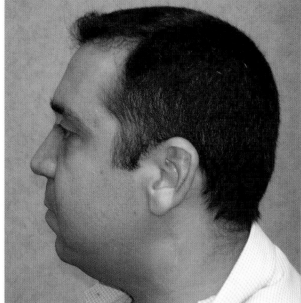

i

Figures 3.8h and 3.8i. At 3 years postoperatively he displays resolution of the disease.

79

and inflammatory cells (Qi, Liu, and Wang 2005). A sialoendoscopic procedure may address any or all of these problems, thereby sparing the gland (Figure 3.7). If pain and swelling become intolerable for the patient, or if special imaging studies reveal abscess formation in the parotid gland, then nerve-sparing parotidectomy is the treatment of choice (Figure 3.8).

CHRONIC RECURRENT JUVENILE PAROTITIS

Recurrent juvenile parotitis is commonly noted prior to puberty and is manifested by numerous episodes of painful enlargements of the parotid gland. Chronic recurrent parotitis in children is ten times more common than chronic recurrent parotitis in adults (Baurmash 2004). Several etiologies have been offered including congenital abnormalities or strictures of Stenson's duct, trauma, foreign bodies within the duct, or a history of viral mumps. Many cases will resolve prior to the onset of puberty such that conservative measures are recommended. These include long-term antibiotics and analgesia. Spontaneous regeneration of salivary function has been reported (Galili and Marmary 1985).

BARTONELLA HENSELAE (CAT SCRATCH DISEASE)

Cat scratch disease (CSD) is a granulomatous lymphadenitis that most commonly results from cutaneous inoculation caused by a scratch from a domestic cat. The causative microorganism is *Bartonella henselae*, a Gram-negative bacillus. Approximately 90% of patients who have cat scratch disease have a history of exposure to cats, and 75% of these patients report a cat scratch or bite (Arrieta and McCaffrey 2005). Dogs have been implicated in 5% of these cases. This disease process begins in the preauricular and cervical lymph nodes as a chronic lymphadenitis and may ultimately involve the salivary glands, most commonly the parotid gland by contiguous spread (English, Wear, and Margileth et al. 1988).

The diagnosis of CSD has changed with advances in serologic and molecular biologic techniques. These methods have replaced the need for the Rose Hanger skin test previously used. Testing for the presence of antibodies to *Bartonella henselae*

is now the most commonly used test to confirm the diagnosis. The two methods used for antibody detection are the indirect fluorescent antibody (IFA) and the enzyme immunoassay (EIA). When tissue is removed for diagnosis, histologic examination might demonstrate bacilli with the use of Warthin-Starry staining or a Steiner stain. Lymph node involvement shows reticular cell hyperplasia, granuloma formation, and occasionally a stellate abscess.

In most cases, no active therapy is required. The patient should be reassured that the lymphadenopathy is self-limited and will spontaneously resolve in 2–4 months. Antibiotic therapy is indicated when patients are symptomatic. Antibiotics reported to be most effective include rifampin, erythromycin, gentamycin, azithromycin, and ciprofloxacin. Surgery becomes necessary when the diagnosis is equivocal, or when incision and drainage is indicated (Figure 3.9).

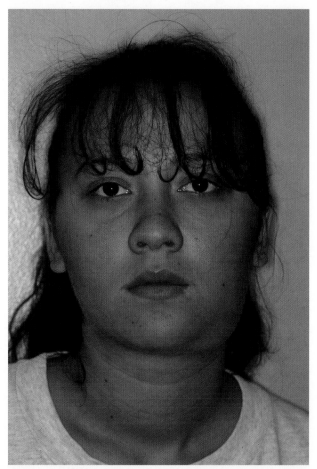

Figure 3.9a. A 21-year-old woman with a 2-week history of left submandibular pain and swelling. A history of animal scratch was provided.

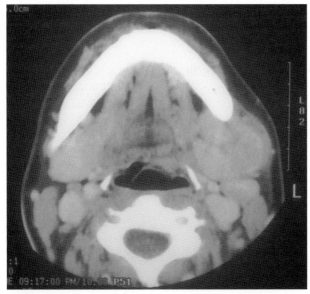

Figure 3.9b. Computerized tomograms revealed a mass of the left submandibular gland. The patient was taken to the operating room, where excision of the submandibular gland and mass was performed.

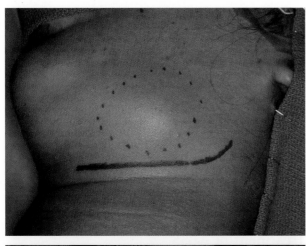

c

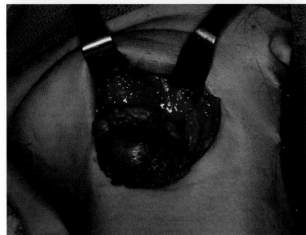

d

Figures 3.9c and 3.9d. Wide access was afforded (c) and the mass was exposed (d).

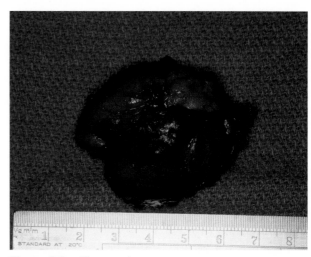

Figure 3.9e. The specimen.

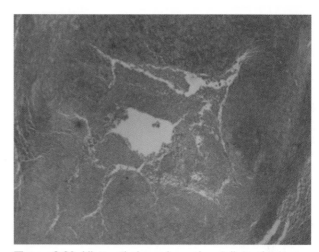

Figure 3.9f. Histopathology showed a stellate abscess.

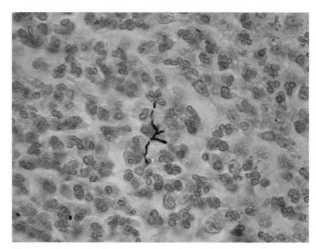

Figure 3.9g. A Steiner stain showed Bartonella (gram negative bacillus).

81

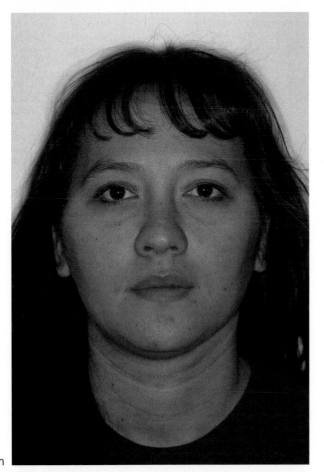 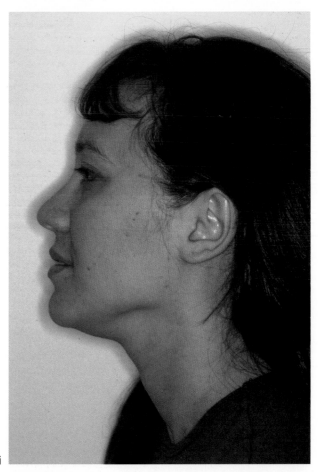

h   i

Figures 3.9h and 3.9i. Her disease resolved without long-term antibiotics as seen in 5-year postoperative images.

ACUTE BACTERIAL SUBMANDIBULAR SIALADENITIS (ABSS)

Acute bacterial submandibular sialadenitis is usually associated with physical obstruction of Wharton's duct. Since sialolithiasis, the likely cause of obstruction of the duct, is discussed in chapter 5, it is only briefly mentioned here. Suffice it to say that the submandibular ductal system is prone to stone formation. The common features of ABSS are swelling in the submandibular region associated with prandial pain. ABSS is a community acquired disease that less frequently is associated with dehydration and hospitalization as compared to ABP. Purulence may be expressed from the opening of Wharton's duct, but in many cases complete obstruction to pus and saliva occurs.

Treatment of ABSS

Treatment of ABSS consists of antibiotic therapy, hydration, avoidance of anti-sialogogues, and removal of a sialolith, if one is identified. Empiric antibiotics used to treat ABSS are similar to ABP, including an extended-spectrum penicillin, a first-generation cephalosporin, clindamycin, or a macrolide. Patients are also encouraged to use sialogogues, such as sour ball candies.

CHRONIC RECURRENT SUBMANDIBULAR SIALADENITIS

Chronic recurrent submandibular sialadenitis usually follows ABSS and is associated with recurrent sialolithiasis. Chronic recurrent submandibular sialadenitis occurs more commonly than chronic recurrent bacterial parotitis. Initial treatment for chronic recurrent submandibular sialadenitis begins with antibiotic therapy, sialogogues, and hydration. Sialoendoscopic intervention may also be of benefit

in the treatment of chronic recurrent submandibular sialadenitis prior to subjecting the patient to sialadenectomy. Ultimately, removal of the submandibular gland is often necessary (Figure 3.10).

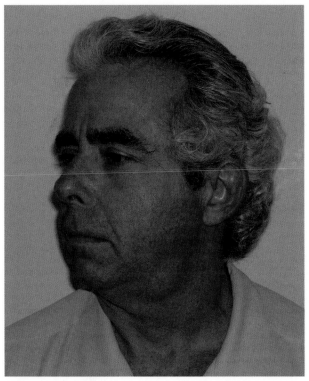

Figure 3.10a. A 52-year-old man with a 1-year history of vague discomfort in the left upper neck.

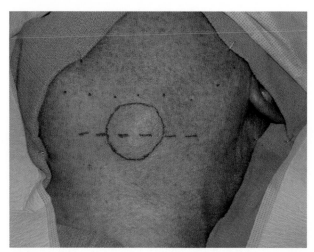

Figure 3.10c. His diagnosis was chronic submandibular sialadenitis and he was prepared for left submandibular gland excision.

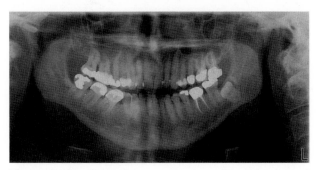

Figure 3.10b. Screening panoramic radiograph showed no evidence of a sialolith.

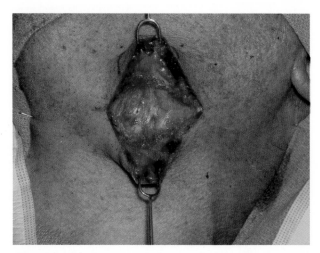

Figure 3.10d. The surgery was carried through anatomic planes, including the investing layer of the deep cervical fascia.

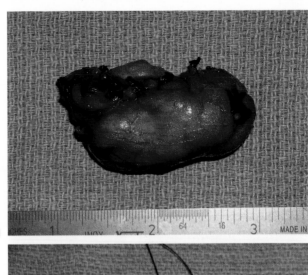

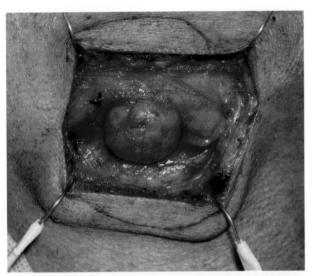

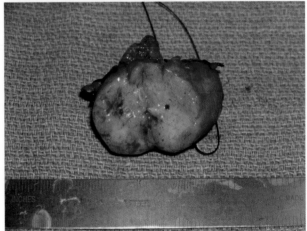

Figure 3.10e. The dissection is carried deep to this layer since a cancer surgery is not being performed that would require a dissection superficial to the investing fascia. Exposure of the gland demonstrates a small submandibular gland due to scar contracture.

Figures 3.10g and 3.10h. The specimen (g) is bivalved (h), which allows for the appreciation of scar within the gland.

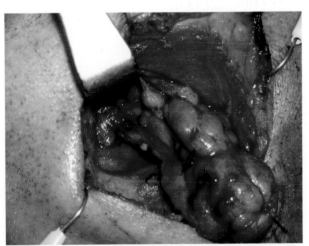

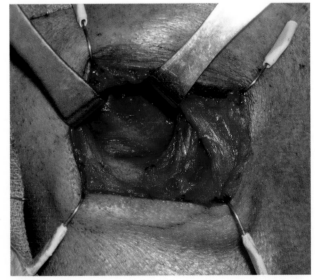

Figure 3.10f. Inferior retraction of the gland allows for identification and preservation of the lingual nerve.

Figure 3.10i. The resultant tissue bed shows the hypoglossal nerve, which is routinely preserved in excision of the submandibular gland.

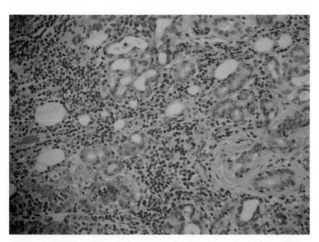

Figure 3.10j. Histopathology shows a sclerosing sialadenitis.

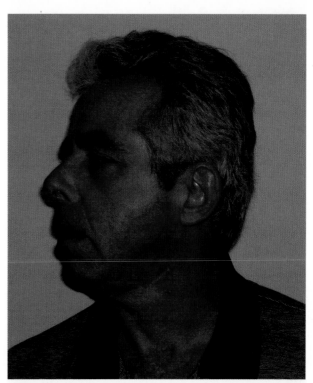

Figure 3.10k. The patient's symptoms were eliminated postoperatively, and he healed uneventfully, as noted at 1 year following the surgery.

TUBERCULOUS MYCOBACTERIAL DISEASE

The most common head and neck manifestation of mycobacterium tuberculosis is infection of the cervical lymph nodes. Tuberculous infection of the salivary glands is generally seen in older children and adults. The infection is believed to originate in the tonsils or gingiva and most commonly ascends to the parotid gland via its duct (Arrieta and McCaffrey 2005). Secondary infection of the salivary glands occurs by way of the lymphatic or hematogenous spread from the lungs. Clinically, tuberculous salivary gland infection presents in two different forms. The first is an acute inflammatory lesion with diffuse glandular edema that may be confused with an acute sialadenitis or abscess. The chronic lesion occurs as a slow-growing mass that mimics a tumor.

NONTUBERCULOUS MYCOBACTERIAL DISEASE

Nontuberculous mycobacterial disease has become an important entity in the pediatric population. It has been estimated that greater than 92% of mycobacterial cervicofacial infections in children are a result of nontuberculous mycobacteria (Arrieta and McCaffrey 2005). The disease primarily affects children younger than 5 years of age. The specific organisms are *M. Kansasii*, *M. avium-intracellulare*, and *M. scrofulaceum*. The typical clinical presentation is that of a rapidly enlarging and persistent parotid and/or neck mass that has failed to resolve with antibiotic therapy (Figure 3.11). A characteristic violaceous discoloration to the skin develops. The treatment of choice is surgical removal of the involved salivary gland and associated lymph nodes.

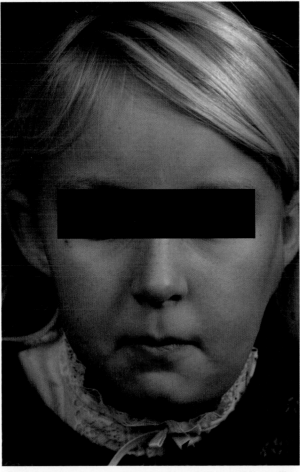

Figure 3.11a. 9-year-old girl with a left parotid swelling with overlying erythema of skin but no signs of acute infection. Reprinted from: J. Cranio-Max.-Fac. Surg volume 16, Mitchell DA, Ord RA, Atypical mycobacterial infection presenting as a parotid mass in a child, 221–223, 1988, Georg Thieme Verlag Stuttgart, New York.

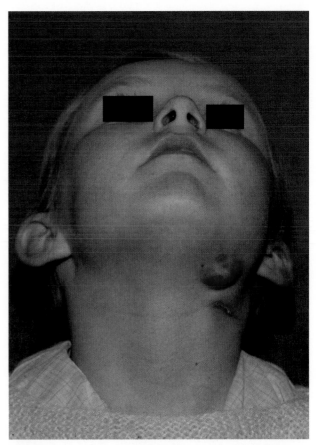

Figure 3.11c. Two months following the parotidectomy, a left submandibular lymph node became enlarged and was treated with medical therapy. Reprinted from: J. Cranio-Max.-Fac. Surg volume 16, Mitchell DA, Ord RA, Atypical mycobacterial infection presenting as a parotid mass in a child, 221–223, 1988, Georg Thieme Verlag Stuttgart, New York.

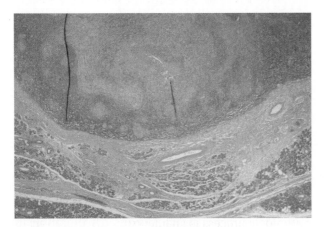

Figure 3.11b. The patient underwent left superficial parotidectomy and excision of a submandibular lymph node. Histopathology showed non-caseating granulomas, and cultures showed mycobacterium avium intracellulare. Reprinted from: J. Cranio-Max.-Fac. Surg volume 16, Mitchell DA, Ord RA, Atypical mycobactevial infection presenting as parvotid mass in a child, 221–223, 1988, Georg Thieme Verlag Stuttgart, New York.

Viral Salivary Gland Infections

MUMPS

Viral mumps is an acute, nonsuppurative communicable disease that often occurs in epidemics during the spring and winter months. The term "mumps" is derived from the Danish "mompen," which refers to mumbling, thereby describing the difficulty with speech because of inflammation and trismus (Arrieta and McCaffrey 2005; McQuone 1999). The nearly routine administration of the measles-mumps-rubella (MMR) vaccination has decreased the incidence of mumps in industrialized nations. Since the introduction of the live attenuated vaccine in the United States in 1967 and its administration as part of the MMR vaccine, the yearly incidence of mumps cases has declined from 76 to 2 cases per 100,000 (Murray, Kobayashi, and Pfaller 1994). Mumps characteristically occurs in the parotid glands. Although the disease is typically seen in children between 6 and 8 years of age, it may occur in adults who have avoided childhood infection as well, and displays an equal sex predilection. The disease is caused most commonly by a paramyxovirus, a ribonucleic acid virus related to the influenza and parainfluenza virus groups. Several other nonparamyxoviruses may cause mumps, including coxsackie A and B viruses, Epstein-Barr virus, influenza and parainfluenza viruses, enteric cytopathic human orphan (ECHO) virus, and human immunodeficiency virus (HIV). Mumps is transmitted by infected saliva and urine. The incubation period between exposure and the development of signs and symptoms is 15–18 days. A prodromal period occurs that lasts 24–48 hours and involves fever, chills, headache, and preauricular tenderness. Following the prodromal period, rapid and painful unilateral or bilateral swelling of the parotid glands occurs. Features that distinguish sialadenitis due to mumps vs. bacteria include a lack of purulent discharge, positive serum titers for mumps, and a relative lymphocytosis in mumps. The diagnosis is made by demonstrating complement-fixing soluble (S) antibodies to the nucleoprotein core of the virus, which are the earliest antibodies to appear. These antibodies peak at 10 days to 2 weeks and disappear within 8–9 months. The S antibodies are therefore associated with active infection. The complement-fixing viral (V) antibodies are against outer surface hemagglutinin and appear later than S antibodies but persist at low levels for years. The diagnosis may also be made by isolating the virus from urine, which is possible up to 6 days prior and 13 days after the salivary gland symptoms occur (Rice 1998). Serum amylase levels may be elevated regardless of an associated pancreatitis. Abdominal pain is often indicative of mumps pancreatitis. Mumps orchitis occurs in 20% of adult males who have mumps parotitis (Goldberg and Bevilacqua 1995). Approximately half of these males will experience secondary testicular atrophy that may result in sterility if the testicular atrophy occurs bilaterally. Other rare complications of mumps include mumps hepatitis, mumps myocarditis, and mumps thyroiditis.

Treatment of mumps is supportive as spontaneous resolution of the disease occurs within 5–10 days. Such supportive care includes bedrest, proper hydration, and dietary modifications to minimize glandular activity. Persistent or recurrent parotid swelling may indicate the presence of sialadenitis.

HUMAN IMMUNODEFICIENCY VIRUS

HIV infection is associated with numerous pathologic processes involving the salivary glands, with the parotid gland being the most common. "HIV-associated salivary gland disease" (HIV-SGD) is a term used to describe the diffuse enlargement of the salivary glands. HIV-SGD may affect patients throughout all stages of the infection, and may be the initial manifestation of HIV infection (Schiodt, Dodd, and Greenspan et al. 1992).

Patients with HIV-SGD present with a history of nontender swelling of one or more of the salivary glands (Figure 3.12). These swellings may fluctuate but are generally persistent. Imaging studies are generally beneficial so as to diagnose lymphoepithelial cysts in this patient population that may clinically resemble the nontender swellings of the parotid glands in this population. Decreased salivary gland function results in xerostomia and sicca symptoms. This sicca symptom complex mimics Sjogren's syndrome and has resulted in the classification of another HIV-related salivary gland process known as the diffuse infiltrative lymphocytosis syndrome (DILS). This pathologic process is characterized by the presence of persistent circulating CD8 lymphocytes and infiltration of organs by CD8 lymphocytes that occur predominantly in the salivary glands and

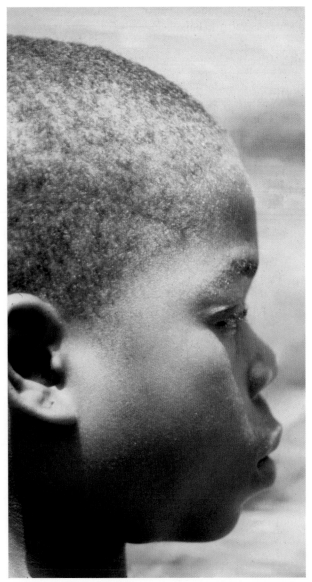

Figure 3.12. A 6-year-old African female with AIDS showing involvement of the right parotid gland by diffuse infiltrative lymphocytosis syndrome (DILS).

lungs. While DILS appears similar to Sjogren's syndrome, it can be differentiated by the presence of extraglandular involvement of the lungs, kidneys, and gastrointestinal tract. In addition, Sjogren's autoantibodies will be absent in patients with DILS.

Medical management of HIV-SGD involves the use of antiretrovirals, observing meticulous oral hygiene, and the use of sialogogues. Corticosteroids may also be of use.

Collagen Sialadenitis

All of the collagen vascular diseases may affect the salivary glands, including polymyositis, dermatomyositis, and scleroderma; however, systemic lupus erythematosus is most commonly responsible. This disease is most frequently seen in fourth- and fifth-decade women. Any of the salivary glands may become involved, and a slowly enlarging gland is the presentation. The diagnosis is made by identification of the underlying systemic disorder, and salivary chemistry levels will reveal sodium and chloride ion levels that are elevated two to three times normal levels (Miloro and Goldberg 2002). The treatment of collagen sialadenitis involves treatment of the responsible systemic disease.

Summary

- Sialadenitis is an infection of salivary glands that has numerous etiologies including microorganisms and autoimmune diseases.
- Staphylococcal and streptococcal species are involved in community acquired acute bacterial parotitis, and Pseudomonas, Klebsiella, Prevotella, Fusobacterium, Hemophilus, and Proteus species are cultured from hospital acquired cases of acute bacterial parotitis. Methicillin resistant *Staphylococcal aureus* may be cultured from cases of community acquired and hospital acquired acute bacterial parotitis.
- The clinician must rule out a neoplastic process in a prompt fashion during the course of treating the sialadenitis.
- The presence of a sialolith must be considered in the initial workup of patients with a clinical diagnosis of sialadenitis. A screening panoramic radiograph or occlusal radiograph should be obtained.
- The parotid and submandibular glands are the most commonly affected salivary glands by sialadenitis.
- The purpose of initial treatment for sialadenitis is to provide medical therapy for the disorder, with surgical therapy being introduced if the disorder becomes refractory to medical treatment.
- Minimally invasive strategies have a role to play in the surgical treatment of sialadenitis, as well as surgical removal of the salivary gland.

References

Andrews JC, Abemayor E, Alessi DM et al. 1989. Parotitis and facial nerve dysfunction. *Arch Otolaryngol Head Neck Surg* 115:240–242.

Arrieta AJ, McCaffrey TV. 2005. Inflammatory disorders of the salivary glands. In: Cummings CW (ed.), Cummings Otolaryngology: Head and Neck Surgery (4th ed.). Philadelphia: Elsevier Mosby, pp. 1323–1338.

Baurmash HD. 2004. Chronic recurrent parotitis: A closer look at its origin, diagnosis, and management. *J Oral Maxillofac Surg* 62:1010–1018.

Brodie, BC. 1834. Inflammation of the parotid gland and salivary fistulae. *Lancet* 1:450–452.

English CK, Wear DJ, Margileth AM et al. 1988. Cat-scratch disease. *JAMA* 259:1347–1352.

Galili D, Marmary Y. 1985. Spontaneous regeneration of the parotid salivary gland following juvenile recurrent parotitis. *Oral Surg* 60:605–606.

Goldberg M, Harrigan W. 1965. Acute suppurative parotitis. *Oral Surg* 20:281–286.

Goldberg MH, Bevilacqua RG. 1995. Infections of the salivary glands. In: Carlson, ER (ed.), The Comprehensive Management of Salivary Gland Pathology. Philadelphia: W.B. Saunders, pp. 423–430.

Guralnick W, Donoff R, Galdabini J. 1968. Parotid swelling in a dehydrated patient. *J Oral Surg* 26:669–675.

Hasson O. 2007. Sialoendoscopy and sialography: Strategies for assessment and treatment of salivary gland obstructions. *J Oral Maxillofac Surg* 65:300–304.

Katz J, Fisher D, Levine S. 1990. Bacterial colonization of the parotid duct in xerostomia. *Int J Oral Maxillofac Surg* 19:7–9.

McQuone SJ. 1999. Acute viral and bacterial infections of the salivary glands. *Otolaryngol Clin North Am* 32:793–811.

Miloro M, Goldberg MH. 2002. Salivary gland infections. In: Topazian RG, Goldberg MH, Hupp JR (eds.), Oral and Maxillofacial Infections (4th ed.). Philadelphia: W.B. Saunders, pp. 279–293.

Mitchell DA, Ord RA. 1988. Atypical mycobacterial infection presenting as a parotid mass in a child. *J. Cranio-Max.-Fac. Surg.* 16:221–223.

Murray PR, Kobayashi GS, Pfaller KS. 1994. Paramyxoviruses. In: Medical Microbiology (2nd ed.). St. Louis: Mosby, pp. 629–640.

Nahlieli O, Nakar LH, Nazarian Y, Turner MD. 2006. Sialoendoscopy: A new approach to salivary gland obstructive pathology. *JADA* 137:1394–1400.

Patey DH. 1965. Inflammation of the salivary glands with particular reference to chronic and recurrent parotitis. *Ann R Col Surg Engl* 36:26–44.

Petersdorf R, Forsyth B, Bernanke D. 1958. Staphylococcal parotitis. *N Engl J Med* 259:1250–1254.

Qi S, Liu X, Wang S. 2005. Sialoendoscopic and irrigation findings in chronic obstructive parotitis. *Laryngoscope* 115:541–545.

Rice DH. 1998. Diseases of the salivary glands—nonneoplastic. In: Bailey, BJ (ed.), Head and Neck Surgery—Otolaryngology (2nd ed.). Philadelphia: Lippincott Raven Publishers, pp. 561–570.

Robinson JR. 1955. Surgical parotitis, vanishing disease. *Surgery* 38:703–707.

Schiodt M, Dodd C, Greenspan D, et al. 1992. Natural history of HIV-associated salivary gland disease. *Oral Surg Oral Med Oral Pathol* 74:326–331.

Chapter 4
Cysts of the Salivary Glands

Outline

Introduction

Cysts of the salivary glands may originate as benign non-neoplastic entities or in association with benign and malignant tumors of the salivary glands. Cystic development as part of specific neoplasms of the salivary glands is well recognized, including those that occur in the pleomorphic adenoma, Warthin's tumor, mucoepidermoid carcinoma, acinic cell carcinoma, and the adenoid cystic carcinoma. The histologic features of these neoplasms are sufficiently distinctive; however, non-neoplastic salivary gland cysts do require differentiation from cystadenoma, mucoepidermoid carcinoma, and acinic carcinoma (Dardick 1996). Many cysts of the salivary glands may be generically attributed to an obstructive process. They can occur as a result of traumatic severance of salivary gland ducts, partial or complete blockage of the excretory ducts, or stasis of salivary flow in ducts. For the purpose of this chapter, salivary cysts are categorized in many ways, including those that originate directly from the salivary gland and those

entities that are associated with the salivary glands. In addition, there are those salivary cysts that exhibit a true cystic epithelium and those that are lined with a non-epithelial lining, that is, pseudocysts. Finally, it is possible to categorize these lesions as acquired (obstructive due to stricture, neoplasms, sialoliths, or trauma) and developmental (dermoid, branchial cleft, branchial pouch, and ductal). It is the purpose of this chapter to discuss those salivary gland cysts that are developmental and acquired in a non-neoplastic nature (see Table 4.1).

Mucous Escape Reaction

The mucous escape reaction can be defined as a pooling of salivary mucus within a connective tissue lining. This concept is defined by a number of names including mucocele, ranula, mucous retention phenomenon, and mucous retention cyst. Of these, mucocele and ranula are the two best-known entities to clinicians diagnosing and managing pathology in the head and neck region. It was once believed that the lesion developed as a result of obstruction of a salivary gland's excretory duct with the subsequent formation of an epithelially lined cyst (Thoma 1950). Early studies investigated the result of ligation of the excretory ducts of the submandibular and sublingual glands (Bhaskar, Bolden, and Weinmann 1956a). A mucous escape reaction did not result, thereby leading to further investigation. The complete obstruction of a salivary duct by the presence of a sialolith without the development of a mucous escape reaction substantiates the lack of a cause and effect relationship. Subsequent studies determined that severance of the excretory duct was required to produce extravasation of salivary mucin into the surrounding tissues with the development

Table 4.1. Cystic lesions of the salivary glands—nomenclature and classification.

Nomenclature
  Mucous escape reaction
  Mucous retention cysts
  Lymphoepithelial cysts
    HIV-associated lymphoepithelial cysts
  Developmental cysts
    Branchial cleft cysts
    Dermoid cysts
    Polycystic (dysgenetic) disease
Classification
 I. Etiology
   a. Origination from salivary gland tissue
     i. Mucous escape reaction
     ii. Mucous retention cyst
   b. Association with salivary gland tissue
 II. Lining
   a. True cystic lining
     i. Mucous retention cyst
   b. Non-epithelial lining (pseudocyst)
     i. Mucous escape reaction
 III. Occurrence
   a. Acquired
     i. Mucous escape reaction
     ii. Mucous retention cyst
   b. Developmental

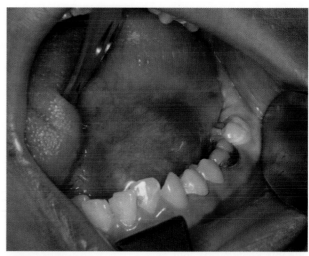

Figure 4.1. The typical appearance of a ranula of the floor of the mouth. The characteristic raised nature of the lesion, as well as its blue hue, are appreciated.

of a lesion histologically identical to the mucous escape reaction observed in humans (Bhaskar, Bolden, and Weinmann 1956b). It is now accepted that severance of a salivary duct with resultant pooling of mucus into surrounding tissues is the pathophysiology of the mucous escape reaction. The fibrous connective tissue encasing the pooled saliva is presumably due to the foreign body nature of the saliva. The occasional report of an epithelial-like lining can be explained as a misinterpretation of compressed macrophages resembling a layer of cuboidal-shaped cells (van den Akker, Bays, and Becker 1978). When these lesions occur in the floor of the mouth, a designation of ranula is given, while a similar lesion in the lower lip carries a designation of mucocele.

CLINICAL FEATURES AND TREATMENT OF THE MUCOUS ESCAPE REACTION

The mucous escape reaction may develop from a major or minor salivary gland but seems to be more commonly observed in the minor glands. Armed Forces Institute of Pathology data of 2,339 cases indicates that the minor glands are the site of predilection of this lesion, with 2,273 (97.2%) of the 2,339 lesions occurring in these glands. The lip accounted for 1,502 of these lesions (64.2%), with the lower lip being the most common site (98.8% when the site was specified). This figure is consistent with other series that indicate a predilection of lower lip lesions (Cataldo and Mosadomi 1970). The major glands showed a nearly equal distribution of occurrence in the parotid, submandibular, and sublingual glands, and collectively accounted for only 2.9% of the 2,339 cases.

Most investigators consider these lesions to be most common in children and young adults, with a mean age of 25 years. No significant sex predilection has been offered. The clinical appearance of these lesions differs depending on their depth within surrounding soft tissues. Superficial lesions present as blue, raised soft tissue swellings with a fluctuant character on palpation (Figure 4.1). The blue hue is generally reflective of the color of pooled saliva at the mucosal surface. Lesions that are located more deeply in the soft tissues take on the color of the surrounding soft tissues; however, they may retain their fluctuant character. The most common clinical course of mucous escape reactions is that of a painless mucosal swelling that develops during a period of between a few days to 1 week and ruptures with

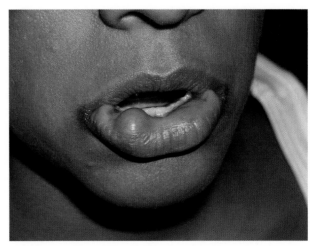

Figure 4.3. The classic appearance of a mucocele of the lower lip. Similar to a ranula of the floor of the mouth, it shows an elevated blue lesion.

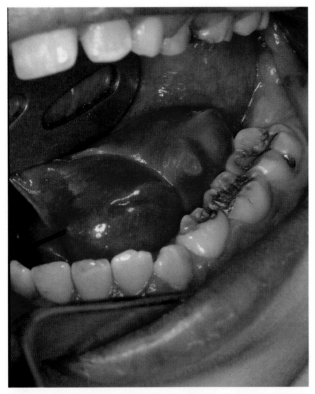

Figure 4.2. This ranula has resulted in significant pain experienced by the patient. The size of the ranula has resulted in obstruction of the sublingual gland.

apparent resolution with subsequent recurrence occurring within 1 month later. Mild symptoms of pain may accompany mucous escape reactions if secondary trauma or inflammation occurs. Pain may also occur in the rare event that the mucous escape reaction impedes the flow of saliva due to obstruction (Figure 4.2).

Mucocele

Mucoceles are common lesions of the oral mucosa, and perhaps the most common benign salivary gland lesion in the oral cavity. The incidence of mucoceles is understandable due to the prevalence of minor salivary gland tissue in the oral cavity and the frequent occurrence of trauma to these tissues, which results in their formation. These lesions are painless, freely movable, smooth, and fluctuant. Their appearance is so characteristic that the clinical diagnosis is most frequently confirmed by subsequent histopathologic diagnosis following removal (Figure 4.3). As such, an incisional biopsy is not required for proper surgical treatment of

the mucocele. Clearly, the most common location for these lesions is the lip, and specifically the lower lip. This notwithstanding, mucoceles occur on the buccal mucosa, tongue, and palate. Patients often give a history of the lesions spontaneously bursting with predictable recurrence. Mucoceles occur most commonly in children and young adults, probably due to the relatively high incidence of oral trauma in younger patients. Treatment with surgical excision of the mucocele and its associated minor salivary gland tissue is highly curable.

Ranula

The ranula represents the prototypical mucous escape reaction occurring in the floor of the mouth. Its nomenclature stems from its derivation from the Latin diminutive "rana," or frog, which refers to its resemblance to the belly of a frog (Figure 4.4). The lesion has a characteristic appearance and history, commonly exhibiting a blue color and displaying periods of bursting of the lesion with liberation of saliva, only to relapse some time thereafter (Figure 4.5). The development of a cervical component of the ranula has been a subject of fascination for centuries (Catone 1995). The oral and cervical mucous escape reactions may exist simultaneously (Figure 4.6), or they may occur independently of one another. As such, it was once considered possible that they had different etiologies, with the oral lesion being derived from the sublingual gland and the cervical lesion being derived from the submandibular gland. Some

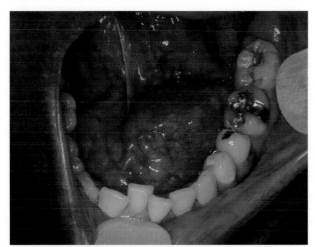

Figure 4.4. A ranula of the left floor of the mouth. While the lesion is clearly elevated, only subtle signs of its blue color exist.

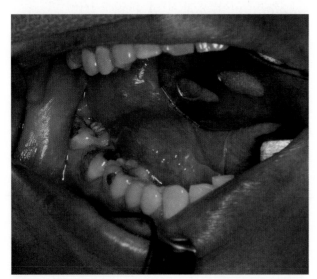

Figure 4.5. A ranula of the right floor of the mouth. Classic signs of elevation and the blue discoloration are present.

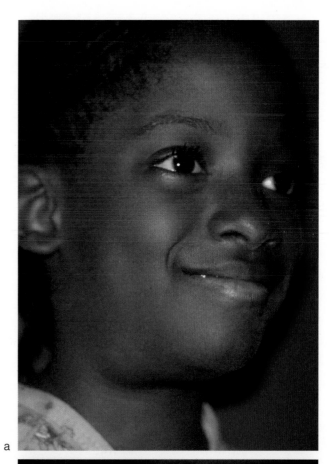

a

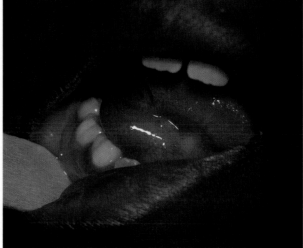

b

Figures 4.6a and 4.6b. An 8-year-old girl with obvious right submandibular swelling (a), as well as simultaneous clinical evidence of a ranula in the right floor of the mouth (b).

observed that the neck mass was often preceded by repeated spontaneous evacuations or surgical drainages of the oral lesion. This was perhaps the first explanation that scar tissue formation in the mucosa of the floor of the mouth was responsible for the development of the cervical mass, as it descended through the cleft of the posterior extent of the mylohyoid muscle as a path of least resistance (Figure 4.7) (Braun and Sotereanos 1982). It has also been demonstrated that approximately one-third of the population has discontinuities of the mylohyoid muscle such that direct invasion of the pseudocyst through these defects of the muscle permits extension into the neck (McClatchey et al. 1984). Perhaps equally controversial is the concept of how it is most appropriate to treat the ranula.

If anything has been learned by reading the scientific literature on this topic, it is the common pathogenesis of three clinical entities: the mucocele, the oral ranula, and the plunging ranula. Specifically, it is their lack of an epithelial lining and their association with a salivary gland, whether major or minor. If the offending salivary gland is not removed, the lesion has a statistical likelihood of recurrence (Catone, Merrill, and Henny 1969). This notwithstanding, there are several published papers adamantly recommending that more conservative procedures be performed as first-line therapy (Baurmash 1992, 2007). One such proce-

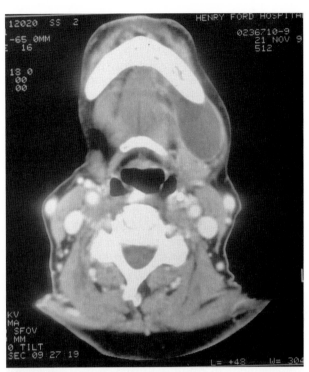

Figure 4.7b. Computerized tomograms of the neck show a fluid-filled lesion of the submandibular region.

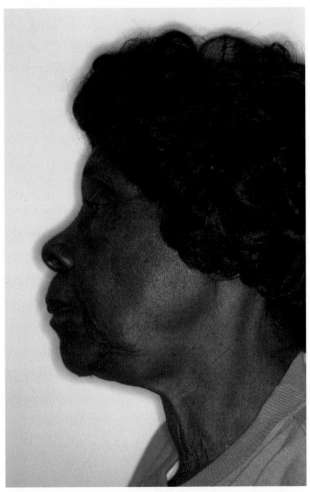

Figure 4.7a. This elderly woman shows left submandibular swelling. Her history includes numerous aspirations of fluid within a ranula of the left floor of the mouth.

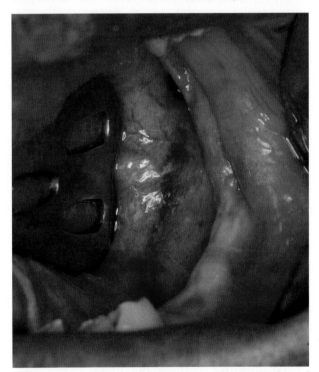

Figure 4.7c. A diagnosis of plunging ranula was made and the patient underwent left sublingual gland excision. Examination of the left floor of the mouth did not show signs of ranula in this region. Scar tissue formation from her previous aspirations resulted in the development of a plunging ranula.

dure is marsupialization with packing (Baurmash 1992). The author contends that routine sublingual removal is inappropriate therapy for several reasons. The first is that the term "ranula" is loosely applied to any cyst-like structure of the floor of the mouth. He believes that some of these lesions are unrelated to the sublingual gland, such that its removal is not indicated. Specifically, he cites the existence of mucoceles arising from the mucous-secreting incisal gland in the anterior floor of the mouth, single or multiple retention cysts involving the openings of the ducts of Rivinus, and retention cysts at Wharton's duct orifice that can resemble the sublingual gland associated ranula but that would possibly not be cured with sublingual gland removal. Moreover, the author states that sublingual gland excision is potentially associated with significant morbidity such as injury to Wharton's duct with resultant salivary obstruction or salivary leakage, and lingual nerve injury (Baurmash 1992). Zhao and his group presented an objective assessment of complications associated with surgical management of ranulas treated with a variety of procedures (Zhao, Jia, and Jia 2005). These included 9 marsupializations, 28 excisions of the ranula only, 356 sublingual gland excisions, and 213 excisions of both the sublingual gland and ranula. A total of 569 sublingual gland excisions were performed in 571 patients undergoing 606 operations. Injury to Wharton's duct occurred in 11 of 569 patients who underwent excision of the sublingual gland with or without excision of the ranula, compared to 0 of 37 patients who did not undergo sublingual gland excision. Injury to the lingual nerve occurred in 21 of the patients who underwent sublingual gland excision, compared to 0 patients who did not undergo sublingual gland excision. Of particular note is that recurrence of the ranula occurred in 1.2% of patients who underwent excision of their sublingual glands, compared to 60% of patients who underwent marsupialization or excision of the ranula only. Baurmash laments that simple marsupialization has fallen into disfavor because of the excessive number of failures associated with this procedure (Baurmash 1992). The recurrence patterns have been confirmed by other authors, as well (Yoshimura et al. 1995). As such, he recommends packing the cystic cavity with gauze for 7–10 days. In so doing, he reports that the recurrence rate is reduced to 10–12% (Baurmash 2007). McGurk points out that the downside of this procedure is that the results are unpredictable and that the packing is uncomfortable for the patient

(McGurk 2007). He concludes by stating that reliable eradication of the ranula comes from removal of the sublingual gland. It is true that the surgery is somewhat anatomically demanding, such that some surgeons may wish to defer the sublingual gland excision for recurrences. Unfortunately, the development of scar tissue in the floor of the mouth is such that the anatomy may be more obscured related to a recurrence after a marsupialization and packing procedure. With this issue in mind, a sublingual gland excision should probably be performed from the outset (Figure 4.8). While the

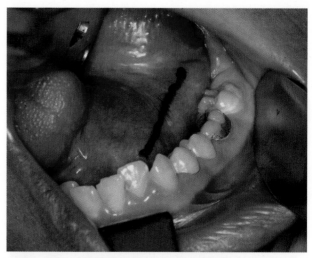

Figure 4.8a. The excision of the sublingual gland and associated ranula from Figure 4.1. An incision is designed over the prominence of the sublingual gland and ranula, and lateral to Wharton's duct.

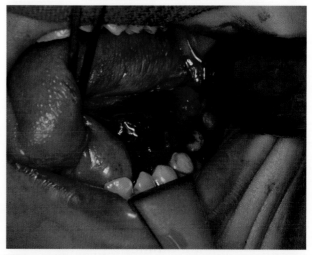

Figure 4.8b. Careful dissection allows for separation of the mucosa from the underlying pseudocystic membrane.

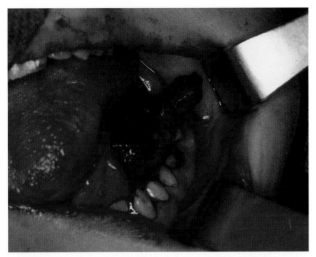

Figure 4.8c. The dissection continues to separate the sublingual gland from surrounding tissues, including the underlying Wharton's duct and the lingual nerve beneath Wharton's duct.

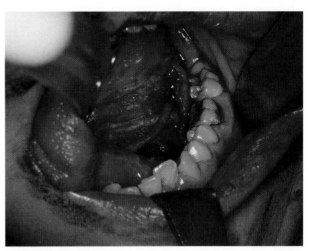

Figure 4.8g. The remaining tissue bed shows the anatomic relationship of the preserved superficial Wharton's duct and underlying lingual nerve. Wharton's duct originates posteriorly in a medial position to the lingual nerve and terminates in a position lateral to the nerve. The sublingual vein can be visualized in the tissue bed lateral to the anterior aspect of Wharton's duct.

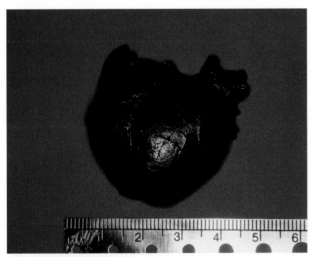

Figure 4.8d. The specimen and ranula are able to be delivered en bloc.

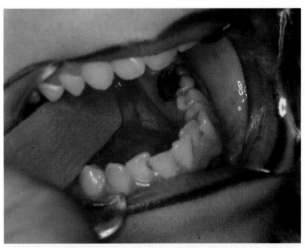

Figure 4.8h. Healing is uneventful as noted in the 1-month postoperative image.

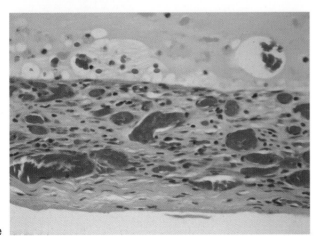

e

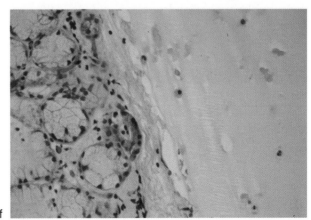

f

Figures 4.8e and 4.8f. If the pseudocyst bursts intraoperatively, no compromise in cure exists as long as the sublingual gland is completely excised. The histopathology shows the non-epithelial lining (e) and the intimate association of the sublingual gland and mucous escape reaction (f).

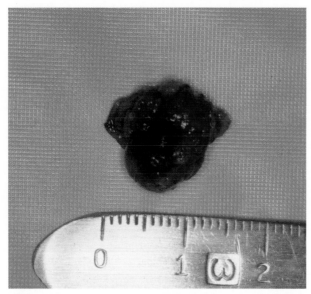

Figure 4.9. The specimen from the excision of the muco-cele seen in Figure 4.3. The minor salivary gland tissue remains attached to the mucous escape reaction.

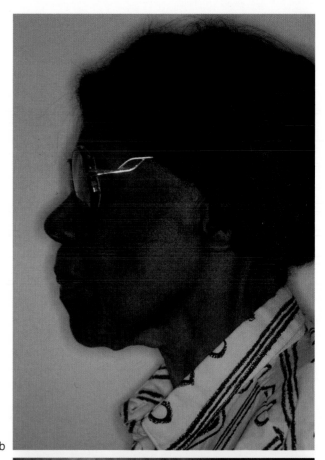

b

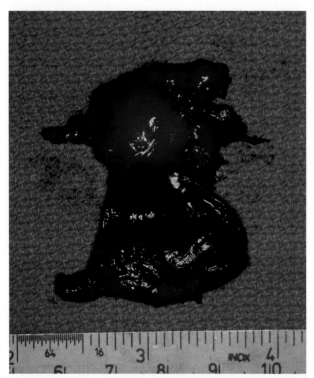

Figure 4.10a. The patient seen in Figure 4.7 underwent excision of her left sublingual gland for her plunging ranula. The specimen includes the sublingual gland and associated mucous escape reaction.

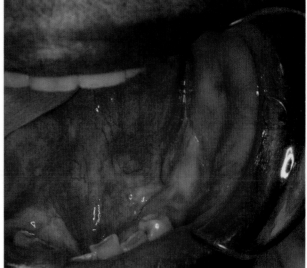

c

Figures 4.10b and 4.10c. Her 2-year postoperative examination shows no mass in the submandibular region (b) and a normal oral examination without recurrence of the ranula (c).

anatomy of the floor of the mouth might be considered foreign and intimidating to some surgeons, preservation of the lingual nerve and Wharton's duct is not a difficult task, and treatment of this pathologic process with sublingual excision should be a curative procedure. One pathologic and clinical similarity of the ranula and mucocele is their derivation from salivary gland tissue. There does not seem to be a dispute among clinicians as to the best surgical therapy for the mucocele, with complete surgical excision of the etiologic minor salivary tissue along with the mucous escape reaction being highly accepted (Figure 4.9). As such, it is advisable to apply the same approach to the ranula that only differs from the mucocele in the anatomic region in which it occurs. With regard to the ranula and plunging ranula, even the most extensive lesions are predictably treated for cure with excision of the offending sublingual gland. While it is not essential to remove the non-epithelial lined pseudocyst with the sublingual gland, it is common for the tightly adherent pseudocyst to be delivered with the sublingual gland specimen (Figure 4.10). As such, documentation of a plunging component to the ranula serves a matter of medical completeness rather than implications for treatment.

Cyst of Blandin and Nuhn's Gland

On rare occasions, the mucosa of the ventral surface of the tongue may become a source for the

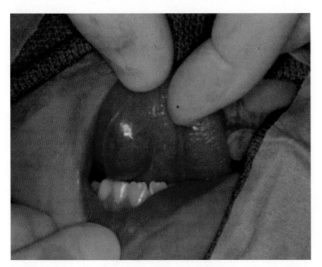

Figure 4.11. A cyst of Blandin and Nuhn's gland of the ventral surface of the tongue. Simple excision of the cyst and associated minor salivary gland tissue is curative for this mucous escape phenomenon.

development of a mucous escape reaction. This process is referred to as a cyst of Blandin and Nuhn's gland (Figure 4.11). This designation is a misnomer, as this process represents a mucous escape reaction, rather than a true cyst. In this sense, then, it represents a ranula of the tongue. Simple excision of the "cyst" and the associated gland of Blandin and Nuhn is the treatment of choice with recurrence being uncommon.

Mucous Retention Cyst

The mucous retention cyst is less common than the mucous escape reaction. This entity is a true cyst that is lined by epithelium. The exact classification of this lesion seems to be in question. Some prefer to simply include it with the more common mucous escape reaction, whereas others describe it as a separate entity (Koudelka 1991). The pathogenesis seems to be related to partial obstruction of a duct, as opposed to complete severance of the salivary duct that is seen in the mucous escape reaction. The increased pressure in the salivary duct causes dilatation without rupture such that proliferation of the ductal epithelium occurs. The Armed Forces Institute of Pathology reviewed 178 cases of mucous retention cysts, accounting for 0.9% of all salivary gland pathology cases in their files (Koudelka 1991). One hundred seventy-one cases (96%) occurred in the major salivary glands, with 156 (87.6%) occurring in the parotid gland (Figure 4.12), 14 cases (7.8%) occurring in the submandibular gland, and only 1 case occurring in the sublingual gland. Only 1 case was specifically documented as occurring in the minor salivary glands. The mean age of patients was late 40s, with a nearly equal gender predilection. The clinical presentation of the mucous retention cyst is that of a slowly enlarging, painless, fluctuant soft tissue swelling that may persist from months to years. These cysts vary in their size, and the color of the overlying tissues depends on their depth within the soft tissue. Superficial lesions are blue in color, whereas deep lesions take on the same color of the overlying tissue. Some pathologists have split the mucous retention cysts into separate categories. Eversole has categorized these lesions as mucous retention cysts, reactive oncocytoid cysts, and mucopapillary cysts (Eversole 1987.) In his series of 121 mucous retention cysts, he found 70 mucous retention cysts, 41 reactive oncocytoid

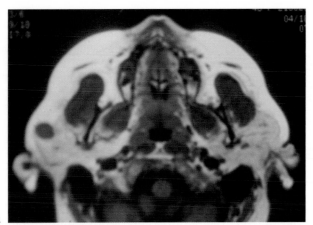
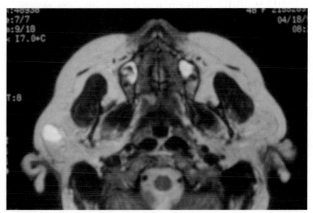

a b

Figures 4.12a and b. A mucous retention cyst of the parotid gland as noted on MRI (T1 images, a; T2 images, b). The patient underwent a superficial parotidectomy due to the concern for a cystic neoplasm.

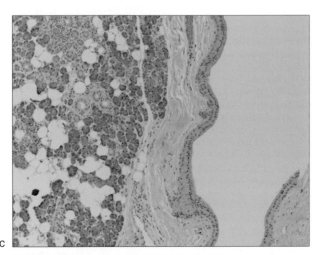
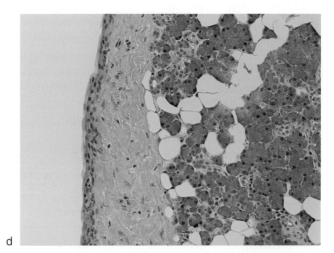

c d

Figures 4.12c and 4.12d. Histopathology showed a parotid cyst lined by columnar epithelium in one section of the cyst (c) and squamoid epithelium in another section (d).

cysts, and 10 mucopapillary cysts. From a pathologic and surgical standpoint, perhaps the most striking piece of information in this report was the need to distinguish the mucopapillary cyst from the low-grade mucoepidermoid carcinoma.

Treatment of mucous retention cysts is most commonly conservative surgical excision (Figure 4.12). Cysts within or closely associated with a salivary gland should include that salivary gland with the excision. Some mucous retention cysts, however, may be removed without the inclusion of the salivary gland, a distinct departure from the recommendations associated with mucous escape reactions.

Parotid Cysts Associated with Human Immunodeficiency Virus Infection

Infection with the human immunodeficiency virus has been shown to manifest in a variety of ways. Symptoms related to the head and neck have historically been encountered in this disease. It has been reported that 41% of patients with acquired immunodeficiency syndrome (AIDS) initially presented with signs or symptoms of head and neck disease (Marcussen and Sooy 1985). Salivary gland diseases include the enlargement of major salivary glands with or without hypofunction and xerostomia (Owotade, Fatusi, and Adebiyi et al. 2005). In early lesions the submandibular and sublingual glands are often initially affected and enlarged. As the disease progresses, however, parotid gland swelling is more commonly noted. As many as 5–10% of patients with HIV-1 infection have been reported to have parotid swelling with the incidence increasing to approximately 20% in AIDS patients (Owotade, Fatusi, and Adebiyi et al. 2005). Ryan and his group were the first to describe salivary gland involvement in HIV disease as intrasalivary gland lymphadenopathy (Ryan, Ioachim, and Marmer et al. 1985). Shortly thereafter, parotid gland cysts were reported and were noted to resemble the benign lymphoepithelial lesion (BLL) histologically (Colebunders, Francis, and Mann et al. 1988). The BLL is a benign sialadenopathy associated with Sjogren's syndrome with pathognomonic

epimyoepithelial islands. It is felt to represent an autoimmune reaction in Sjogren's syndrome, but the BLL is felt to be of unknown pathogenesis in HIV (Sperling, Lin, and Lucente 1990). It remains unclear whether lymphoepithelial cysts within parotid glands in HIV/AIDS patients develop from pre-existing salivary gland inclusions in intraparotid lymph nodes or from a lymphoepithelial lesion of the parenchyma of the salivary gland.

Treatment of lymphoepithelial cysts of the parotid gland in HIV/AIDS patients is a function of the size of the cysts, the patient's concern for cosmetics, and compliance with medical therapy. Following their original description, these cysts were managed in a variety of ways including periodic aspirations, simple excision of the cysts, and nerve-sparing superficial parotidectomy (Figure 4.13). Shaha and his group reported an early experience with 50 patients with lymphoepithelial cysts of the

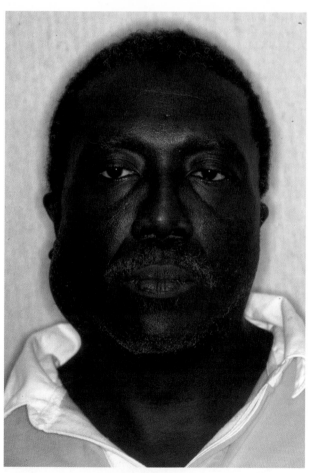

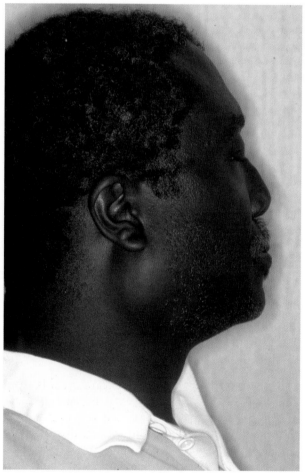

a   b

Figures 4.13a and 4.13b. A 50-year-old HIV positive male presented in 1994 with obvious right parotid swelling. This time period pre-dated the development of HAART. Examination of the bilateral parotid gland regions revealed a large mass of the right parotid gland, and a smaller mass of the left parotid gland.

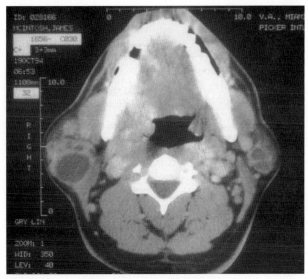

Figure 4.13c. Computerized tomograms confirmed the findings of the physical examination. A clinical diagnosis of bilateral lymphoepithelial cysts was made. The patient requested removal of these cysts.

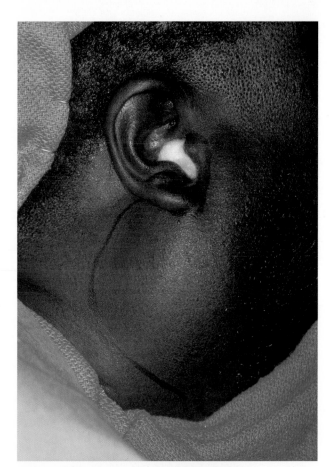

Figure 4.13d. A standard incision was made.

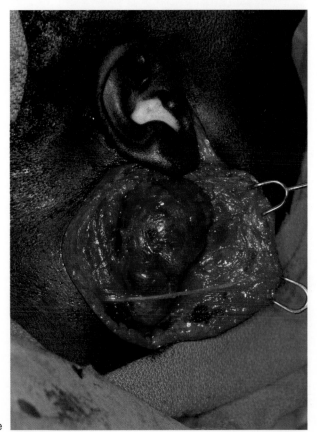

e

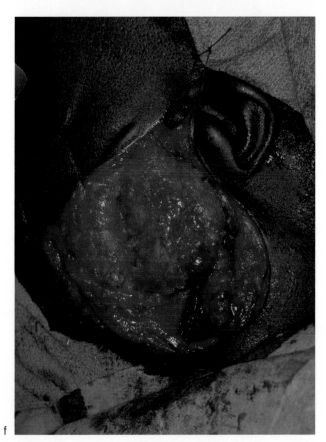

f

Figures 4.13e and 4.13f. This permitted unroofing of the large cyst in the right parotid gland (e) and the smaller cysts in the left parotid gland (f).

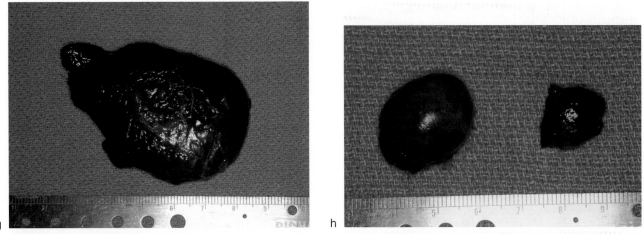

g
h

Figures 4.13g and 4.13h. The specimen from the right parotid gland (g) and the left parotid gland (h) showed typical gross signs of lymphoepithelial cysts.

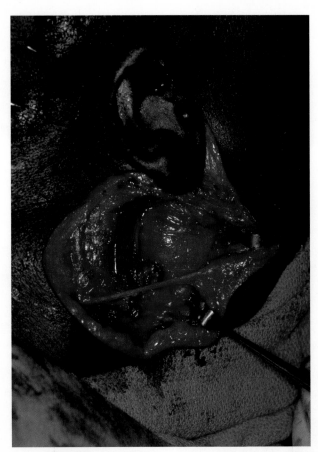

Figure 4.13i. The resultant right parotid tissue bed is noted.

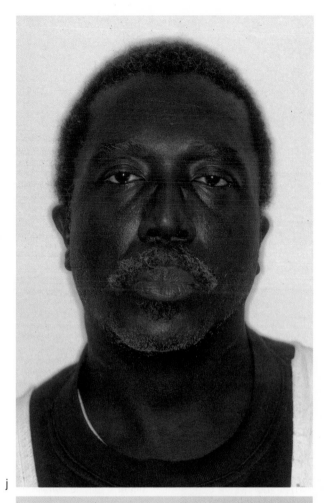

j

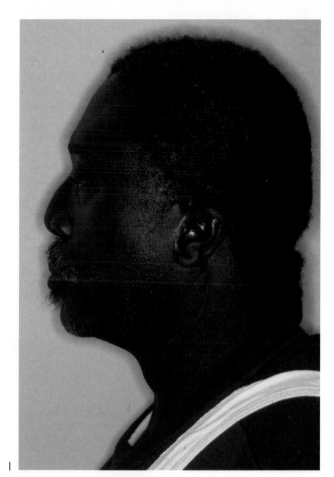

l

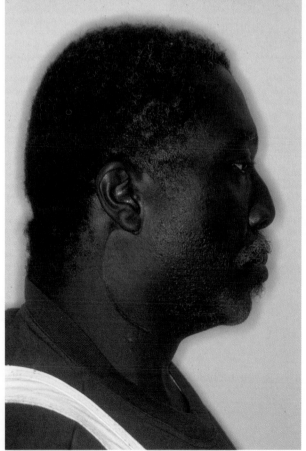

k

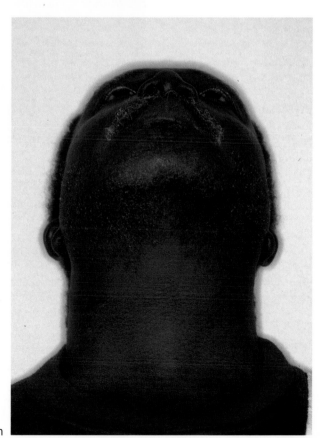

m

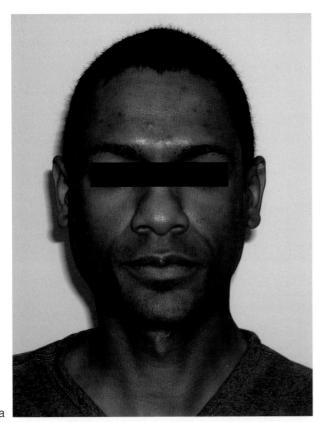

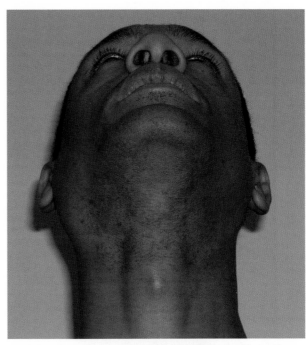

a   b

Figures 4.14a and 4.14b. A 35-year-old HIV positive man presented in 2005 with a complaint of bilateral parotid swellings. He admitted to non-compliance with his HAART. His CD4/CD8 was 0.69 at the time of initial consultation. Physical examination revealed an obvious right parotid swelling and a subtle mass of the left parotid gland.

bilateral parotid glands (Shaha, DiMaio, and Webber et al. 1993). Their initial approach involved superficial parotidectomy with identification and preservation of the facial nerve. They subsequently performed excision of the cyst only. Ferraro and his group recommended against superficial parotidectomy due to possible recurrence in the deep lobe at a later date (Ferraro et al. 1993). They indicated that aspiration is usually ineffective as a long-term solution because of the high rates of recurrence, in addition to the inability to obtain a tissue diagnosis of the cyst wall. Their solution for recurrence of the cyst was a second enucleation procedure.

Improved and evolving pharmacologic therapy of HIV/AIDS has changed the manage-ment of these cysts. Highly active antiretroviral therapy (HAART) uses combinations of drugs to maximize viral suppression and minimize selection of drug-resistant strains. Most commonly, HAART consists of a backbone of two nucleoside analog reverse transcriptase inhibitors in combination with either a protease inhibitor or a non-nucleoside reverse transcriptase inhibitor. Gland enlargement has been shown to be significantly and positively associated with viral load in a linear fashion (Mulligan, Navazesh, and Komaroff et al. 2000). Compliance with HAART, therefore, has led to the observation that this therapy will result in these cysts subsiding without the need for surgery (Figure 4.14).

Figures 4.13j, 4.13k, 4.13l, and 4.13m. Six months postoperatively, the patient showed well-healed surgical sites without signs of recurrent lymphoepithelial cysts.

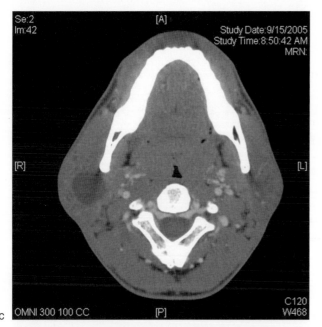
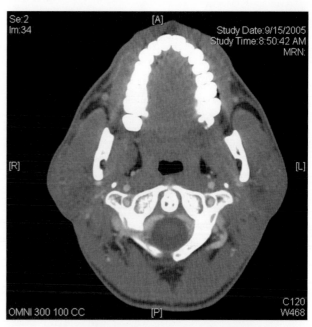

Figures 4.14c and 4.14d. Computerized tomograms confirmed these findings. A fine needle aspiration biopsy was performed that yielded thick white fluid. A diagnosis of lymphoepithelial cysts was made.

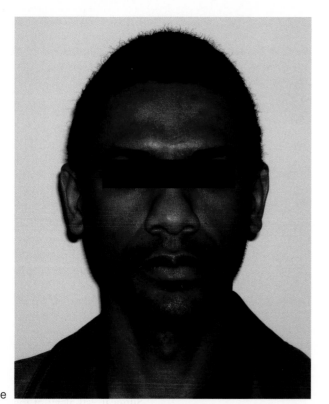
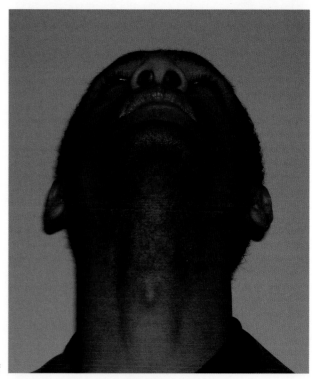

Figures 4.14e and 4.14f. The patient resumed his HAART and the cysts regressed, as noted on an examination 4 months later. His CD4/CD8 was 1.12 at this time.

Branchial Cleft Cysts

Patients with first branchial anomalies usually present with a unilateral painless swelling of the parotid gland. Bilateral swelling is rare. Work has classified these cysts as types I and II (Work 1977). Type I branchial defects are duplication anomalies of the membranous external auditory canal. These defects are composed of ectoderm only. They are located within the preauricular soft tissues and parotid gland and present as sinus tracts or areas of localized swelling near the anterior tragus. Complete surgical removal is curative. Type II branchial anomalies are less common than type I anomalies. This defect is a duplication anomaly consisting of an anomalous membranous and cartilaginous external auditory canal. Unlike type I cysts, type II cysts are composed of ectoderm and mesoderm. They commonly present in the upper neck and are located posterior or inferior to the angle of the mandible and can extend into the external auditory canal or middle ear cavity. Sinus tracts are common and abscess formation may also occur. Complete surgical excision during an asymptomatic period is the treatment of choice. The reader is directed to chapter 13 for a more detailed discussion and illustration of these pathologic processes.

Summary

- Cysts of the salivary glands may be associated with neoplasms or occur independently.
- While these lesions are collectively referred to as cysts, many are not actually lined by epithelium.
- The ranula and mucocele are examples of mucous escape reactions that are not lined by epithelium.
- Severance of a salivary duct due to trauma with resultant pooling of mucus into surrounding tissues is the pathophysiology of the mucous escape reaction.
- Excision of the salivary gland with or without the associated mucous escape reaction represents curative therapy for this process.
- The mucous escape reaction is most commonly seen in the minor salivary glands.
- Mucous retention cysts are lined by epithelium, but are very rare.
- When mucous retention cysts do occur, they seem to be most common in the major salivary glands, particularly the parotid gland. Simple excision is the treatment of choice.
- As many as 5–10% of patients with HIV-1 infection have been reported to have parotid swelling with the incidence increasing to approximately 20% in AIDS patients. Lymphoepithelial cysts account for the majority of these swellings.

References

Baurmash HD. 1992. Marsupialization for treatment of oral ranula: A second look at the procedure. *J Oral Maxillofac Surg* 50:1274–1279.

Baurmash HD. 2007. A case against sublingual gland removal as primary treatment of ranulas. *J Oral Maxillofac Surg* 65:117–121.

Bhaskar SN, Bolden TE, Weinmann JP. 1956a. Experimental obstructive adenitis in the mouse. *J Dent Res* 35:852–862.

Bhaskar SN, Bolden TE, Weinmann JP. 1956b. Pathogenesis of mucoceles. *J Dent Res* 35:863–874.

Braun TW, Sotereanos GC. 1982. Cervical ranula due to an ectopic sublingual gland. *J Max Fac Surg* 10:56–58.

Cataldo E, Mosadomi A. 1970. Mucoceles of the oral mucous membrane. *Arch Otolaryngol* 91:360–365.

Catone GA. 1995. Sublingual gland mucous escape: Pseudocysts of the oral-cervical region. In: Carlson, ER (ed.). The Comprehensive Management of Salivary Gland Pathology. Philadelphia: W.B. Saunders, pp. 431–477.

Catone GA, Merrill RG, Henny FA. 1969. Sublingual gland mucus-escape phenomenon—treatment by excision of sublingual gland. *J Oral Surg* 27:774–786.

Colebunders R, Francis H, Mann JM et al. 1988. Parotid swelling during human immunodeficiency virus infection. *Arch Otolaryngol Head Neck Surg* 114:330–332.

Dardick I. 1996. Mucocele and sialocysts. In: Color Atlas/Text of Salivary Gland Tumor Pathology. New York: Igaku-Shoin Medical Publishers, pp. 131–141.

Eversole LR. 1987. Oral sialocysts. *Arch Otolaryngol Head Neck Surg* 113:51–56.

Ferraro FJ, Rush BF, Ruark D, Oleske J. 1993. Enucleation of parotid lymphoepithelial cyst in patients who are human immunodeficiency virus positive. *Surg Gyn Obstet* 177:525–527.

Koudelka BM. 1991. Obstructive disorders. In: Ellis GL, Auclair PL, Gnepp DR (eds.). Surgical Pathology of the Salivary Glands. Philadelphia: W.B. Saunders, pp. 26–38.

Marcussen DC, Sooy CD. 1985. Otolaryngologic and head and neck manifestations of acquired immunodeficiency syndrome (AIDS). *Laryngoscope* 95:401–405.

McClatchey KD, Appelblatt NH, Zarbo RJ, Merrel DM. 1984. Plunging ranula. *Oral Surg* 57:408–412.

McGurk M. 2007. Management of the ranula. *J Oral Maxillofac Surg* 65:115–116.

Mulligan R, Navazesh M, Komaroff et al. 2000. Salivary gland disease in human immunodeficiency virus-positive women from the WIHS study. *Oral Surg Oral Med Oral Pathol Oral Radiol Endod* 89:702–709.

Owotade FJ, Fatusi OA, Adebiyi KE et al. 2005. Clinical experience with parotid gland enlargement in HIV infection: A report of five cases in Nigeria. *J Contemp Dent Pract* 15:136–145.

Ryan JR, Ioachim HL, Marmer J et al. 1985. Acquired immune deficiency syndrome—related lymphadenopathics presenting in the salivary gland lymph nodes. *Arch Otolaryngol Head Neck Surg* 111:554–556.

Shaha AR, DiMaio T, Webber C et al. 1993. Benign lymphoepithelial lesions of the parotid. *Am J Surg* 166:403–406.

Sperling NM, Lin P, Lucente FE. 1990. Cystic parotid masses in HIV infection. *Head & Neck* 12:337–341.

Thoma KH. 1950. Cysts and tumors of the salivary and mucous glands. In: Oral Pathology: A Histological, Roentgenological, and Clinical Study of the Diseases of the Teeth, Jaws, and Mouth (3rd ed.). St. Louis: C.V. Mosby Co., pp. 1260–1265.

van den Akker HP, Bays RA, Becker AE. 1978. Plunging or cervical ranula: Review of the literature and report of 4 cases. *J Max Fac Surg* 6:286–293.

Work WP. 1977. Cysts and congenital lesions of the parotid gland. *Otlaryngol Clin North Am* 10:339–343.

Yoshimura Y, Obara S, Kondoh T, Naitoh S. 1995. A comparison of three methods used for treatment of ranula. *J Oral Maxillofac Surg* 53:280–282.

Zhao YF, Jia J, Jia Y. 2005. Complications associated with surgical management of ranulas. *J Oral Maxillofac Surg* 63:51–54.

Chapter 5
Sialolithiasis

Introduction

Sialolithiasis is a relatively common disorder of the salivary glands characterized by the development of calculi. Sialolithiasis is thought to affect approximately 1% of the population based on autopsy studies (Williams 1999). It has been estimated to represent more than 50% of major salivary gland diseases and is the most common cause of acute and chronic salivary gland infections (Escudier 1998). Sialadenitis (see chapter 3) and sialolithiasis are disorders of the salivary glands that go hand in hand. Some consider sialolithiasis to be both a consequence and cause of sialadenitis (Berry 1995). For example, in some cases, the presence of a sialolith may cause obstruction such that the salivary gland is predisposed to retrograde infection. In other cases, the presence of sialadenitis may result in a change in the characteristics of the saliva, thereby favoring the deposition of calcium and subsequent formation of a sialolith. In addition, the development of edema within a salivary duct can exacerbate existing obstruction when a small sialolith is present. As such, sialadenitis and sialolithiasis should be considered together. Which of these pathologic processes is the instigating causative factor, however, is unknown (Williams 1999). This chapter will therefore discuss sialolithiasis and review some important concepts of sialadenitis previously discussed in chapter 3.

Pathophysiology of Sialolithiasis

Sialolithiasis results from the deposition of calcium salts within the ductal system of salivary glands. The salivary stones are comprised primarily of calcium phosphate with traces of magnesium and ammonia with an organic matrix consisting of carbohydrates and amino acids. Historically, it has been taught that salivary stones develop around a central nidus of any number of elements, including desquamated epithelial cells, foreign bodies, micro-organisms, and mucous plugs (Bodner 1993). Progression occurs once the nidus becomes lodged within the salivary ductal system. Stagnation of saliva enhances the development of the sialolith and occurs secondary to either the nidus itself, or due to the tortuosity of the ductal system. The nidus subsequently becomes bathed in a solution supersaturated with respect to calcium and phosphate and slowly calcifies. This pathophysiologic mechanism has been empirically accepted for decades, while a paucity of evidence exists on the specific cause of sialolith formation. Kasaboglu et al. (2004) analyzed the chemical composition and micromorphology of sialoliths using X-ray diffraction analysis (EDX) and scanning electron microscopy (SEM). In their six cases reported, X-ray diffraction analysis determined that the sialoliths were comprised completely of multiple and polymorphous hydroxyapatite crystals. In their SEM evaluation, no foreign body or organic material and no signs of micro-organism-dependent core formation were detected.

109

There are several reasons for sialolithiasis being observed most commonly in the submandibular system. First, the submandibular gland lies inferior to Wharton's duct such that the flow of saliva must travel against the forces of gravity. The physical characteristics of Wharton's duct, specifically its length and two acute bends, also theoretically predispose the ductal system to the development of sialolithiasis. The relatively long duct increases the transit time of saliva in the ductal system. The first bend occurs as the gland courses posterior to the mylohyoid muscle, and the second occurs just proximal to the exit of the duct superiorly into the anterior floor of the mouth. While the anatomic nature of Wharton's duct has been considered to be etiologic in the genesis of sialoliths in this system, the angle of the genu of the duct has been investigated as to whether it represents a significant contributory factor (Drage, Wilson, and McGurk 2002). Specifically, these researchers retrospectively studied this issue using sialograms in 23 patients with sialadenitis, 61 patients with sialolithiasis, and a control group of 18 patients. There were no statistical differences in the angle of the genu in the three groups, suggesting that the difference in the angle of the genu of the submandibular duct in the sagittal plane is not of etiologic significance in the formation of sialoliths. The authors indicated that the *length* of the duct might be of significance in the formation of stones; however, that parameter was not investigated in their study. One final issue related to submandibular sialolithiasis is the alkaline nature of the saliva, its viscosity, and its relatively high content of calcium salts, specifically phosphates, carbonates, and oxalates that make the submandibular saliva more prone to sialolithiasis than the other major glands (see Table 5.1). All of these features contribute to salivary stasis, crystallization of precipitated calcium salts with calculus formation, obstruction to salivary flow, and infection. Interestingly, *partial* obstruction appears to be of great importance in the development of sialoliths. A completely obstructed gland, although possessing salivary stagnation, does not result in an increase in stone formation (Williams 1999). In completely obstructed glands, the calcium secretory granules in the acini become depleted and the saliva is less likely to produce stones. Baurmash has stated that salivary stasis and salivary viscosity, rather than the calcium content of the salivary secretion, determine the development of sialoliths (Baurmash 2004).

Table 5.1. Composition of normal adult saliva.

	Submandibular Gland	Parotid Gland
Calcium	3.6 mEq/L	2.0 mEq/L
Phosphate	4.5 mEq/L	6.0 mEq/L
Bicarbonate	18 mEq/L	20 mEq/L
Sodium	21 mEq/L	23 mEq/L
Potassium	17 mEq/L	20 mEq/L
Chloride	20 mEq/L	23 mEq/L
Magnesium	0.3 mEq/L	0.2 mEq/L
Urea	7.0 mEq/L	15 mEq/L
Proteins	150 mg/dL	250 mg/dL
Amino acids	<1 mg/dL	1.5 mg/dL
Fatty acids	<1 mg/dL	1 mg/dL
Glucose	<1 mg/dL	<1 mg/dL

Clinical Features of Sialolithiasis

Approximately 85% of sialoliths occur in the submandibular gland, 10% in the parotid gland, 5% in the sublingual gland, and the incidence of this pathology is extremely rare in the minor salivary glands (Miloro 1998). When involved, minor salivary gland sialoliths occur in the buccal mucosa or upper lip, forming an indurated nodule that may mimic a neoplastic process. Sialolithiasis occurs more often in males, with a peak occurrence between 20 and 50 years of age (Lustmann, Regev, and Melamed 1990). The left submandibular gland is more often affected than the right gland, and bilateral involvement in the absence of another systemic disorder is rare. In fact, stone formation is not highly associated with systemic abnormalities of calcium metabolism (King, Ridgley, and Kabasela 1990). Gout is the only systemic disease known to predispose to salivary stone formation. These stones are primarily made up of uric acid. Multiple occurrences of sialolith formation independent of systemic illness in the same gland, however, are common. While salivary stones are single in 70–80% of cases (Figure 5.1), two calculi occur in 20% of cases, and more than two calculi occur in 5% of cases (Miloro and Goldberg 2002; Williams 1999) (Figure 5.2). Sialolithiasis of the parotid gland is rare. When stones occur in the parotid gland, they are smaller than submandibular gland stones, and more often multiple (Figure 5.3). With regard to location, submandibular stones are located in the duct 75–85% of the time, while

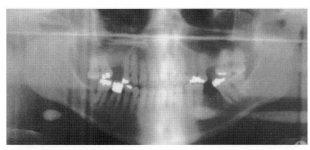

Figure 5.1. A single sialolith noted within the right submandibular gland. Isolated stones are most common in the submandibular system.

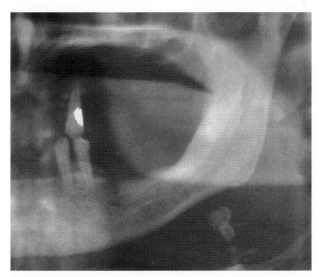

Figure 5.2. This panoramic radiograph close-up shows two sialoliths within the left submandibular gland.

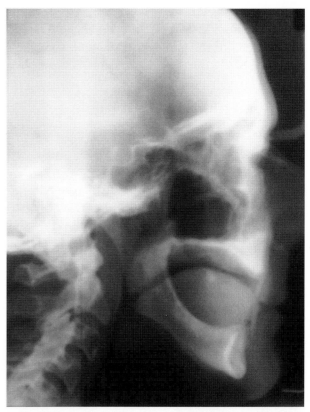

Figure 5.3. This lateral cephalometric radiograph shows a single stone located within Stenson's duct.

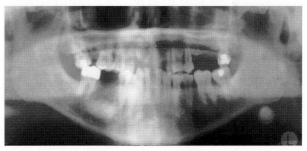

Figure 5.4. This panoramic radiograph shows an oval sialolith of the left submandibular gland.

parotid stones are located in the hilum or gland parenchyma in at least half of the cases (Williams 1999). Submandibular stones located within the gland are oval in shape (Figure 5.4) and elongated in shape when they occur in the duct. When present for long periods of time, these stones may become quite large (Figure 5.5). Bilateral salivary stones are quite rare; however, they have been observed (Lutcavage and Schaberg 1991) (Figure 5.6).

Sialolithiasis most commonly presents with painful swelling, although painless swelling or pain only are occasionally reported as symptoms. Lustmann's study showed swelling to be present in 94% of their 245 cases of sialolithiasis, while pain occurred in 65.2%, pus secretion in 15.5%, and an absence of symptoms in 2.4% of their patients (Lustmann, Regev, and Melamed 1990).

When symptoms do occur, their magnitude seems to vary according to the gland involved and the location and size of the sialolith. A small sialolith may be asymptomatic and serendipitously discovered during routine dental radiographic examination. Once the stone increases in size, salivary flow will be impaired, and spasmodic pain occurs during eating. Purulent infection may accompany sialolithiasis.

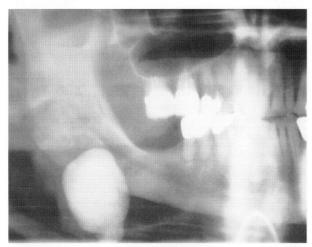

Figure 5.5a. This very large sialolith is associated with the right submandibular gland as seen on panoramic radiograph.

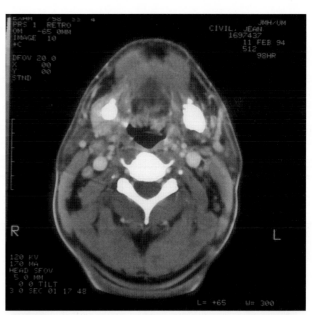

Figure 5.6. This axial section of computerized tomograms shows the presence of bilateral sialoliths of the submandibular glands.

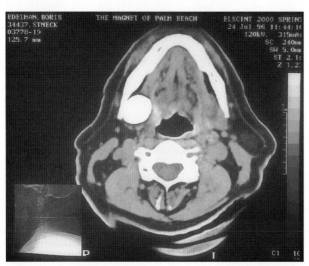

Figure 5.5b. Due to its size, it might be confused with an osteoma of the mandible such that computerized tomograms help to identify its presence within the submandibular gland.

Differential Diagnosis and Diagnosis of Sialolithiasis

Patients with sialolithiasis most commonly present with clinical and historical evidence of salivary calculi. A history of submandibular swelling, prandial pain, and bouts of sialadenitis are highly suggestive of a diagnosis of sialolithiasis. This notwithstanding, many patients are asymptomatic such that only a panoramic radiograph may allow for the diagnosis of submandibular sialolithiasis, as it may reveal calcifications within the submandibular triangle. It has been observed that submandibular stones located anteriorly are more often symptomatic than those lodged in the intraglandular portion of the duct (Karas 1998). While such calcifications may lead to a diagnosis of submandibular sialolithiasis, it is important for the clinician to consider other diagnoses that present with submandibular calcifications, particularly when pain is absent. Among these are calcified lymph nodes associated with mycobacterial adenitis (scrofula) (Figure 5.7), phleboliths associated with oral/facial hemangiomas (Figure 5.8), and a mandibular osteoma as might occur in Gardner's syndrome (Figure 5.9). All of these calcifications may, at first glance, appear similar to submandibular sialolithiasis. Close examination of panoramic radiographs may, however, allow for the clinician to establish a radiographic diagnosis other than submandibular sialolithiasis (Mandel 2006). Most submandibular calculi contain smooth borders when they exist within the gland. Calcified lymph nodes generally show irregular borders, and osteomas of the mandible are larger than most salivary

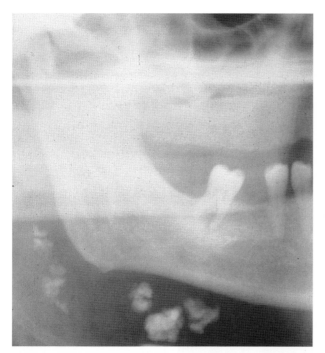

Figure 5.7a. A close-up of a panoramic radiograph obtained in a patient with a chief complaint of right submandibular pain. The calcifications noted on this radiograph are located in the retromandibular region as well as the submandibular gland area.

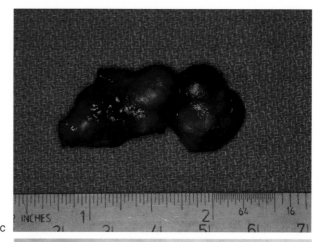

c

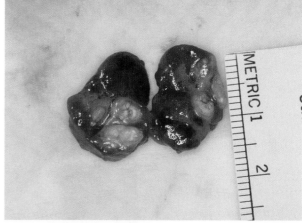

d

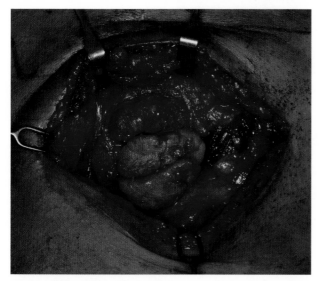

Figure 5.7b. Exploration of the neck showed indurated lymph nodes present in association with the right submandibular gland, but clearly not sialoliths.

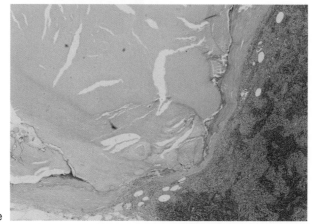

e

Figures 5.7c, 5.7d, and 5.7e. The lymph nodes were removed (c) and bisected, showing macroscopic (d) and microscopic evidence of caseous necrosis (e). A diagnosis of tuberculous adenitis was therefore established. The patient was subjected to a purified protein derivative (PPD) skin test that was positive.

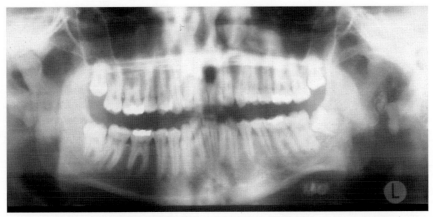

Figure 5.8a. A panoramic radiograph demonstrating calcifications within the left submandibular region.

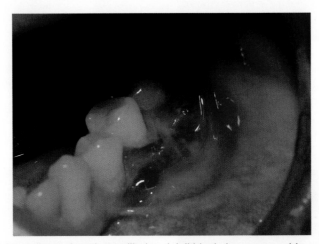

Figure 5.8b. At first glance of the radiograph, submandibular sialolithiasis is a reasonable consideration. Close examination of the radiograph reveals multicentric lamellated calcifications in the submandibular and preauricular regions, as well as a calcification superimposed on the left mandibular second molar roots. A complete physical examination revealed signs consistent with a hemangioma associated with the left mandibular gingiva. As such, the calcifications are presumed to represent phleboliths, and are not removed. It is important, therefore, to diagnose sialolithiasis based on a review of a radiograph as well as a physical examination.

114

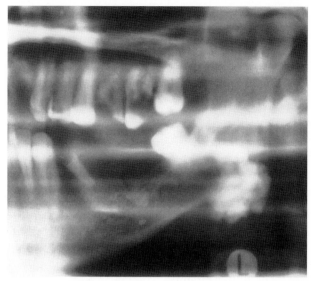

Figure 5.9a. This panoramic radiographic close-up shows an irregular mass associated with the left submandibular region.

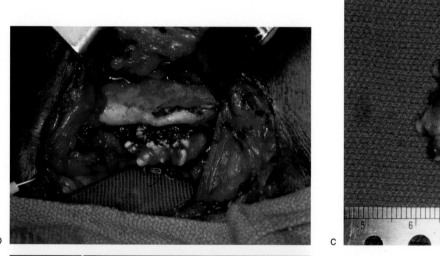

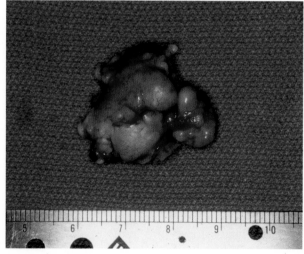

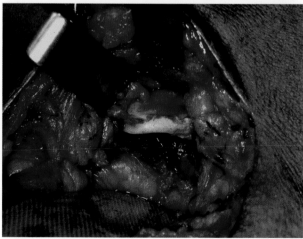

b

c

d

Figures 5.9b, 5.9c, and 5.9d. Computerized tomograms were not obtained preoperatively, and a differential diagnosis of submandibular sialolithiasis was established. The calcification, however, does not show typical radiographic signs of a sialolith, including its irregular borders. The patient underwent exploration of the left submandibular region, whereupon the calcified mass was identified as a distinct entity from the left submandibular gland (b). The mass was removed (c) and the left submandibular gland remained in the tissue bed (d). A histopathologic diagnosis of osteoma was made. A subsequent diagnosis of Gardner's syndrome was made, and the patient underwent colectomy when a diagnosis of adenocarcinoma of the colon was established.

115

gland stones and are intimately associated with the mandible. Phleboliths are commonly multiple in number and also exist within the neck outside of the submandibular triangle. They are scattered and have a classic lamellated appearance with a lucent core. Finally, phleboliths are smaller than sialoliths and demonstrate an oval shape, compared to the sialolith, whose elliptical shape has been created by a salivary duct (Mandel and Surattanont 2004). One further entity worthy of mention is calcified atheromas of the carotid artery, which is sufficiently distant from the submandibular triangle so as to not be confused with a submandibular sialolith. These are most commonly located inferior and posterior to the mandibular angle adjacent to the intervertebral space between cervical vertebrae 3 and 4 (Friedlander and Freymiller 2003).

While the diagnosis of sialolithiasis is frequently confirmed radiographically, it is important for the clinician to not obtain radiographs prior to performing a physical examination. Bimanual palpation of the floor of the mouth may reveal evidence of a stone in a large number of patients. Similar palpation of the gland may also permit detection of a stone as well as the degree of fibrosis present within the gland. Examining the opening of Wharton's duct for the flow of saliva or pus is an important aspect of the evaluation. It has been estimated that approximately one-quarter of symptomatic submandibular glands that harbor stones are non-functional or hypofunctional. Radiographs should be obtained and may reveal the presence of a stone. It has been reported that 80% of submandibular stones are radio-opaque, 40% of parotid stones are radio-opaque, and 20% of sublingual gland stones are radio-opaque (Miloro 1998).

Treatment of Sialolithiasis

General principles of management of patients with sialolithiasis include conservative measures such as effective hydration, the use of heat, gland massage, and sialogogues that might result in flushing a small stone out of the duct. A course of oral antibiotics may also be beneficial. These measures may be particularly appropriate since some patients may carry a clinical diagnosis of sialadenitis in case of a radiolucent sialolith. As such, the treatment is the same in the initial management of both diagnoses.

SUBMANDIBULAR SIALOLITHIASIS

The treatment of salivary calculi of the submandibular gland is a function of the location and size of the sialolith (Figure 5.10). For example, sialoliths present within the duct may often be retrieved with a transoral sialolithotomy procedure and sialodochoplasty. In general terms, if the stone can be palpated transorally, it can probably be removed transorally. A review of 172 patients who underwent intraoral sialolithotomy of a submandibular stone assessed results as to complete removal, partial removal, and failure (Park, Sohn, and Kim 2006). The effect of location, size, presence of infection, and palpability of the calculi on the results was assessed. Univariate analysis showed that palpability and the presence of infection were statistically significant factors affecting transoral sialolithotomy. Palpability was the only significant factor after multivariate analysis. This study provides scientific evidence supporting intraoral removal of extraglandular submandibular gland stones regardless of location, size, presence of infection, or recurrence of calculi as long as the calculi are palpable. This procedure involves excising Wharton's duct overlying the stone, thereby permitting its retrieval (Figure 5.11). Reconstruction of the duct in the form of a sialodochoplasty permits shortening of the duct and enlargement of salivary outflow, thereby preventing recurrence and allowing for healing of the gland (Rontal and Rontal 1987). A properly performed sialodochoplasty ensures effective flow of saliva from the gland in hopes of maintaining the health of the salivary gland. This procedure involves suturing the edges of the duct's mucosa to the surrounding oral mucosa (Figure 5.11). The number of sutures placed is arbitrary; however, a sufficient number of sutures is required so as to stabilize the reconstructed duct to the floor of the mouth. Proper postoperative hydration of the patient with free flowing saliva maintains patency of the sialodochoplasty, thereby enhancing the potential for reversal or stabilization of the underlying sialadenitis. Chronic submandibular obstructive sialolithiasis clearly leads to chronic sialadenitis with presumed parenchymal destruction. After removal of the sialolith, however, the apparent resiliency of the submandibular gland usually results in no adverse symptoms (Baurmash 2004). As such, the ability to effectively retrieve a sialolith usually refutes the need to also remove the affected salivary gland.

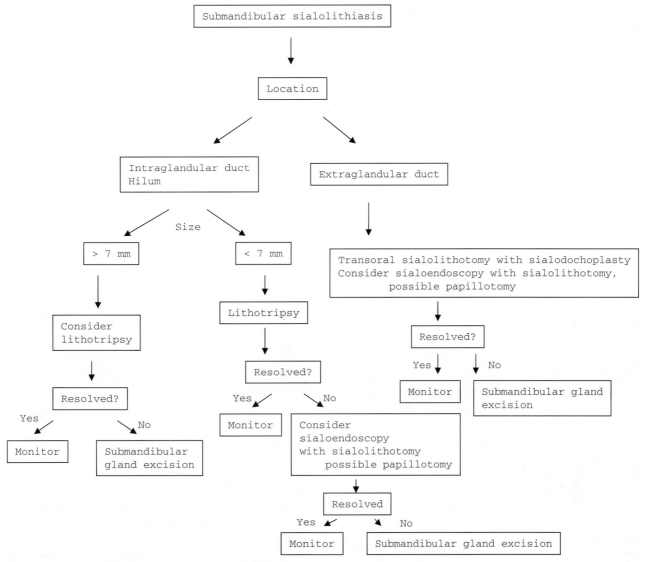

Figure 5.10. Algorithm for submandibular sialolithiasis.

Sialoliths located within the submandibular gland or its hilum are most commonly managed with submandibular gland excision (Figure 5.12). This controversial statement is made based on the relative difficulty to retrieve stones from this anatomic region of the gland, rather than based on the assumption that proximal stones cause permanent structural damage to the gland that results in the need for removal of the gland. To this end, a study examined a series of 55 consecutive patients who underwent transoral removal of stones from the hilum of the submandibular gland (McGurk, Makdissi, and Brown 2004). Stones were able to be retrieved in 54 patients (98%), but four glands

(8%) required subsequent removal due to recurrent obstruction. The authors emphasized that it was necessary for the stone to be palpable and no limitation of oral opening should exist in order for patients to undergo their technique. They reported an acceptable incidence of complications associated with their technique, although they lamented that it remained to be seen if the asymptomatic nature of their patients would be maintained over time.

Shock wave lithotripsy has been reported as a primary form of treatment for submandibular salivary gland stones. Salivary stone lithotripsy requires a gland to be functional by virtue of production of

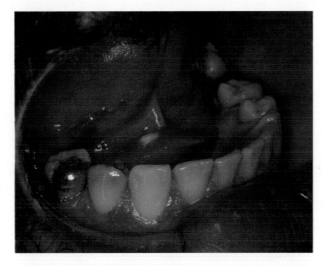

Figure 5.11a. A sialolith is noted at the opening of the right Wharton's duct. Since this stone was able to be palpated on oral examination, it was removed transorally without necessitating the removal of the right submandibular gland. Reprinted from: Berry, RL. Sialadenitis and sialolithiasis. Diagnosis and management. In: The Comprehensive Management of Salivary Gland Pathology, Carlson ER (ed), Oral and Maxillofacial Surgery Clinics of North America, WB Saunders, Philadelphia, 407–503.

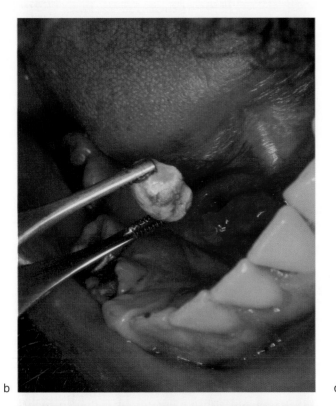

b

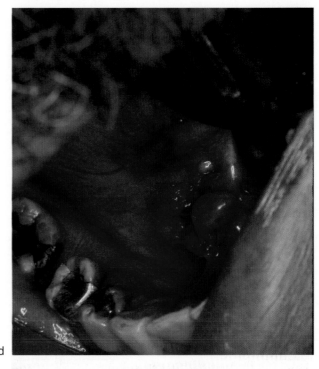

d

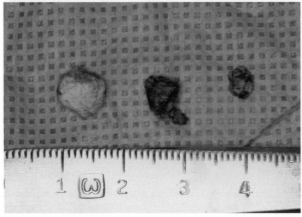

c

Figures 5.11b, 5.11c, and 5.11d. The main stone was removed (b), after which time exploration of the proximal duct revealed two additional stones that were also removed (c). A sialodochoplasty was performed to widen and shorten the right Wharton's duct (d). A sialodochoplasty performed near the papilla of Wharton's duct is termed a "papillotomy." Reprinted from: Berry, RL. Sialadenitis and sialolithiasis. Diagnosis and management. In: The Comprehensive Management of Salivary Gland Pathology, Carlson ER (ed), Oral and Maxillofacial Surgery Clinics of North America, WB Saunders, Philadelphia, 407–503.

118

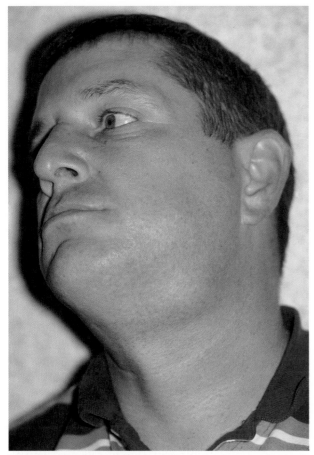

Figure 5.12a. The clinical appearance of a man with pain and left submandibular swelling.

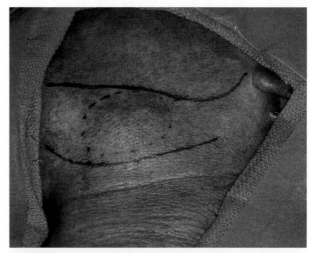

Figure 5.12c. A standard transcutaneous approach was followed to submandibular gland excision.

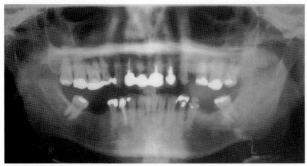

Figure 5.12b. His panoramic radiographic shows a sialolith in the left submandibular gland.

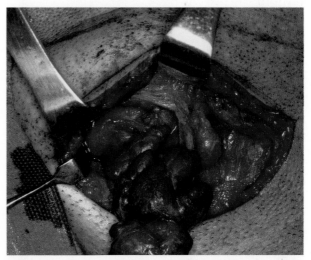

Figure 5.12d. A subfascial dissection of the gland was performed. Inferior retraction on the gland allowed for preservation of the marginal mandibular branch of the facial nerve.

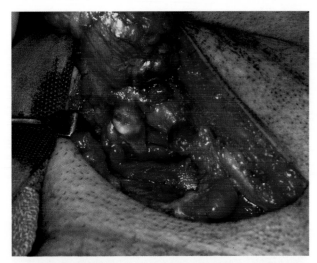

Figure 5.12e. Superior and anterior retraction of the gland allowed for identification of the sialolith that was located at the hilum of the gland.

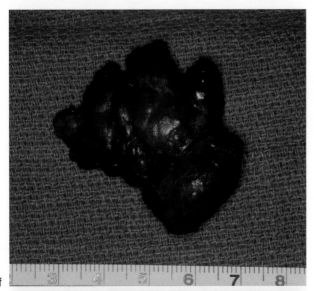

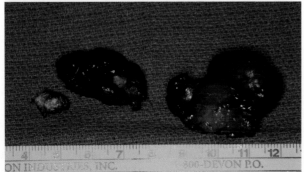

Figures 5.12f and 5.12g. The excised gland (f) was bisected (g) and demonstrated significant scar tissue formation.

saliva in order for the stone fragments to be eliminated from the duct. Some authors have implemented a sour gum test prior to performing extracorporeal lithotripsy (Williams 1999). This test involves the patient chewing sour gum while the clinician looks for swelling of the gland. The development of swelling indicates that the gland is functional such that extracorporeal lithotripsy may be attempted. In the absence of swelling, extracorporeal lithotripsy is contraindicated, and the gland is planned for removal. Two techniques of salivary lithotripsy have been developed, including extracorporeal sonographically controlled lithotripsy and intracorporeal endoscopically guided lithotripsy (Escudier 1998). Extracorporeal shockwave lithotripsy was first used to treat renal stones in the early 1980s. The shockwaves can be generated by electromagnetic, piezoelectric, and electrohydraulic mechanisms and the resultant waves are brought to a focus through acoustic lenses. They then pass through a water-filled cushion to the stone, where stress and cavitation act to fracture the stone. At the sialolith-water interface a compressive wave is propagated through the stone, thereby subjecting it to stress. Cavitation occurs when reflected energy at the sialolith-water interface results in a rebounding tensile or expansion wave that induces bubbles. When these bubbles collapse a jet of water is projected through the bubble onto the stone's surface. This force is sufficient to pit the stone and break it. Extracorporeal lithotripsy for submandibular gland stones is somewhat less successful than that of parotid stones (Williams 1999). Ottaviani and his group evaluated the results of 52 patients treated with electromagnetic extracorporeal lithotripsy for calculi of the submandibular gland (n = 36 patients) and parotid gland (n = 16 patients). Complete disintegration was achieved in 46.1% of patients, including 15 with submandibular sialolithiasis and 9 with parotid sialolithiasis. Elimination of the stones was confirmed by sonogram. Residual concrements were detected by ultrasound in 30.8% of patients, including 9 with submandibular stones and 7 with parotid stones. Four patients with residual submandibular stones required surgical retrieval. The authors concluded by indicating that if hilar and intraglandular duct stones are smaller than 7 mm in size, they may be successfully treated with lithotripsy (Williams 1999). The surgeon should proceed with submandibular gland excision if this trial of lithotripsy is not successful, or if stones larger than 7 mm are identified.

Intracorporeal lithotripsy techniques are now used in which a miniature endoscope is utilized to manipulate the stone under direct vision. In this technique, shockwaves are applied directly to the surface of the stone under endoscopic guidance. The shockwave may be derived from an electro-hydraulic source, a pneumoballistic source, or from a laser. Pneumoballistic energy has been shown to produce calculus fragmentation with greater efficiency than lasertripsy (Arzoz et al. 1996). The disadvantage of these techniques is that the size of the endoscope and probe requires that the duct be incised so as to facilitate entry.

Finally, interventional sialoendoscopy has been developed that may permit the use of a fine sialoendoscope to retrieve salivary stones (Nakayama, Yuasa, and Beppu et al. 2003) (Figure 5.13). The size of some sialoliths, however, is such that an incision of the papilla may be necessary for their delivery. Interventional sialoendoscopy may be used with lithotripsy to fragment large

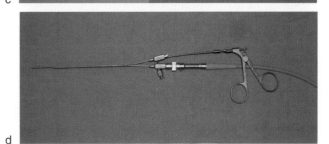

c

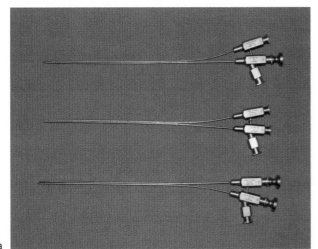

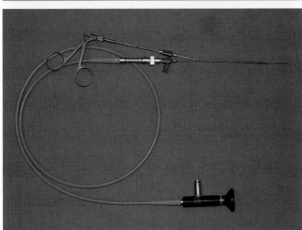

a

b

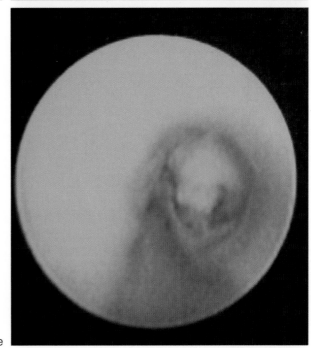

d

e

Figures 5.13a and 5.13b. Interventional sialoendoscopic instrumentation for retrieval of salivary calculus, including the operating sheaths (a) that accept the miniature endoscope (Karl Storz Endoscopy-America, Inc., Culver City, California) in the *telescope* channel (b).

Figures 5.13c, 5.13d, and 5.13e. The grasping forceps (c), are placed within the *working* channel of the operating sheaths (d), and are able to retrieve stones that may be identified on diagnostic sialoendoscopy (e). Figure 5.13e courtesy of Dr. Maria Troulis, Boston, Massachusetts.

stones so as to achieve a completely non-invasive therapeutic sialoendoscopy.

McGurk, Escudier, and Brown (2004) assessed the efficacy of extracorporeal shock wave lithotripsy, basket retrieval as part of interventional sialoendoscopy, and intraoral surgical removal of salivary calculi. Three hundred twenty three patients with submandibular calculi were managed. Extracorporeal shockwave lithotripsy was successful in 43 of 131 (32.8%) patients, basket retrieval was successful in 80 of 109 (73.4%) patients, and surgical removal was successful in 137 of 143 (95.8%) patients with submandibular stones.

PAROTID SIALOLITHIASIS

Sialoliths of the parotid gland are divided anatomically into those that are located within the intrag-landular duct and the extraglandular duct (Figure 5.14). Extraglandular duct sialoliths may be removed surgically through an intraoral approach (Figure 5.15). In this procedure, a C-shaped incision is made anterior to Stenson's papilla. Dissection is performed deep (lateral) to the duct such that it is included in the mucosal flap so that the duct is separated from the more lateral soft tissues. A retraction suture may be placed at the anterior aspect of the mucosal aspect of the flap. The duct is dissected from anterior to posterior so as to identify the stone within the duct. Once the stone is located, the duct is incised longitudinally, thereby allowing for retrieval of the sialolith. The mucosal flap is reapproximated; however, the incision in the duct is not sutured. These longitudinal incisions placed in the duct do not appear to result in the formation of strictures, although transverse

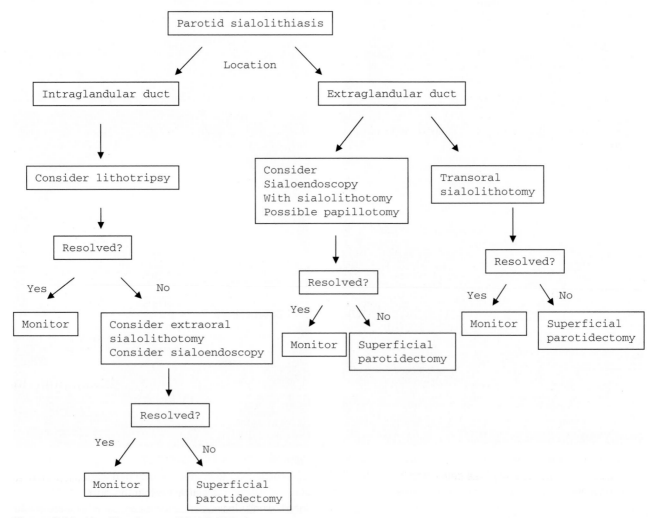

Figure 5.14. Algorithm for parotid sialolithiasis.

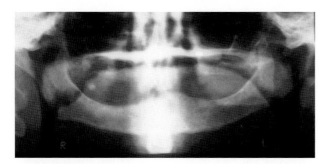

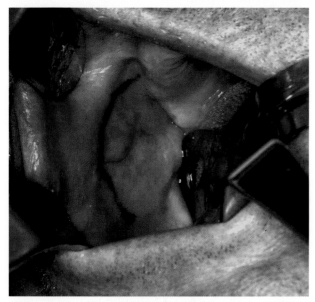

Figure 5.15a. Management of an extraglandular parotid duct sialolith. The panoramic radiograph demonstrates a small sialolith in the right Stenson's duct.

Figure 5.15b. The approach for this transoral sialolithotomy involved a mucosal incision anterior to Stenson's papilla.

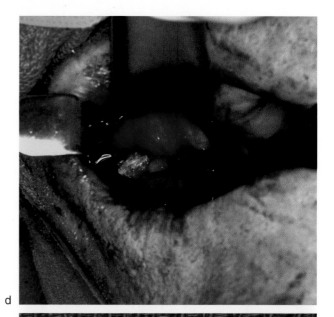

d

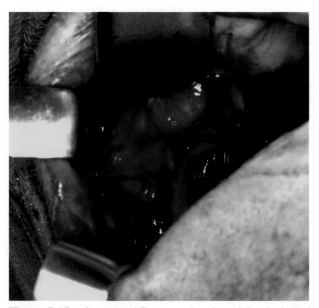

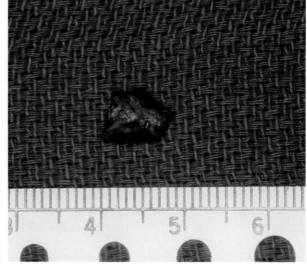

e

Figure 5.15c. A mucosal flap was developed that included Stenson's duct such that the dissection occurred lateral to the duct.

Figures 5.15d and 5.15e. Continued dissection allowed for palpation of the sialolith within the duct. The duct was longitudinally incised over the sialolith (d), such that the stone was able to be removed (e).

123

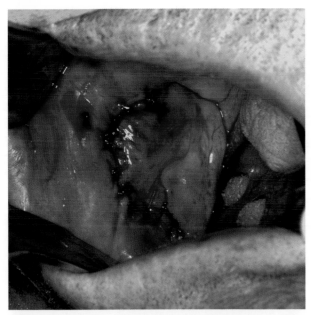

Figure 5.15f. The mucosal flap was sutured without reapproximating the incision in Stenson's duct.

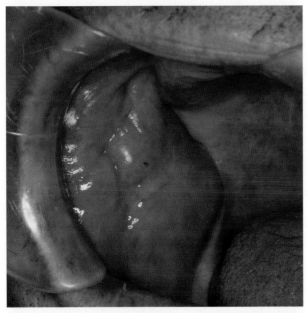

Figure 5.15g. Patent salivary flow was re-established as noted 2 months postoperatively. No further treatment of the gland was required.

incisions in the duct may result in stricture formation (Berry 1995; Seward 1968). Strictures in the parotid duct will respond favorably to intermittent dilation; however, submandibular duct strictures usually require surgical intervention.

Parotid sialoliths located within the intraglandular portion of the ductal system may be addressed through an extraoral approach. Two options exist, one involving a traditional parotidectomy approach (without performing a parotidectomy) with a curvilinear skin incision in the preauricular and upper neck regions (Berry 1995), and the other involving a horizontal incision over the duct in the cheek region (Baurmash and Dechiara 1991). In the former approach, the skin flap is elevated superficial to the parotid fascia, and the duct is identified at the point where it exits the anterior border of the gland. The placement of a lacrimal probe within Stenson's duct may permit accurate identification of the duct. Once the duct is located, it is dissected posteriorly into the gland and the stone is identified. A longitudinal incision is made over the duct and the stone is retrieved (Figure 5.16). As in the case of a transoral sialolithotomy, the incision in Stenson's duct is not closed at the conclusion of the surgery. Sialolithotomy performed with a transcutaneous approach in the cheek may also be accomplished for a diagnosis of parotid sialolithiasis (Figure 5.17).

Extracorporeal lithotripsy seems to be quite effective for the treatment of intraparotid stones. With three outpatient treatments, 50% of patients have been reported to be rendered free of calculus (Williams 1999). Half of the remaining patients may be rendered free of symptoms but having small fragments left in the ductal system. In Ottaviani's cohort of 16 patients with parotid stones, all were relieved of their symptoms with extracorporeal lithotripsy (Ottaviani, Capaccio, and Campi et al. 1996). Nine of their 16 patients experienced complete disintegration and elimination of stones, and 7 patients showed residual stone fragments that were able to be flushed out spontaneously or with salivation induced by citric acid.

McGurk, Escudier, and Brown (2004) found extracorporeal shock wave lithotripsy to be successful in 44 of 90 (48.9%) patients with parotid sialoliths, and basket retrieval was successful in 44 of 57 (77.2%) patients with parotid sialoliths. Interestingly, no patients with parotid stones underwent transoral surgical removal.

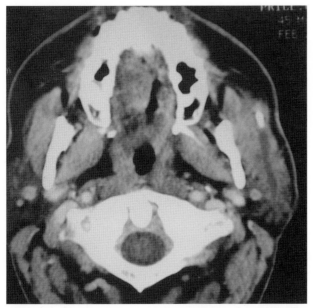

Figure 5.16a. Axial CT scan demonstrating a parotid sialolith at the hilum with proximal dilatation of the duct due to obstruction of salivary flow.

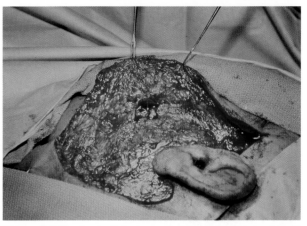

Figure 5.16b. A parotidectomy approach to stone retrieval was performed without parotidectomy.

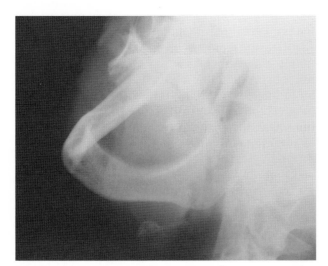

Figure 5.17a. A lateral oblique plain film demonstrating two sialoliths of Stenson's duct.

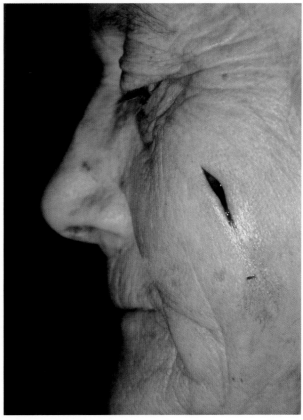

Figure 5.17b. An incision through skin was placed in a resting tension line of the cheek.

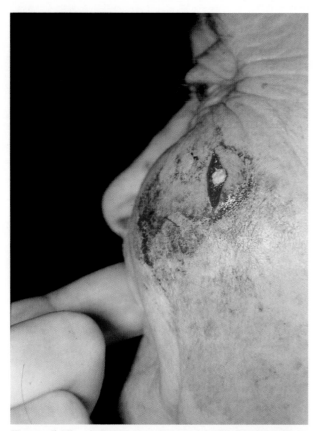

Figure 5.17c. A finger was inserted in the oral cavity to create better access to the duct, thereby permitting stone retrieval.

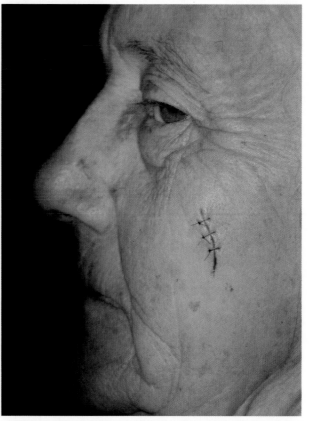

Figure 5.17d. A primary closure was obtained. Reprinted with permission from Ord RA. 2000. Salivary gland disease. In: Fonseca R (ed.), Oral and Maxillofacial Surgery, Volume 5, Surgical Pathology. Philadelphia: W.B. Saunders Co., pp. 273–293.

Miscellaneous Sialolithiasis

The incidence of sialolithiasis of the sublingual gland and the minor salivary glands is very rare. In McGurk, Escudier, and Brown's (2004) study of 455 cases of salivary calculi, no cases were present in the sublingual gland or minor salivary glands. As such, swellings of these glands are most likely to engender a clinical diagnosis of neoplastic disease, with the diagnosis of sialolithiasis made only after final histopathologic analysis of the gland occurs (Figure 5.18). One report examining sialolithiasis of the minor salivary glands found that only 20% of cases were correctly clinically diagnosed as sialolithiasis (Anneroth and Hansen 1983). The paucity of accurate diagnosis may also stem from the frequent spontaneous resolution of

the problem due to ejection of the calculus (Lagha, Alantar, and Samson et al. 2005). Two stages of minor salivary gland sialolithiasis have been described, including an acute stage characterized by inflamed overlying soft tissue whereby the most common clinical diagnosis is cellulitis of the soft tissue. The chronic stage follows and calls to mind a differential diagnosis of neoplasm, irritation fibroma, or foreign body. An anatomic distribution of 126 cases of sialolithiasis of the minor salivary glands identified a significant majority occurring in either the upper lip or the buccal mucosa. As such, sialolithiasis should be included on the differential diagnosis of an indurated submucosal nodule of the upper lip or buccal mucosa, and surgical excision should be performed.

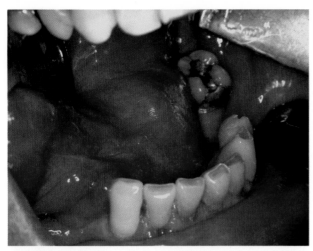

Figure 5.18a. Floor of the mouth swelling present in a 55-year-old woman. Reprinted from: Berry BL. Sialadenitis and sialolithiasis. Diagnosis and management. In: The Comprehensive Management of Salivary Gland Pathology, Carlson ER (ed), Oral and Maxillofacial Surgery Clinics of North America, WB Saunders, Philadelphia, 479–503.

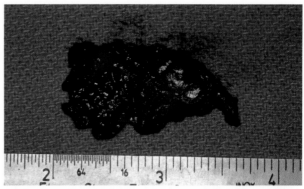

Figure 5.18c. The specimen exhibited mild induration without signs of ranula, such that a neoplastic process was favored while the possibility of a mucous escape reaction was discarded. Reprinted from: Berry BL. Sialadenitis and sialolithiasis. Diagnosis and management. In: The Comprehensive Management of Salivary Gland Pathology, Carlson ER (ed), Oral and Maxillofacial Surgery Clinics of North America, WB Saunders, Philadelphia, 479–503.

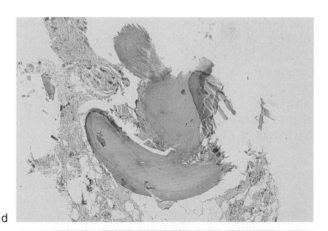

d

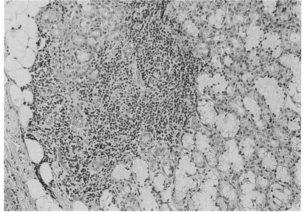

e

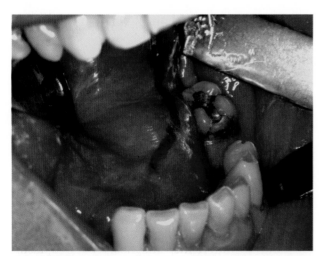

Figure 5.18b. A diffuse mass is noted beneath the surface mucosa that is smooth and of normal color. A presumptive diagnosis of ranula vs. neoplasm was established. A left sublingual gland excision was performed in the standard fashion. Reprinted from: Berry BL. Sialadenitis and sialolithiasis. Diagnosis and management. In: The Comprehensive Management of Salivary Gland Pathology, Carlson ER (ed), Oral and Maxillofacial Surgery Clinics of North America, WB Saunders, Philadelphia, 479–503.

Figures 5.18d and 5.18e. Final histopathology showed a sialolith (d) in the background of sialadenitis (e). Reprinted from: Berry BL. Sialadenitis and sialolithiasis. Diagnosis and management. In: The Comprehensive Management of Salivary Gland Pathology, Carlson ER (ed), Oral and Maxillofacial Surgery Clinics of North America, WB Saunders, Philadelphia, 479–503.

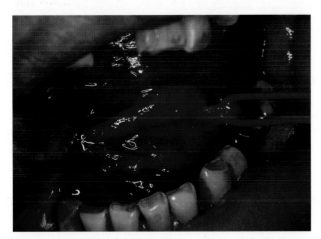

Figure 5.18f. The tissue bed is noted, particularly the lingual nerve (retracted with the vessel loop) and Wharton's duct. Reprinted from: Berry BL. Sialadenitis and sialolithiasis. Diagnosis and management. In: The Comprehensive Management of Salivary Gland Pathology, Carlson ER (ed), Oral and Maxillofacial Surgery Clinics of North America, WB Saunders, Philadelphia, 479–503.

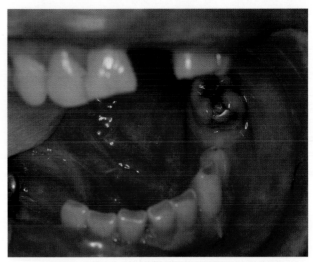

Figure 5.18g. A 6-month postoperative evaluation showed acceptable healing. Reprinted from: Berry BL. Sialadenitis and sialolithiasis. Diagnosis and management. In: The Comprehensive Management of Salivary Gland Pathology, Carlson ER (ed), Oral and Maxillofacial Surgery Clinics of North America, WB Saunders, Philadelphia, 479–503.

Summary

- Sialoliths are calcium phosphate stones that develop within the ductal system of salivary glands.
- Sialolithiasis is thought to affect approximately 1% of the population based on autopsy studies.
- It has been estimated to represent more than 50% of major salivary gland disease and is the most common cause of acute and chronic salivary gland infections.
- Approximately 85% of sialolithiasis occurs in the submandibular gland, 10% in the parotid gland, 5% in the sublingual gland, and the incidence of this pathology is rare in the sublingual gland and minor salivary glands.
- 80% of submandibular sialoliths are radio-opaque, while 40% of sialoliths of the parotid gland are radio-opaque.
- Systemic disorders of calcium metabolism do not seem to represent predisposing factors to sialolithiasis. The one exception to this rule is gout, where a higher incidence of uric acid stones has been observed.
- 75–85% of submandibular stones are located in the duct, while parotid stones are located in the hilum or gland parenchyma in at least half of cases.
- Several "great imitators" of submandibular sialolithiasis exist, including scrofula, phleboliths, osteomas, and occasionally carotid plaques.
- Numerous techniques are available to treat sialolithiasis including surgical sialolithotomy with or without sialodochoplasty, sialoendoscopy with sialolithotomy, intracorporeal or extracorporeal lithotripsy, or gland removal.

References

Anneroth G, Hansen LS. 1983. Minor salivary gland calculi. A clinical and histopathological study of 49 cases. *Int J Oral Maxillofac Surg* 12:80–89.

Arzoz E, Santiago A, Esnal F, Palomero R. 1996. Endoscopic intracorporeal lithotripsy for sialolithiasis. *J Oral Maxillofac Surg* 54:847–850.

Baurmash HD. 2004. Submandibular salivary stones: Current management modalities. *J Oral Maxillofac Surg* 62:369–378.

Baurmash H, Dechiara SC. 1991. Extraoral parotid sialolithotomy. *J Oral Maxillofac Surg* 49:127–132.

Berry RL. 1995. Sialadenitis and sialolithiasis: Diagnosis and management. *Oral Maxillofac Surg Clin North Am* 7:479–503.

Bodner L. 1993. Salivary gland calculi: Diagnostic imaging and surgical management. *Compend Contin Educ Dent* 14:572–584.

Drage NA, Wilson RF, McGurk M. 2002. The genu of the submandibular duct—is the angle significant in salivary gland disease? *Dentomaxillofacial Radiology* 31:15–18.

Escudier MP. 1998. The current status and possible future for lithotripsy of salivary calculi. *Atlas Oral Maxillofac Surg Clin North Am* 6:117–132.

Friedlander AH, Freymiller EG. 2003. Detection of radiation-accelerated atherosclerosis of the carotid artery by panoramic radiography. *JADA* 134:1361–1365.

Karas ND. 1998. Surgery of the salivary ducts. *Atlas of the Oral Maxillofac Surg Clin North Am* 6:99–116.

Kasaboglu O, Er N, Tumer C, Akkocaoglu M. 2004. Micromorphology of sialoliths in submandibular salivary gland: A scanning electron microscope and x-ray diffraction analysis. *J Oral Maxillofac Surg* 62:1253–1258.

King CA, Ridgley GV, Kabasela K. 1990. Sialolithiasis of the submandibular gland: A case report. *Compend Contin Educ Dent* 11:262–264.

Lagha NB, Alantar A, Samson J et al. 2005. Lithiasis of minor salivary glands: Current data. *Oral Surg Oral Med Oral Pathol* 100:345–348.

Lustmann J, Regev E, Melamed Y. 1990. Sialolithiasis: A survey on 245 patients and a review of the literature. *Int J Oral Maxillofac Surg* 19:135–138.

Lutcavage GJ, Schaberg SJ. 1991. Bilateral submandibular sialolithiasis and concurrent sialadenitis: A case report. *J Oral Maxillofac Surg* 49:1220–1222.

Mandel L. 2006. Tuberculous cervical node calcifications mimicking sialolithiasis: A case report. *J Oral Maxillofac Surg* 64:1439–1442.

Mandel L, Surattanont F. 2004. Clinical and imaging diagnoses of intramuscular hemangiomas: The wattle sign and case reports. *J Oral Maxillofac Surg* 62:754–758.

McGurk M, Escudier MP, Brown JE. 2004. Modern management of salivary calculi. *Br J Surg* 92:107–112.

McGurk M, Makdissi J, Brown JE. 2004. Intra-oral removal of stones from the hilum of the submandibular gland: Report of technique and morbidity. *Int J Oral Maxillofac Surg* 33:683–686.

Miloro M. 1998. The surgical management of submandibular gland disease. *Atlas Oral Maxillofac Surg Clin North Am* 6:29–50.

Miloro M, Goldberg MH. 2002. Salivary gland infections. In: Topazian RG, Goldberg MH, Hupp JR (eds.), Oral and Maxillofacial Infections (4th ed.). Philadelphia: W.B. Saunders, pp. 279–293.

Nakayama E, Yuasa K, Beppu M et al. 2003. Interventional sialendoscopy: A new procedure for noninvasive insertion and a minimally invasive sialolithectomy. *J Oral Maxillofac Surg* 61:1233–1236.

Ottaviani F, Capaccio P, Campi M et al. 1996. Extracorporeal electromagnetic shock-wave lithotripsy for salivary gland stones. *Laryngoscope* 106:761–764.

Park JS, Sohn JH, Kim JK. 2006. Factors influencing intra-oral removal of submandibular calculi. *Otolaryngol Head Neck Surg* 135:704–709.

Rontal M, Rontal E. 1987. The use of sialodochoplasty in the treatment of benign inflammatory obstructive submandibular gland disease. *Laryngoscope* 97:1417–1421.

Seward GR. 1968. Anatomic surgery for salivary calculi. I: Symptoms, signs, and differential diagnosis. *Oral Surg Oral Med Oral Pathol* 25:150–157.

Williams MF. 1999. Sialolithiasis. *Otolaryngol Clin North Am* 32:819–834.

Chapter 6
Systemic Diseases Affecting the Salivary Glands

Outline

Introduction

A number of systemic diseases result in infiltration of the salivary glands. These include immune-modulated or idiopathic diseases such as sarcoidosis, Sjogren's disease, sialosis, and lymphoepithelial lesions, as well as lymphoma, a malignant proliferation of B or T lymphocytes. Each of these processes involves multiple physiologic systems and may be diagnosed at an early stage with salivary gland biopsy. It is the purpose of this chapter to describe the clinical features of salivary gland involvement of systemic diseases.

Sjogren's Syndrome

Sjogren's syndrome is an inflammatory autoimmune disease that manifests as a chronic, slowly progressive disease characterized by keratoconjunctivitis sicca and xerostomia. Since 1965, it has been defined as a triad of dry eyes, dry mouth, and rheumatoid arthritis or other connective tissue diseases (Daniels 1991). This process may evolve from an exocrine organ–specific disorder to an extraglandular multisystem disease affecting the lungs, kidneys, blood vessels, and muscles (Table 6.1). These features are believed to be the result of immune system activation with the production of various autoantibodies with lymphocyte invasion of the salivary and lacrimal glands and other affected organs. The autoantibodies include those produced to the ribonucleoprotein particles SS-A/Ro and SS-B/La, and these are thought to interfere with muscarinic receptors (Garcia-Carrasco, Fuentes-Alexandro, and Escarcega et al. 2006). One study identified IgG from patients with primary Sjogren's syndrome containing autoantibodies capable of damaging saliva production and contributing to xerostomia (Dawson, Stanbury, and Venn et al. 2006). Other mechanisms of glandular dysfunction include destruction of glandular elements by cell-mediated mechanisms; secretion of cytokines that activate pathways bearing the signature of type 1 and 2 interferons; and secretion of metalloproteinases (MMP) that interfere with the interaction of the glandular cell with its extracellular matrix (Garcia-Carrasco, Fuentes-Alexandro, and Escarcega et al. 2006). In addition, increased MMP-3 and MMP-9 expression has been found to be responsible for acinar destruction in Sjogren's syndrome (Perez, Kwon, and Alliende et al. 2005). These substantial increases in MMP expression in diseased labial salivary glands may be potentiated by moderate decreases in tissue inhibitors of matrix metalloproteinases (TIMP).

Primary Sjogren's syndrome is designated when it is not associated with other connective tissue diseases. This notwithstanding, evidence exists that shows genetic aggregation of autoim-

Table 6.1. Frequency of extraglandular findings in primary Sjogren's syndrome.

Clinical Involvement	Percent
Arthritis	60
Kidney	9
Liver	6
Lung	14
Lymphadenopathy	14
Lymphoma	6
Myositis	1
Peripheral neuropathy	5
Raynaud's phenomenon	35
Splenomegaly	3

mune diseases in families of patients with primary Sjogren's syndrome (Anaya et al. 2006). The suggestion is that autoimmune diseases in general may aggregate as a trait favoring a common immunogenetic origin for diverse autoimmune phenotypes, such that a risk factor exists for the development of primary Sjogren's syndrome and other autoimmune diseases. Secondary Sjogren's syndrome is defined when the disease is associated with other clinically expressed autoimmune processes, specifically rheumatoid arthritis, systemic lupus erythematosus, myositis, biliary cirrhosis, systemic sclerosis, chronic hepatitis, cryoglobulinemia, thyroiditis, and vasculitis. Following rheumatoid arthritis, Sjogren's syndrome is the second most common autoimmune rheumatic disorder (Moutsopoulos 1993). Eight to 10 years are generally required for the disorder to progress from initial symptoms to the development of the syndrome. Although typically seen in middle-aged women, Sjogren's syndrome can occur in all ages and in males. It has been estimated that 80–90% of patients are women, and that the mean age at diagnosis is 50 years (Daniels 1991).

CLINICAL MANIFESTATIONS OF SJOGREN'S SYNDROME

Most patients with Sjogren's syndrome develop symptoms related to decreased salivary gland and lacrimal gland function. Primary Sjogren's syndrome patients generally complain of dry eyes, often described as a sandy or gritty feeling under the eyelids. Other symptoms such as itching of the eyes, eye fatigue, and increased sensitivity to light can accompany the primary symptoms. Many of these symptoms are due to the destruction of corneal and bulbar conjunctival epithelium and come under the diagnosis of keratoconjunctivitis sicca. This disorder is assessed by tear flow and composition. Tear flow is measured using the Schirmer test, while tear composition can be determined by tear break-up time or tear lysozyme content. The Schirmer test is considered positive when filter paper wetting of less than 5 mm occurs in 5 minutes, and suggests clinically significant keratoconjunctivitis sicca (Moutsopoulos 1993). There are, nonetheless, numerous false positive and negative results, such that the predictive value is limited. The integrity of the corneal and bulbar conjunctiva may be assessed using the Rose Bengal staining procedure and slip lamp examination. Punctate corneal ulcerations and attached filaments of corneal epithelium indicative of corneal and bulbar conjunctival epithelial destruction are noted on slip lamp examination in Sjogren's patients.

Xerostomia is the second principal symptom of Sjogren's syndrome. Xerostomia can be documented by salivary flow measurements, parotid sialography, and salivary scintigraphy. Salivary flow measurements must be adjusted for age, time of day, gender, and concomitant medications. Patients with dry mouths complain of a burning oral discomfort and difficulty in chewing and swallowing dry foods. Xerostomia is commonly associated with changes in taste and the inability to speak continuously for longer than several minutes.

Salivary gland enlargement occurs in as many as 30% of patients with Sjogren's syndrome during the course of their illness, with the parotid gland being most often enlarged (Figure 6.1) (Kulkarni 2005). Bilateral painful submandibular glands have been described as a presenting symptom of this syndrome (Kulkarni 2005). While the parotid glands are most commonly enlarged, they may be the last glands to be affected in patients with Sjogren's syndrome from the standpoint of decreased saliva production (Pijpe, Kalk, and Bootsma et al. 2007). The parotid glands have a longer-lasting secretory capacity in patients with Sjogren's syndrome, and therefore are the last glands to manifest hyposalivation during the disease. In the more advanced stages of the disease, both unstimulated and stimulated submandibular, sublingual, and parotid func-

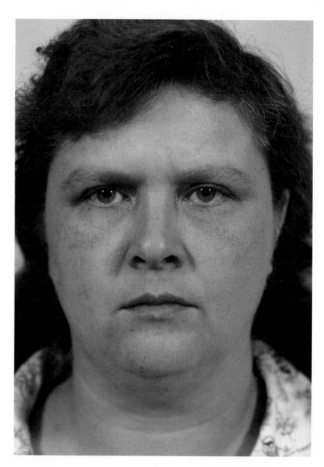

Figure 6.1. A 36-year-old woman with a known history of Sjogren's syndrome associated with rheumatoid arthritis. She described a recent history of painful swelling of the right parotid gland such that an incisional parotid biopsy was recommended.

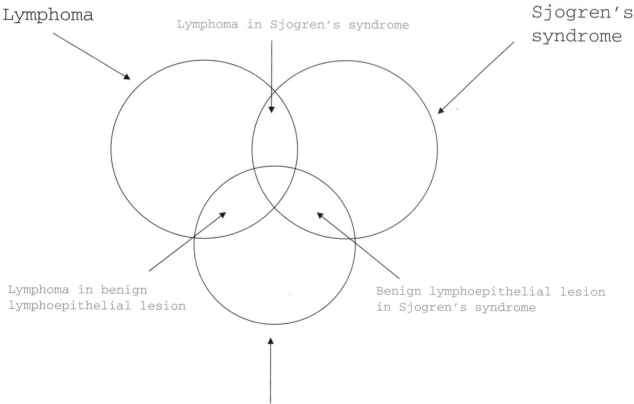

Figure 6.2. The association between the lymphoepithelial lesion, Sjogren's syndrome, and lymphoma.

tions fall to a low level. The accelerated development of dental caries is also noted. Enlargement of the lacrimal glands is uncommon. Even when the salivary glands are not enlarged, they always exhibit lymphohistiocyte-mediated acinar destruction (Marx 1995). When enlarged, however, they show features of the benign lymphoepithelial lesion (BLL) in almost all cases. These lesions may occur in patients who do not have Sjogren's syndrome. Furthermore, they may undergo malignant transformation to lymphomas in patients with or without Sjogren's syndrome (Figure 6.2). This concept, as well as the entity Mikulicz's disease, is clearly worthy of additional discussion.

MIKULICZ'S DISEASE AND THE BENIGN LYMPHOEPITHELIAL LESION

The pathologic entity known as the benign lymphoepithelial lesion was once referred to as Mikulicz's disease. The German surgeon Johann Mikulicz first described the benign lymphoepithelial lesion in 1888 in a report of a single case of lacrimal gland involvement (Daniels 1991). The lacrimal gland enlargement was followed by enlargement of the submandibular and parotid glands, as well as minor salivary gland tissue. The term "Mikulicz's disease" was subsequently applied to a variety of cases of bilateral salivary or lacrimal gland enlargement, including those caused by sarcoidosis, lymphoma, tuberculosis, or syphilis. The term "lymphoepithelial lesion" was proposed by Godwin in 1952 to describe parotid gland lesions previously called Mikulicz's disease, adenolymphoma, chronic inflammation, lymphoepithelioma, or lymphocytic tumor (Godwin 1952). One year later, Morgan and Castleman observed numerous similarities of the benign lymphoepithelial lesion to the histopathology of Sjogren's syndrome and proposed that Mikulicz's disease is not a distinct clinical and pathologic entity but rather one manifestation of the symptom complex of the syndrome (Morgan and Castleman 1953). The benign lymphoepithelial lesion may become large enough to present as a mass resembling a parotid tumor (Figure 6.3).

Acinar degeneration and hyperplasia and metaplasia of the ducts led to the formation of the pathognomonic epimyoepithelial islands, which define the condition. Whether myoepithelial cells or ductal basal cells are responsible for these islands has been questioned. An immunohistochemical investigation has shown that myoepithelial cells do not play a role in the formation of these islands and they should be designated lymphoepithelial metaplasia (Ihrler, Zietz, and Sendelhofert et al. 1999). The condition is often a manifestation of Sjogren's syndrome or other immunological abnormality but may occur outside the Sjogren's disease process. Usually the lesion starts unilaterally but becomes bilateral in the parotids (Figure 6.4). It is less common in the submandibular and minor salivary glands (Figure 6.5).

The lesion may reach a large size, although it is usually asymptomatic. It may be diagnosed by fine needle aspiration if the etiology is uncertain and may require removal by parotidectomy for aesthetic reasons. Sudden growth or pain may be an ominous feature, as a benign lymphoepithelial lesion can undergo malignant change and is perhaps not as benign as its name suggests. The lymphocytic component can undergo change to MALT lymphoma (see chapter 11), particularly in Sjogren's syndrome (Abbondanzo 2001) but also in HIV infections (Del Bono, Pretolesi, and Pontali et al. 2000). Recurrent benign lymphoepithelial lesion may also undergo malignant change of its epithelial component to become an undifferentiated carcinoma with lymphoid stroma (see chapter 8) (Cai, Wang, and Lu 2002).

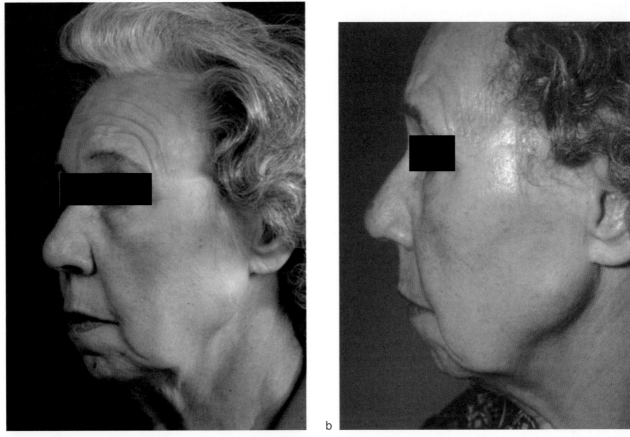

Figures 6.3a and 6.3b. A 75-year-old woman with a left parotid mass. Fine needle aspiration biopsy suggested lymphoma, leading to superficial parotidectomy. Histopathology identified benign lymphoepithelial lesion.

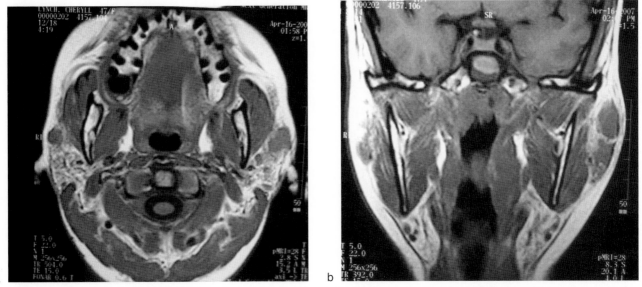

Figures 6.4a and 6.4b. A 45-year-old woman diagnosed with Sjogren's syndrome with bilateral parotid lesions shown on axial (a) and coronal images (b).

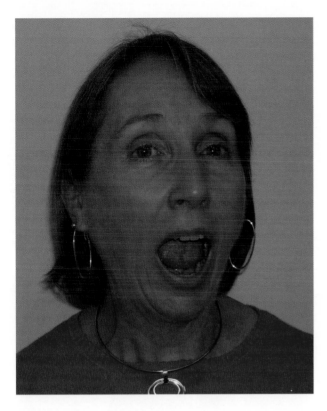

Figure 6.5a. A 55-year-old woman with a 10-year history of a progressively enlarging mass of the left cheek that is able to be visualized inferior to her left zygomatic buttress when she opens her mouth. She reported a history of Sjogren's syndrome.

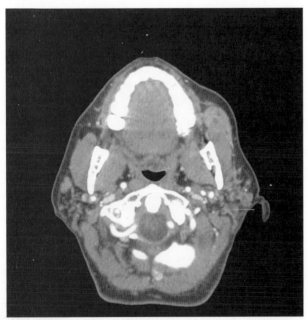

Figure 6.5b. Computerized tomograms identified a heterogenous mass of the left buccal region, associated with minor salivary gland tissue vs. an accessory parotid gland. A salivary gland neoplasm was favored based on clinical and radiographic information.

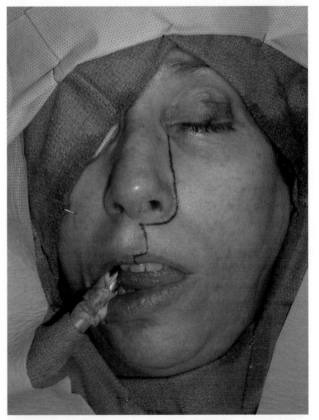

Figure 6.5c. Excision was accomplished with a Weber-Ferguson incision so as to provide access and minimize trauma to Stenson's duct and the buccal branch of the facial nerve.

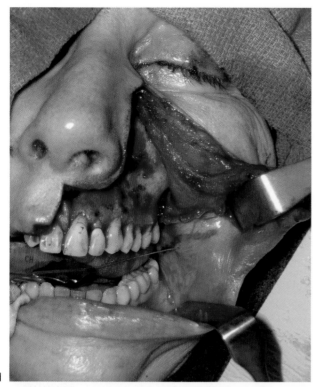

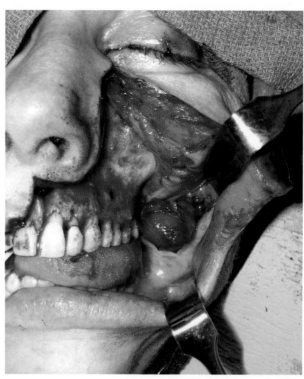

d

e

Figures 6.5d and 6.5e. An incision in the buccal mucosa (d) was also utilized, which permitted effective dissection of the tissue bed (e).

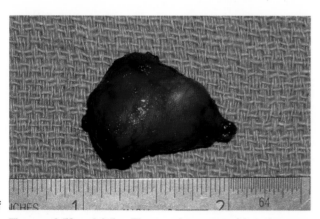

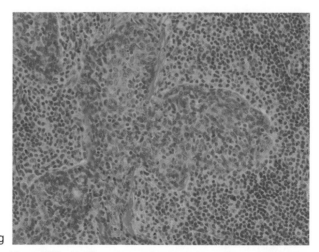

f

g

Figures 6.5f and 6.5g. The specimen was able to be removed without difficulty (f) and was diagnosed as a lymphoepithelial lesion.

DIAGNOSIS OF SJOGREN'S SYNDROME WITH SALIVARY GLAND BIOPSY

Incisional biopsy of minor salivary glands was introduced as a clinical diagnostic procedure for Sjogren's syndrome in 1966. Many studies since that time have examined the value of this biopsy procedure (Marx, Hartman, and Rethman 1988). One study graded inflammation in labial salivary gland biopsy specimens from patients with various rheumatologic diseases and in postmortem specimens (Chisolm and Mason 1968). A grading scheme of lymphocytes and plasma cells per 4 mm^2 was established and has been described by numerous authors since its original description (Greenspan et al. 1974). Grade 0 referred to the absence of these cells, grade 1 showed a slight infiltrate, grade 2 showed a moderate infiltrate or less than one focus per 4 mm^2, grade 3 showed one focus per 4 mm^2, and grade 4 showed more than one focus per 4 mm^2. It has been noted that grade 4 (more than one focus of 50 or more lymphocytes per 4 mm^2 area of gland) is seen only in patients with Sjogren's syndrome and was not seen in postmortem specimens. Due to the strong association with the presence of Sjogren's syndrome, focal sialadenitis in a labial minor salivary gland incisional biopsy specimen with a focus score of more than one focus/4 mm^2 has been proposed as the diagnostic criterion for the salivary component of this disease (Daniels, Silverman, and Michalski et al. 1975). It has been pointed out that the focus score cannot separate early from late disease as chronicity of symptoms and focus score did not show a relationship (Greenspan et al. 1974). The highest focus score, however, was seen in patients with the sicca components of Sjogren's syndrome without associated connective tissue disease. Finally, since variation of disease apparently exists from minor salivary gland lobe to lobe, at least 4–7 lobes of minor salivary gland tissue should be removed and examined microscopically (Greenspan et al. 1974).

Incisional biopsy of the parotid gland has at least theoretical benefit and justification in the diagnosis of Sjogren's syndrome. Previous recommendations for major salivary gland biopsy reported potential complications of facial nerve damage, cutaneous fistula, and scarring of the facial skin when utilizing a parotid biopsy to establish or confirm a diagnosis of Sjogren's syndrome. Incisional parotid biopsy may be performed without assuming any of these complications, except in very rare circumstances (Marx, Hartman, and Rethman 1988). Recent studies, in fact, point to a higher yield of diagnosis when using the parotid biopsy (Marx 1995) (Figure 6.6). In Marx's series of 54 patients with Sjogren's syndrome, 31 (58%) had a positive labial biopsy, while 54 (100%) had a positive parotid biopsy (Marx 1995). He concluded his study by stating that incisional parotid biopsy will confirm and definitively document the diagnosis of Sjogren's syndrome (Figure 6.7). The incisional parotid biopsy will also serve to rule out

the presence of lymphoma, which is observed to develop in approximately 5–10% of patients with Sjogren's syndrome (Daniels 1991; Talal and Bunim 1964). Patients with Sjogren's syndrome are felt to have 47 times greater incidence of lymphoma than that of an age-controlled population (Marx, Hartman, and Rethman 1988). Ten such lymphomas were reported in Marx's study. They developed 4–12 years after the diagnosis of Sjogren's syndrome was made, with a mean of 7.2 years. In 8 of the 10 cases, a rapid change in the size of the parotid enlargement was noted, and all of the patients exhibited a darkening of the skin overlying the enlarged parotid gland. These changes dictated biopsy of the parotid gland in the background of the systemic disease, with the knowledge that lymphoma does not develop in the lower lip in patients with Sjogren's syndrome.

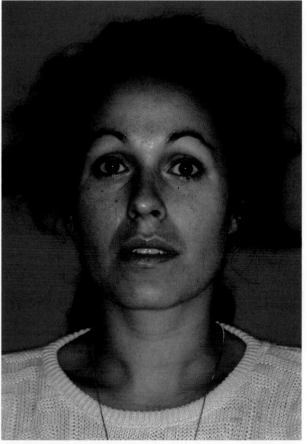

Figure 6.6a. A 32-year-old woman with the recent development of dry eyes and mouth, possibly suggestive of Sjogren's syndrome.

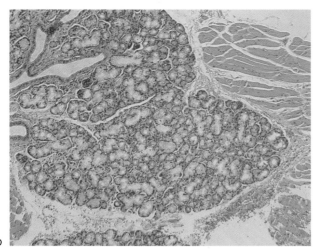 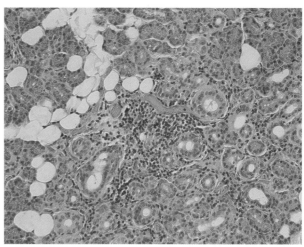

b   c

Figures 6.6b and 6.6c. No swelling of the parotid glands was appreciated on physical examination. An incisional biopsy of the lower lip and right parotid gland were performed. The histopathology showed a normal lower lip biopsy (b) and signs consistent with Sjogren's syndrome on parotid biopsy (c).

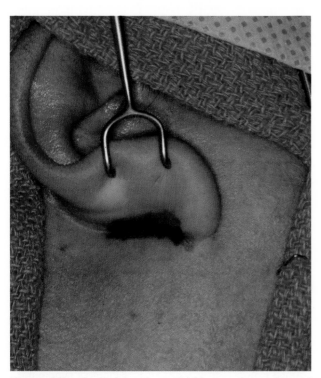 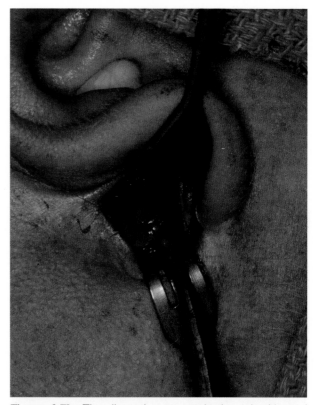

Figure 6.7a. An incisional parotid biopsy was performed on the patient seen in Figure 6.1. The incision is placed behind the right ear, which enables the surgeon to procure sufficient parotid tissue to establish a diagnosis, while also providing a cosmetic scar.

Figure 6.7b. The dissection proceeds through skin and subcutaneous tissue, after which time the parotid capsule is noted. This is incised and a 1 cm² specimen of parotid gland is removed. The closure requires a reapproximation of the parotid capsule so as to avoid a salivary fistula postoperatively.

139

Histopathology of Sjogren's Syndrome

Abnormal salivary gland function is associated with well-defined histologic alterations including clustering of lymphocytic infiltrates as a common feature of all salivary glands and other organs affected by Sjogren's syndrome (Figure 6.8). Histologic evaluation of enlarged parotid or submandibular glands usually reveals the benign lymphoepithelial lesion, with a lymphocytic infiltrate and epimyoepithelial islands. These features are not invariably noted in the major salivary glands, however (Daniels 1991). The characteristic microscopic feature of Sjogren's syndrome in the minor glands is a focal lymphocytic infiltrate, and includes focal aggregates of 50 or more lymphocytes, defined as a focus, that are adjacent to normal appearing acini and the consistent presence of these foci in all or most of the glands in the specimen (Daniels 1991). Epimyoepithelial islands occur uncommonly in minor glands of patients affected by Sjogren's syndrome.

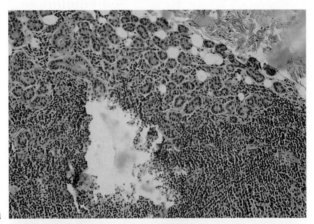

a

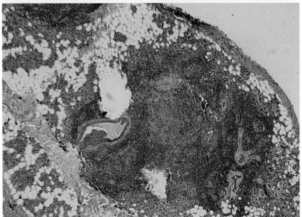

b

Figures 6.8a and 6.8b. The histopathology of the incisional parotid biopsy of the patient in Figure 6.1. Signs consistent with Sjogren's syndrome were noted.

Sarcoidosis

Sarcoidosis is a chronic systemic disease characterized by the production of non-caseating granulomas whose etiology is unknown. It can affect any organ system, thereby mimicking rheumatic diseases causing fever, arthritis, uveitis, myositis, and rash (Table 6.2). The peripheral blood shows a dichotomy of depressed cellular immunity and enhanced humoral immunity. Depressed cellular immunity is manifested by lymphopenia and cutaneous energy. The enhanced humoral immunity is noted by polyclonal gammopathy and autoantibody production.

CLINICAL MANIFESTATIONS OF SARCOIDOSIS

Sarcoidosis occurs most commonly in American blacks and northern European Caucasians. It is eight times more common in American blacks than American Caucasians (Hellmann 1993). Women are affected slightly more frequently than men. Patients with sarcoidosis generally present with one of the following four problems: respiratory symptoms such as dry cough, shortness of breath, and chest pain (40–50%); constitutional symptoms such as fever, weight loss, and malaise (25%); extrathoracic inflammation such as peripheral lymphadenopathy (25%); and rheumatic symptoms such as arthritis (5–10%) (Hellmann 1993).

Respiratory symptoms are the most common presenting chief complaints including those previously mentioned. Regardless of symptoms, greater than 90% of patients with sarcoidosis have an

Table 6.2. Clinical involvement by sarcoidosis.

Clinical Finding	Frequency in Sarcoidosis (%)	Differential Diagnosis
Arthritis	5–10	Rheumatoid arthritis
Parotid gland enlargement	5	Sjogren's syndrome
Upper airway disease	3	Wegener's granulomatosis
Uveitis	22	Spondyloarthropathies
Facial nerve palsy	2	Lyme disease
Keratoconjunctivitis	5	Sjogren's syndrome

abnormal chest radiograph. Four types of radiographic appearance have been described: type 0 is normal; type I shows enlargement of hilar, mediastinal, and occasionally paratracheal lymph nodes; and type II shows the adenopathy seen in type I as well as pulmonary infiltrates (Figure 6.9). Type III demonstrates the infiltrates without the adenopathy. Type II involvement is the most common among patients with sarcoidosis who have respiratory distress.

Two patterns of arthritis are observed in sarcoidosis, and are classified as to whether the arthritis occurs within the first 6 months after the onset of the disease, or late in the course of the disease. The early form of arthritis often begins in the ankles and may spread to involve the knees and other joints. The axial skeleton is typically spared. Monarthritis in the early phase is unusual.

Erythema nodosum, a syndrome of inflammatory cutaneous nodules frequently found on the extensor surfaces of the lower extremities, occurs in about two-thirds of patients and is strikingly associated with early arthritis. *Lofgren's syndrome* involves a triad of hilar lymphadenopathy, erythema nodosum, and arthritis. The late form of arthritis occurs at least 6 months after the onset of sarcoidosis, and is generally less dramatic than the early form. The knees are the most common joints to be involved, followed by the ankles. Monarthritis can occur in the late form of arthritis, and erythema nodosum is not commonly noted.

Other rheumatic manifestations associated with sarcoidosis include involvement of the larynx, nasal turbinates, and nasal cartilage, thereby resembling the clinical presentation of Wegener's granulomatosis (Figure 6.10). Eye involvement

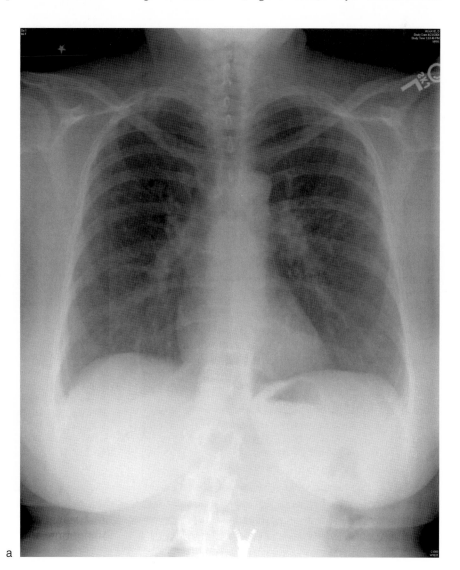

Figures 6.9a and 6.9b. Posterior-anterior (a) and lateral (b) chest radiographs of a patient with type II sarcoidosis. This patient presented with severe shortness of breath.   a

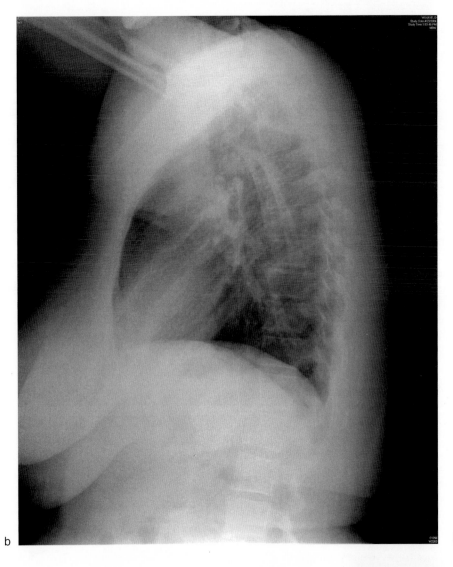

b

Figures 6.9a and 6.9b. *Continued*

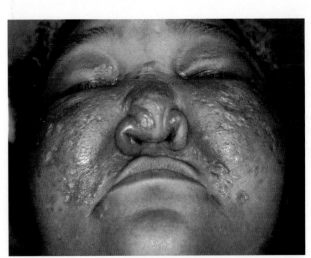

Figure 6.10. Severe nasal cartilage involvement by sarcoidosis in this elderly woman. (Image courtesy of Dr. James Sciubba.)

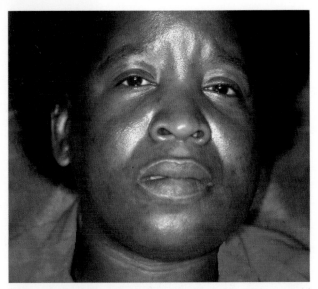

Figure 6.11. Bilateral parotid enlargement in a 50-year-old black woman (left > right) with a known history of sarcoidosis. (Image courtesy of Dr. James Sciubba.)

142

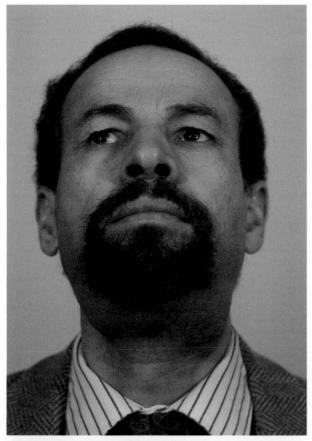

a

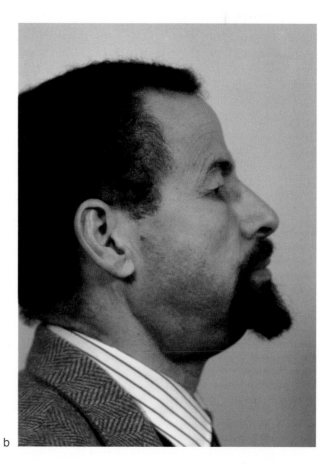

b

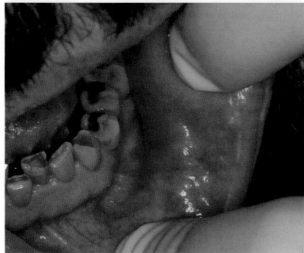

c

Figures 6.12a, 6.12b, and 6.12c. A 55-year-old man with bilateral submandibular gland swellings (a and b), as well as lower lip lesions (c). Excision of the left submandibular gland and biopsy of the lower lip swelling identified non-caseating granulomas. Additional workup identified signs consistent with sarcoidosis.

occurs in 22% of patients, with uveitis being most common (Hellmann 1993). The triad of anterior uveitis in conjunction with parotitis and facial nerve palsy has been referred to as *Heerfordt's syndrome,* also known as uveoparotid fever.

While salivary gland involvement seems to primarily involve the parotid gland (Figure 6.11),

the submandibular gland can also be involved (Vairaktaris, Vassiliou, and Yapijakis et al. 2005; Werning 1991). The Armed Forces Institute of Pathology registry identified 85 cases of sarcoidosis. In the 77 cases in which a gland was specified, parotid involvement occurred in 65% of the cases, while the submandibular gland accounted for 13% of cases (Werning 1991). Submandibular gland enlargement may occur in the absence of parotid swelling, with or without clinical evidence of minor salivary gland involvement (Figure 6.12). Minor salivary gland involvement is occasionally noted histologically in the presence of clinically apparent major salivary gland swelling (Mandel and Kaynar 1994). In fact, enlargement of the major salivary glands may be the first identifiable sign of sarcoidosis (Fatahzadeh and Rinaggio 2006). When this occurs, therefore, it is important to differentiate the parotid swelling associated with sarcoidosis from that of Sjogren's syndrome (Folwaczny et al. 2002). Salivary gland biopsy with histopathologic examination is one means to make this distinction.

DIAGNOSIS OF SARCOIDOSIS WITH SALIVARY GLAND BIOPSY

As with Sjogren's syndrome diagnoses with salivary gland biopsies, early stage disease is perhaps more readily diagnosed with a parotid biopsy rather than a minor salivary gland biopsy. It has been pointed out that cases of sarcoidosis that do not clinically produce parotid enlargement nonetheless show involvement at the microscopic level (Marx 1995). In this review, the labial biopsy was positive in 38% of cases while 88% of parotid biopsies were positive for sarcoidosis. The lesions of sarcoidosis in labial salivary gland biopsies tend to be sparse such that multiple labial glands require excision for microscopic analysis. Another report investigated the yield of minor salivary gland biopsy in the diagnosis of sarcoidosis (Nessan and Jacoway 1979). In this study of 75 patients, non-caseating granulomas were present in minor salivary gland biopsies in 44 patients (58%). There was no correlation with minor salivary gland biopsy yield and stage of the disease. The highest yield for diagnosis of sarcoidosis was found in transbronchial lung biopsies (93%). Nonetheless, the diagnosis of sarcoidosis is one of exclusion, owing to an absence of a diagnostic gold standard. As such, a compatible clinical picture is established based on the patient's symptoms, physical, and radiographic findings. The biopsy of salivary gland tissue or other tissue identifies the presence of non-caseating granulomas such that a provisional diagnosis of sarcoidosis is made. It then becomes necessary to exclude other sources of granulomatous inflammation, such as Crohn's

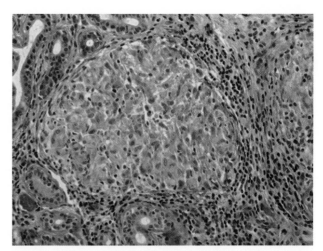

Figure 6.13. Histopathology of sarcoidosis. (Image courtesy of Dr. Joseph A. Regezi.)

disease, deep fungal infections, and others. It is important to point out that there are no pathognomonic diagnostic tests for sarcoidosis. Rather, the salivary biopsy must be considered with an elevated angiotensin converting enzyme (ACE) and lysozyme result, and an altered ratio of CD4/CD8 cells, among others, so as to offer a diagnosis of sarcoidosis (Kasamatsu et al. 2007).

Histopathology of Sarcoidosis

Numerous granulomas may be seen in the salivary gland biopsy. The typical sarcoid granuloma is non-caseating and consists of a tightly packed central focus of histiocytes that is surrounded by lymphocytes and fibroblasts at its periphery (Figure 6.13). The histiocytes may be epithelioid and may join to form multinucleated giant cells, frequently of the Langhans type.

Sialosis

Sialosis, also known as sialadenosis, represents a bilateral enlargement of the parotid gland that is multifactorial in its etiology (Table 6.3). It is not commonly associated with an autoimmune phenomenon, as is the case for Sjogren's syndrome and sarcoidosis, although it can easily be confused with these two pathologic processes due to its clinical presentation (Figure 6.14). Quite commonly, sialosis is caused by nutritional disturbances such as alcoholism, bulimia, or in the rare case of achalasia (Figure 6.15). Chronic alcoholism with or without

Table 6.3. Classification of sialosis.

Malnutritional sialosis
  Achalasia
  Bulemia
  Alcoholism
Hormonal sialosis
  Sex hormonal sialosis
  Diabetic sialosis
  Thyroid sialosis
  Pituitary and adrenocortical disorders
Neurohumoral sialosis
  Peripheral neurohumoral sialosis
  Central neurogenous sialosis
Dysenzymatic sialosis
  Hepatogenic sialosis
  Pancreatogenic (exocrine) sialosis
  Nephrogenic sialosis
  Dysproteinemic sialosis
Mucoviscidosis
Drug-induced sialosis

From Werning 1991.

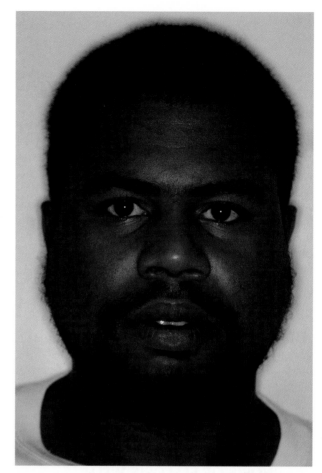

Figure 6.14. A 32-year-old man with a chronic history of bilateral parotid swellings. He gave a history of achalasia. The history suggested that the parotid swellings were consistent with a diagnosis of sialosis. There were no physical or historical findings suggestive of another diagnosis.

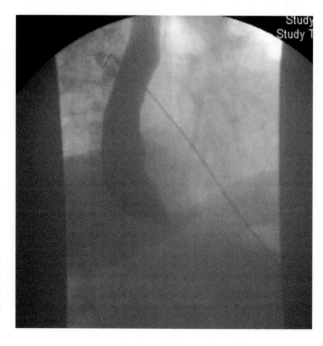

Figure 6.15. The fluoroscopic images of the barium swallow performed in the patient in Figure 6.14. The characteristic "bird's beak" deformity is noted, reflective of failure of the lower esophageal sphincter to relax. This is diagnostic of achalasia.

145

cirrhosis results in asymptomatic enlargement of the parotid glands in 30–80% of these patients (Regezi, Sciubba, and Jordan 2003). In such cases, parotid enlargement has been attributed to protein deficiency. In diabetes mellitus, the mechanism of acinar hypertrophy associated with this condition is unknown. Due to the numerous causes of sialosis, as well as a large number of diagnoses that can clinically resemble sialosis, the patient's history is paramount in such cases so as to properly initiate the diagnostic process. In addition, the treatment for these disorders differs significantly.

CLINICAL MANIFESTATIONS OF SIALOSIS

Sialosis is characterized by chronic, afebrile salivary enlargement. The enlargement is described by patients as slowly evolving and recurrent. A thorough history will most frequently divulge symptoms associated with comorbid disease such as diabetes mellitus, achalasia, alcoholism, or others.

DIAGNOSIS OF SIALOSIS WITH SALIVARY GLAND BIOPSY

The role of salivary gland biopsy in a patient suspected of having sialosis is to rule out Sjogren's syndrome, sarcoidosis, and lymphoma. Sialosis is a disease limited to the major salivary glands such that an incisional biopsy of parotid enlargement is indicated, rather than an incisional biopsy of the lip as might be considered in Sjogren's syndrome or sarcoidosis. As such, a minor salivary gland biopsy is of no value in making a diagnosis of sialosis. While histopathologic confirmation of this process is valuable, it is certainly possible to make a clinical diagnosis of sialosis based on historical findings (Mandel, Vakkas, and Saqi 2005). In addition, once a histopathologic diagnosis of sialosis has been established, the underlying cause of this disorder must be ascertained, if not already known preoperatively. Prompt treatment of the underlying disease process must then occur.

Histopathology of Sialosis

The parotid swelling of sialosis is due to acinar enlargement (Figure 6.16). The diameter of the acinar cell tends to increase by two to three times that of normal. The nuclei tend to be basally situated, and the cytoplasm tends to be packed with granules. There is no correlation between the specific clinical type of sialosis and the histologic appearance. Inflammatory cells tend to be absent. The long-standing nature of the underlying disease may ultimately lead to acinar atrophy and replacement with fat (Werning 1991).

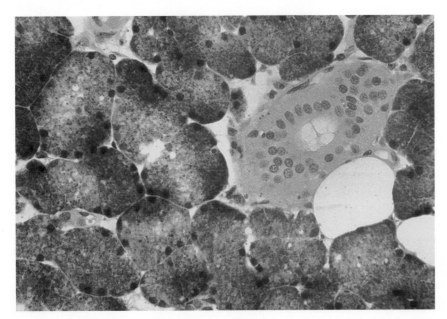

Figure 6.16. The histopathology of the incisional parotid biopsy performed on the patient in Figure 6.14. Acinar hypertrophy is noted. The physical, radiographic, and histologic information confirms a diagnosis of achalasia. He was treated accordingly.

Summary

- A number of systemic diseases may infiltrate salivary gland tissue, including Sjogren's syndrome, sarcoidosis, and sialosis.
- Sjogren's syndrome and sarcoidosis are auto-immune disorders, while sialosis is not.
- Sjogren's syndrome is characterized by keratoconjunctivitis sicca and xerostomia, with or without association with another connective tissue disease.
- Approximately 30% of patients with Sjogren's syndrome will develop salivary gland enlargement, most commonly in the parotid gland.
- A salivary gland biopsy may confirm the patient's diagnosis of Sjogren's syndrome. Either a labial biopsy or parotid gland biopsy may be performed. Disease may be identified more often in a parotid biopsy, even when the patient does not demonstrate parotid swelling.
- Another benefit of parotid biopsy is the identification of lymphoma that is known to develop in 5–10% of patients with Sjogren's syndrome.
- Specific histologic criteria have been established for the diagnosis of Sjogren's syndrome in salivary gland biopsies, specifically referred to as a focus.
- Sarcoidosis is a multisystem disease, with particular proclivity for lung involvement.
- Erythema nodosum represents cutaneous nodules most commonly involving the extensor surfaces of the lower extremities, and occurs in about two-thirds of patients with sarcoidosis.
- Lofgren's syndrome involves a triad of hilar lymphadenopathy, erythema nodosum, and arthritis.
- Approximately 5% of patients with sarcoidosis have parotid gland enlargement.
- The triad of anterior uveitis in conjunction with parotitis and facial nerve palsy has been referred to as Heerfordt's syndrome.
- As with Sjogren's syndrome, there is a higher yield of positive findings to make a diagnosis of sarcoidosis based on parotid biopsy compared to lip biopsy.
- Sialosis is a non-inflammatory, non-neoplastic, non-autoimmune disorder showing enlargement of the salivary glands, most notably the parotid gland.

References

Abbondanzo SL. 2001. Extranodal marginal-zone B-cell lymphoma of the salivary gland. *Ann Diag Pathol* 5(4):246–254.

Anaya JM, Tobon GJ, Vega P, Castiblanco J. 2006. Autoimmune disease aggregation in families with primary Sjogren's syndrome. *J Rheumatol* 33:2227–2234.

Cai YL, Wang ZH, Lu SJ. 2002. Analysis for therapy and prognosis of undifferentiated carcinoma with lymphoid stroma in the salivary gland. *Shanghai Kou Qiang Yi Xue* 11(4):310–313 (in Chinese).

Chisolm DM, Mason DK. 1968. Labial salivary gland biopsy in Sjogren's syndrome. *J Clin Pathol* 21:656–660.

Daniels TE. 1991. Benign lymphoepithelial lesion and Sjogren's syndrome. In: Ellis GL, Auclair PL, Gnepp DR (eds.), Surgical Pathology of the Salivary Glands. Philadelphia: W.B. Saunders, pp. 83–106.

Daniels TE, Silverman S, Michalski JP, et al. 1975. The oral component of Sjogren's syndrome. *Oral Surg Oral Med Oral Pathol* 39:875–885.

Dawson LJ, Stanbury J, Venn N et al. 2006. Antimuscarinic antibodies in primary Sjogren's syndrome reversibly inhibit the mechanism of fluid secretion by human submandibular salivary acinar cells. *Arthritis Rheum* 54:1165–1173.

Del Bono V, Pretolesi F, Pontali E et al. 2000. Possible malignant transformation of benign lymphoepithelial lesions in human deficiency virus-infected patients: Report of three cases. *Clin Infect Dis* 30(6):947–949.

Fatahzadeh M, Rinaggio J. 2006. Diagnosis of systemic sarcoidosis prompted by orofacial manifestations: A review of the literature. *JADA* 137:54–60.

Folwaczny M, Sommer A, Sander CA, Kellner H. 2002. Parotid sarcoidosis mimicking Sjogren's syndrome: Report of a case. *J Oral Maxillofac Surg* 60:117–120.

Garcia-Carrasco M, Fuentes-Alexandro S, Escarcega RO et al. 2006. Pathophysiology of Sjogren's syndrome. *Arch Med Res* 37:921–932.

Godwin JT. 1952. Benign lymphoepithelial lesion of the parotid gland (adenolymphoma, chronic inflammation, lymphoepithelioma, lymphocytic tumor, Mikulicz disease): Report of eleven cases. *Cancer* 5:1089–1103.

Greenspan JS, Daniels TE, Talal N, Sylvester RA. 1974. The histopathology of Sjogren's syndrome in labial salivary gland biopsies. *Oral Surg Oral Med Oral Pathol* 37:217–229.

Hellmann DB. 1993. Sarcoidosis. In: Schumacher HR, Klippel JH, Koopman WJ (eds.), Primer on the Rheumatic Diseases (10th ed.). Atlanta, GA: Arthritis Foundation, pp. 204–205.

Ihrler S, Zietz C, Sendelhofert A et al. 1999. Lymphoepithelial duct lesions in Sjogren-type sialadenitis. *Virchows Arch* 434(4):315–323.

Kasamatsu A, Kanazawa H, Watanabe T, Matsuzaki O. 2007. Oral sarcoidosis: Report of a case and review of literature. *J Oral Maxillofac Surg* 65:1256–1259.

Kulkarni K. 2005. Unusual presentation of Sjogren syndrome. *Southern Med J* 98:1210–1211.

Mandel L, Kaynar A. 1994. Sialadenopathy: A clinical herald of sarcoidosis. Report of two cases. *J Oral Maxillofac Surg* 52:1208–1210.

Mandel L, Vakkas J, Saqi A. 2005. Alcoholic (beer) sialosis. *J Oral Maxillofac Surg* 63:402–405.

Marx RE. 1995. Incisional parotid biopsy for diagnosis of systemic disease. *Oral Maxillofac Surg Clinics of North Am* 7:505–517.

Marx RE, Hartman KS, Rethman KV. 1988. A prospective study comparing incisional labial to incisional parotid biopsies in the detection and confirmation of sarcoidosis, Sjogren's disease, sialosis and lymphoma. *J Rheumatol* 15:621–629.

Morgan WS, Castleman B. 1953. A clinicopathologic study of "Mikulicz's disease." *Am J Pathol* 29:471–503.

Moutsopoulos HM. 1993. In: Schumacher HR (ed.), Primer on the Rheumatic Diseases (10th ed.) Atlanta: Arthritis Foundation, pp. 131–135.

Nessan VJ, Jacoway JR. 1979. Biopsy of minor salivary glands in the diagnosis of sarcoidosis. *New Engl J Med* 301:922–924.

Perez P, Kwon YJ, Alliende C et al. 2005. Increased acinar damage of salivary glands of patients with Sjogren's syndrome is paralleled by simultaneous imbalance of matrix metalloproteinase 3/tissue inhibitor of metalloproteinases 1 and matrix metalloproteinase 9/tissue inhibitor of metalloproteinases 1 ratios. *Arthritis Rheum* 52:2751–2760.

Pijpe J, Kalk WWI, Bootsma H et al. 2007. Progression of salivary gland dysfunction in patients with Sjogren's syndrome. *Ann Rheum Dis* 66:107–112.

Regezi JA, Sciubba JJ, Jordan RCK. 2003. In: Regezi JA, Sciubba JJ, Jordan RCK (eds.), Oral Pathology, Clinical Pathologic Correlations (4th ed.). Philadelphia: W.B. Saunders, pp. 183–217.

Talal N, Bunim J. 1964. The development of malignant lymphoma in the course of Sjogren's syndrome. *Am J Med* 36:529–540.

Vairaktaris E, Vassiliou S, Yapijakis C et al. 2005. Salivary gland manifestations of sarcoidosis: Report of three cases. *J Oral Maxillofac Surg* 63:1016–1021.

Werning JT. 1991. Infectious and systemic diseases. In: Ellis GL, Auclair PL, Gnepp DR (eds.), Surgical Pathology of the Salivary Glands. Philadelphia: W.B. Saunders, pp. 39–59.

Chapter 7
Classification, Grading, and Staging of Salivary Gland Tumors

John J. Sauk, DDS, MS, FAAAS, FAHNS

Outline

Introduction

Scientific classification is a method by which scientists categorize species of organisms. Modern classification has its root in the work of Carolus Linnaeus, also known as Carl von Linné, the Father of Taxonomy, who grouped species according to shared physical characteristics. Accordingly, scientific classification belongs to the science of taxonomy or biological systematics. Molecular systematics, which uses genomic and proteomic expression data, has driven many recent revisions in these systems. In a like manner, surgeons, pathologists, and oncologists have endeavored to symmetrically categorize tumors on the basis of designated characteristics so as to predict probable biological behavior that would help dictate appropriate therapeutic modalities to be employed and to forecast a probable prognosis. As such, the "designated characteristics" upon which

149

tumors have been classified may be in more contemporary terms considered as "biomarkers." In like fashion, genomic and proteomic expression profiles of tumors have thrust pathology and oncology into molecular systematics to develop classifications.

The role of molecular profiling or systematics for clinical decision making and taxonomy has been recently considered, and the classification of tissue or other specimens for diagnostic, prognostic, and predictive purposes based on multiple gene expression and proteomics has been noted to hold major promise for optimizing the management of patients with cancer (Ioannidis 2007). However, assay development and data analysis have been principally investigative, and there exists a lofty potential for the introduction of bias. Most troubling is that standardization of profiles has been the exception. Moreover, classifier performance is typically overinterpreted by conveying the results as p-values or multiplicative effects, whereas the absolute sensitivity and specificity of classification are modest, particularly when tested in large validation samples (Ioannidis 2007). Furthermore, validation has frequently been made with less than favorable consideration for methodology and safeguarding for bias. Most disconcerting is that the postulated classifier performance can be inflated compared to what these profiles can accomplish.

Whether traditional morphological designated characteristics or molecular systematics are employed, the aim of any classification is to demonstrate diagnostic, prognostic, and predictive performance. This can generally be accomplished for any data set by training. However, it is well known that unless training is unsupervised (no knowledge of the correct class is involved), the performance of the system being tested on the training dataset is totally uninformative about its true operation (Ioannidis 2007). Cross-validation and independent validation are two methods to determine whether the proposed scheme is an accurate classifier (Allison et al. 2006). Despite the method employed, different metrics can be used to describe the classifier performance. These may include statistical testing measures, multiplicative effect measures such as likelihood ratios or hazard ratios, or absolute effect measures. Although all information has some value, absolute effect measures (sensitivity and specificity) are the most meaningful from a clinical perspective (Buyse et al. 2006).

Classification Systems for Salivary Gland Neoplasms

The classification system for salivary gland neoplasms has evolved with the accumulation of clinical experience and our understanding of the basis for neoplasia. Although a variety of classifications have been advocated, there has been some regional variation in terminology and classification between European and American authors. Historically, the first and most notable classification was that put forth by Foote and Frazell (1954). Later systems reflect the recognition and description of previously unrecognized entities or the deletion of some terms that were misnomers or were considered meaningless. The succeeding classifications include those by Thackray and Lucas (1974); Evans and Cruickshank (1970); the World Health Organization (WHO); Thackray and Sobin (1972); Batsakis (1979); Seifert et al. (1986); and Ellis and Auclair (Auclair, Ellis, and Gnepp 1991). The most recent fascicle on the subject provides a stepwise evolution of these taxonomies (Ellis and Auclair 1996).

THE CELLULAR CLASSIFICATION OF SALIVARY GLAND NEOPLASMS

Salivary gland neoplasms are noted for their histological variability. Reflecting the anatomy of these glands, benign and malignant salivary gland neoplasms may arise either from epithelial, mesenchymal, or lymphoid origins. The complexity of the classification and the rarity of some of these tumors, some of which display a wide spectrum of morphological patterns within the same tumor and the existence of hybrid lesions, challenge the surgical pathologist with a difficult task in differentiating benign from malignant tumors (Seifert and Donath 1996; Speight and Barrett 2002).

The following cellular classification system reiterates that advocated by the National Cancer Institute (NCI) of the U.S. Public Health Service (USPHS) (www.cancer.gov), which is derived heavily from that published by the Armed Forces Institute of Pathology (AFIP) (Ellis and Auclair 1996) (Table 7.1). Similar to the NCI scheme we also include malignant non-epithelial neoplasms because these lesions embrace a sizable proportion of salivary gland neoplasms. Though less common,

Table 7.1. Cellular classification of salivary gland tumors.

Epithelial neoplasms
  Benign salivary gland neoplasms
    Pleomorphic adenoma or mixed tumor
    Papillary cystadenoma lymphomatosum or Warthin's
      tumor
    Monomorphic adenomas
      Basal cell adenoma
      Canalicular adenoma
      Oncocytoma
      Sebaceous adenoma
      Sebaceous lymphadenoma
    Myoepithelioma
    Cystadenoma
    Ductal papillomas
    Sialoblastoma
  Malignant epithelial neoplasms
    Mucoepidermoid carcinoma
    Adenoid cystic carcinoma
    Adenocarcinomas
      Acinic cell carcinoma
      Polymorphous low-grade adenocarcinoma
      Adenocarcinoma, NOS
      Rare adenocarcinomas
        Basal cell adenocarcinoma
        Clear cell carcinoma
        Cystadenocarcinoma
        Sebaceous adenocarcinoma
        Sebaceous lymphadenocarcinoma
        Oncocytic carcinoma
        Salivary duct carcinoma
        Primary mucinous adenocarcinoma
        Malignant mixed tumors
          Carcinoma ex-pleomorphic adenoma
          Salivary carcinosarcoma
          Metastasizing mixed tumor
      Rare carcinomas
        Primary squamous cell carcinoma
        Epithelial-myoepithelial carcinoma
        Anaplastic small cell carcinoma
        Undifferentiated carcinomas
          Small cell undifferentiated carcinoma
          Large cell undifferentiated carcinoma
          Lymphoepithelial carcinoma
        Myoepithelial carcinoma
        Adenosquamous carcinoma
Non-epithelial neoplasms
  Lymphomas and benign lymphoepithelial lesion
Mesenchymal neoplasms
  Malignant mesenchymal Salivary gland tumors

the inclusion of malignant secondary tumors is presented to be inclusive.

As noted in the introduction, statistics regarding incidence, frequency, and prognosis have varied depending on the study. Moreover, a cursory review of the literature generally reveals that power analyses are rarely performed to access the necessary sample size for many of these studies, and most rudimentary statistical measures are employed to arrive at conclusions. In large part, these deficiencies have stemmed from the general rare incidence of many salivary gland neoplasms. Although the AFIP statistics have been criticized to be biased because of the methods of case accrual as a reference service, these data are probably the most reliable, especially for rare and unusual lesions.

Benign Salivary Gland Neoplasms
Pleomorphic Adenoma
The pleomorphic adenoma or mixed tumor is the most common salivary gland tumor, representing 45–75% of all salivary gland tumors. Clinically, the tumors are smooth, multilobular, and appear encapsulated. However, microscopically, tumor extensions may be seen extending beyond the apparent capsule. The tumor is varied depending on the cellularity and the myxoid content. The presence of both epithelial and mesenchymal-like elements resulting from epithelial cells and myoepithelial cells produces significant diversity in the appearance of these tumors. Notable is that stromal components may encompass myxoid, fibroid, or chondroid features providing the mixed appearance of these lesions (Ellis and Auclair 1996).

Papillary Cystadenoma Lymphomatosum
The papillary cystadenoma lymphomatosum or Warthin's tumor has been regarded as the second most common benign salivary gland neoplasm, and comprises 6–10% of all parotid tumors. These tumors seldom arise in the submandibular or minor salivary glands. Men are more commonly affected than women, with a gender ratio of 5:1. Interestingly, the prevalence increases in smokers and bilateral distribution has been noted in ~12% of cases (Ellis and Auclair 1996).

Monomorphic Adenomas
Basal Cell Adenoma
The basal cell adenoma is a lesion characterized by a monomorphous uniform basiloid pattern and

lacking any myxochondroid features typical of mixed tumors.

Canalicular Adenoma

Canalicular adenomas are benign salivary gland tumors composed of interconnecting and branching cords of columnar cells manifesting as single or double rows of cells.

Oncocytoma

The oncocytoma is a rare benign salivary gland neoplasm composed of large eosinophilic granular cells (oncocytes) containing atypical mitochondria.

Sebaceous Adenoma

The sebaceous adenoma is a rare benign salivary gland neoplasm that demonstrates sebaceous differentiation.

Sebaceous Lymphadenoma

Sebaceous lymphadenoma is believed by some to be a variant of sebaceous adenoma but contains sebaceous glands that are surrounded by lymphoid elements.

Myoepithelioma

Myoepitheliomas are tumors that demonstrate myoepithelial differentiation and are believed to represent a spectrum of mixed tumors but which lack chondroid and myxochondroid features.

Cystadenoma

The cystadenoma is a rare benign tumor that is characterized by unicystic or polycystic growths that contain regions of overgrowth that may at times be papillary in character.

Ductal Papillomas

Ductal papillomas have been categorized by the WHO into three morphological types. These include (a) intraductal papillomas, which are luminal papillary lesions that result in cystic dilatation of a duct; (b) inverted duct papillomas, a papillary proliferation that occurs at the junction of salivary duct and mucosal surface; and (c) sialadenoma papilliferum, an exophytic growth involving the mucosal surface and salivary ductal structures.

Sialoblastoma

Sialoblastoma is a rare neoplasm of major salivary glands. The tumors are either congenital or arise in the prenatal period. It has been suggested that these tumors be divided into benign and malignant lesions based on cytologic features and patterns of growth that include nerve and vascular invasion and necrosis (Batsakis and Frankenthaler 1992; Ellis and Auclair 1996).

Malignant Epithelial Neoplasms
Mucoepidermoid Carcinoma

There still exists some conjecture about whether mucoepidermoid carcinoma exists as only low-grade and high-grade neoplasms (Spiro et al. 1978). The presence of mucoepidermoid carcinoma is usually asymptomatic and presenting as solitary, painless masses. When present, symptoms encompass pain, drainage from the ipsilateral ear, dysphagia, trismus, and facial paralysis (Ellis and Auclair 1996). On rare occasions, mucoepidermoid carcinoma may occur within the mandible or maxilla (3:1) (Brookstone and Huvos 1992). These tumors are referred to as "central mucoepidermoid carcinomas" (Ellis and Auclair 1996).

Mucoepidermoid carcinomas may consist of various proportions of mucous, epidermoid, intermediate, columnar, and clear cells, and are often cystic in pattern. These tumors constitute the majority of malignant neoplasms found in both major and minor salivary glands (Speight and Barrett 2002). Thus, mucoepidermoid carcinoma embodies 29% to 34% of malignant salivary gland tumors residing in both major and minor salivary glands (Ellis and Auclair 1996; Eveson and Cawson 1985; Spiro et al. 1978; Spitz and Batsakis 1984). The best evidence to date indicates that 84–93% of these neoplasms initiate within the parotid glands (Goode, Auclair, and Ellis 1998; Guzzo et al. 2002). Among the minor salivary glands, mucoepidermoid carcinoma has an affinity for the lower lip (Ellis and Auclair 1996). Generally, the mean age for these carcinomas is 47 years; however, there exists a broad age range of 8 years to 92 years, and this is one of the few salivary gland malignancies occurring in childhood (Ellis and Auclair 1996). Notably, previous exposure to ionizing radiation has been suggested to significantly increase the risk of mucoepidermoid carcinomas of the major salivary glands (Ellis and Auclair 1996; Guzzo et al. 2002).

The level of microscopic grading of mucoepidermoid is of paramount importance to establish the prognosis (Auclair, Goode, and Ellis 1992; Goode, Auclair, and Ellis 1998; Speight and Barrett 2002). These tumors may be graded as low grade, intermediate grade, or high grade. The grade of a lesion is ascertained as a sum of five parameters. Sums that are 0–4 are regarded as low grade, those that are 5–6 are considered intermediate grade, and sums 7–14 are regarded as high-grade cancers. The five parameters considered are

1. Intracystic component (+2).
2. Neural invasion present (+2).
3. Necrosis present (+3).
4. Mitosis (≥ 4 per 10 high-power field (+3).
5. Anaplasia present (+4).

Importantly, retrospective reviews of mucoepidermoid carcinoma of the major salivary glands have revealed a statistical correlation between this point-based grading system and outcome for parotid tumors; however, similar rigor was not deemed useful for tumors of the submandibular glands (Goode, Auclair, and Ellis 1998) or minor salivary glands (Guzzo et al. 2002). When more emphasis on features of tumor invasion was employed, better correlations were obtained, indicating that tumor staging may be a better indicator of prognosis (Ellis and Auclair 1996). These results reinforce the need for analyses that encompass absolute effect measures (Brandwein et al. 2001).

Adenoid Cystic Carcinoma

Adenoid cystic carcinoma, in earlier times known as "cylindroma," is a slow-growing but nevertheless aggressive neoplasm with a notable capacity for recurrence (Brookstone and Huvos 1992). Three growth patterns have been acknowledged: cribriform, tubular, and a solid (basaloid) pattern. The tumors are classified according to the predominant pattern (Batsakis, Luna, and el-Naggar 1990; Brookstone and Huvos 1992; Ellis and Auclair 1996). The cribriform pattern is the most common, while the solid pattern is the least common (Perzin, Gullane, and Clairmont 1978). Solid adenoid cystic carcinoma is a high-grade lesion with reported recurrence rates of as much as 100%, compared with 50–80% for the tubular and cribriform variants (Ellis and Auclair 1996).

Reports from the AFIP indicate that adenoid cystic carcinoma is the fifth most common malignant epithelial tumor of the salivary glands after mucoepidermoid carcinomas; adenocarcinomas, NOS (not otherwise specified); acinic cell carcinomas; and polymorphous low-grade adenocarcinomas (PLGAs)(Ellis and Auclair 1996). The peak incidence for this tumor is stated to be in the fourth through sixth decades of life (Ellis and Auclair 1996).

These neoplasms characteristically progress as slow-growing lesions in the preauricular or submandibular region. Not infrequently, pain and facial paralysis are noted with progressive growth of the tumors, which may be attributed to their propensity to invade nerves (Ellis and Auclair 1996). Adenoid cystic carcinomas have a tendency to have an extended course resulting in a poor clinical result. The 10-year survival for these tumors is considered to be less than 50% (Speight and Barrett 2002). In that these carcinomas characteristically repeatedly recur and spur late distant metastases, clinical staging of these lesions appears to be a more superior prognostic indicator than histologic grade (Friedrich and Bleckmann 2003; Hamper et al. 1990; Speight and Barrett 2002.)

Adenocarcinomas
Acinic Cell Carcinoma
The acinic cell carcinoma, also referred to as "acinic cell adenocarcinoma," is a malignant epithelial neoplasm in which the tumor cells convey acinar serous differentiation as opposed to mucous acinar cells (Ellis and Auclair 1996). AFIP data has indicated that acinic cell carcinoma is the third most common salivary gland epithelial neoplasm after mucoepidermoid carcinoma and adenocarcinoma, NOS. Moreover, acinic cell carcinoma comprised 17% of primary malignant salivary gland tumors with more than 80% occurring in the parotid gland. Women are generally more affected than males, with a mean age of 44 years. However, others have reported a 0–19% frequency of acinic cell carcinoma among malignant salivary gland neoplasms (Ellis and Auclair 1996). Patients usually present with a slowly increasing mass in the parotid. Pain is a symptom in approximately 33% of patients. Again, staging appears to be a better prognostic predictor than histologic grading (Ellis and Auclair 1996).

Polymorphous Low-Grade Adenocarcinoma (PLGA)

Polymorphous low-grade adenocarcinoma is a malignant tumor that is predominately restricted to minor salivary glands. The tumors are distinguished by bland, uniform nuclear features; varied but distinctive architecture; invasive growth; and perineural infiltration (Ellis and Auclair 1996). PLGAs have been reported to represent ~11% of all tumors of salivary glands and ~26% of malignant neoplasms. PLGAs characteristically emerge as solid, nontender swellings of the mucosa of the hard and soft palates, buccal mucosa, or upper lip. Soreness, hemorrhage, telangiectasia, or ulceration have been associated with these lesions (Ellis and Auclair 1996). These tumors are slowly progressive salivary gland neoplasms with an apparent survival approaching 80% at 25 years (Evans and Luna 2000). Noteworthy is that since some of these tumors may behave capriciously, the qualifying term "low-grade" may be deceptive and the term "polymorphous adenocarcinoma" is preferable (Speight and Barrett 2002).

The average age of patients has been 59 years, with the vast majority of cases occurring between the ages of 50 and 79 years. The gender predisposition is in favor of females in a ratio of ~2:1. Among minor gland tumors, PLGA is two times as frequent as adenoid cystic carcinoma (Ellis and Auclair 1996). The AFIP series indicates that >60% of PLGAs occur in the mucosa of either the soft or hard palates, the next most frequent sites being buccal mucosa (16%) and the upper lip (12%).

Adenocarcinoma, NOS (Not Otherwise Specified)

Adenocarcinoma, NOS demonstrates glandular or ductal differentiation but does not have any of the distinct morphologic features that typify the other, more explicit carcinoma types. The diagnosis of adenocarcinoma, NOS is fundamentally one of elimination. Adenocarcinoma, NOS has been suggested to be only second to mucoepidermoid carcinoma in frequency among malignant salivary gland neoplasms (Ellis and Auclair 1996). However, reports have shown a varied incidence from 4% to 10% (Speight and Barrett 2002). The AFIP reports the mean patient age of 58 years with roughly 40% and 60% of tumors occurring in the major and minor salivary glands, correspondingly,

with 90% of tumors occurring in the parotid gland (Ellis and Auclair 1996). Adenocarcinoma, NOS is graded according to the degree of differentiation as low-grade, intermediate-grade, and high-grade tumors (Ellis and Auclair 1996; Speight and Barrett 2002). Some reports have indicated that survival is more superior for patients with tumors of the oral cavity than for those with tumors of the major glands (Ellis and Auclair 1996; Matsuba et al. 1988).

Rare Adenocarcinomas

Basal Cell Adenocarcinoma

Basal cell adenocarcinoma, also known as basaloid salivary carcinoma, carcinoma ex monomorphic adenoma, malignant basal cell adenoma, malignant basal cell tumor, and basal cell carcinoma, is an epithelial neoplasm that is cytologically similar to basal cell adenoma but is infiltrative and has a small potential for metastasis (Ellis and Auclair 1996). In AFIP case files spanning almost 11 years, basal cell carcinoma comprised 1.6% of all salivary gland neoplasms and 2.9% of salivary gland malignancies (Ellis and Auclair 1996). Nearly 90% of tumors occurred in the parotid gland (Muller and Barnes 1996). The average age of patients is reported to be 60 years (Ellis and Auclair 1996).

Similar to most salivary gland neoplasms, swelling is typically the only sign or symptom experienced (Muller and Barnes 1996). A sudden increase in size may occur in a few patients (Ellis and Auclair 1996). Basal cell carcinomas are low-grade carcinomas that are infiltrative, locally destructive, and tend to recur. They occasionally metastasize. In a retrospective series of 29 cases, there were recurrences in 7 and metastases in 3 (Muller and Barnes 1996). In another retrospective review of 72 cases, 37% involved local recurrences (Ellis and Auclair 1996). The overall prognosis for patients with this tumor is good (Ellis and Auclair 1996; Muller and Barnes 1996).

Clear Cell Carcinoma

Clear cell carcinoma, also known as clear cell adenocarcinoma, is a very rare, malignant epithelial neoplasm composed of a monomorphous population of cells that have optically clear cytoplasm with standard hematoxylin and eosin stains and that lack features of other specific neoplasms. Because of inconsistencies in the methods of reporting salivary gland neoplasms, meaningful incidence rates for this tumor are difficult to derive from the literature (Ellis and Auclair 1996). Most cases involve the minor salivary glands. In the AFIP case files, the mean age of patients is approximately 58 years (Ellis and Auclair 1996).

In most patients, swelling is the only symptom. Clear cell adenocarcinoma is a low-grade neoplasm. As of 1996, the AFIP reported that no patient is known to have died as a result of this tumor (Ellis and Auclair 1996).

Cystadenocarcinoma

Cystadenocarcinoma, also known as malignant papillary cystadenoma, mucus-producing adenopapillary, or nonepidermoid, carcinoma, low-grade papillary adenocarcinoma of the palate, and papillary adenocarcinoma, is a rare, malignant epithelial tumor characterized histologically by prominent cystic and frequently papillary growth but lacking features that characterize cystic variants of several more common salivary gland neoplasms. Cystadenocarcinoma is the malignant counterpart of cystadenoma (Ellis and Auclair 1996).

In a review of 57 cases, the AFIP found that men and women are affected equally; the average patient age was about 59 years; and about 65% occurred in the major salivary glands, and primarily in the parotid. Most patients present with a slowly growing asymptomatic mass. Clinically, this neoplasm is rarely associated with pain or facial paralysis. Cystadenocarcinoma is considered to be a low-grade neoplasm (Ellis and Auclair 1996).

Sebaceous Adenocarcinoma

Sebaceous adenocarcinoma is an uncommon malignant epithelial neoplasm that is generally regarded as an intermediate grade neoplasm. The tumors have been noted to be comprised of islands and sheets of cells with areas of sebaceous differentiation. The cells of these tumors possess atypical nuclear morphology and manifest an infiltrative pattern of growth (Ellis and Auclair 1996). Clinical presentation as a painless, slow-growing, asymptomatic swelling has been reported; however, lesions may be painful or result in facial nerve involvement with paralysis. Approximately one-third of these tumors have been reported to have a recurrence potential (Gnepp 1983). The vast majority of examples of this neoplasm have been limited to the parotid gland with the mean age of

occurrence being 69 years (Ellis and Auclair 1996; Gnepp 1983).

Sebaceous Lymphadenocarcinoma

Sebaceous lymphadenocarcinoma is a particularly uncommon malignant low-grade neoplasm with a good prognosis (Gnepp and Brannon 1984). These neoplasms are believed to correspond to carcinomatous transformation of sebaceous lymphadenoma. The carcinoma portion of the tumor has been reported as sebaceous adenocarcinoma, however, other forms of salivary gland carcinomas have been recognized (Ellis and Auclair 1996). In that merely 3 cases, all associated with the parotid gland in elderly patients, have been reported, there is little information on these neoplasms (Ellis and Auclair 1996; Gnepp and Brannon 1984).

Oncocytic Carcinoma

Oncocytic carcinoma, or oncocytic adenocarcinoma, is a rare high-grade carcinoma, salivary neoplasm with predominantly oncocytic features. The oncocytic carcinomas constitute <1% of the cases of salivary gland tumors accessioned to the AFIP files (Ellis and Auclair 1996). The majority of reported cases have been in the parotid gland, where they present as painful lesions or are associated with paralysis (Sugimoto et al. 1993). Similar to other parotid gland carcinomas, tumors that are less than 2 cm have a better prognosis than larger tumors. Thus, TNM (T = tumor size, N = number of nodes, M = metastasis) staging correlates with the prognosis (Goode, Auclair, and Ellis 1998). The AFIP series reports that the average age of patients with these neoplasms has been 63 years (Ellis and Auclair 1996).

Salivary Duct Carcinoma

Salivary duct carcinoma, or salivary duct adenocarcinoma, is a high-grade malignant epithelial neoplasm comprised of elements that bear a resemblance to expanded salivary gland ducts. The AFIP files indicate that salivary duct carcinomas represent only 0.2% of all epithelial salivary gland neoplasms, with ~85% of cases affecting the parotid gland and with a male gender predominance of 75% and mean incidence occurring in the seventh and eighth decades of life (Ellis and Auclair 1996). Parotid swelling has generally been the most common presenting symptom. However, facial nerve involvement has been noted in ~25% of patients. Although a low-grade variant of this tumor has been described, high-grade variants of this neoplasm have been regarded as one of the most aggressive types of salivary gland carcinoma. One review has revealed that one-third of patients with these neoplasms developed local recurrence and 46% developed distant metastasis (Ellis and Auclair 1996). The high-grade lesions are epitomized by local invasion, hematogenous and lymphatic metastasis, and a dismal prognosis (Delgado, Klimstra, and Albores-Saavedra 1996; Ellis and Auclair 1996; Guzzo et al. 2002).

Primary Mucinous Adenocarcinoma

Primary mucinous adenocarcinoma of salivary glands is an uncommon low-grade malignant neoplasm distinguished by significant quantities of extracellular epithelial mucin. The tumors generally are organized as cords, nests, and/or appear as solitary epithelial cells. Almost all known cases of these lesions have presented with minimal symptoms and have been limited to the major salivary glands. Interestingly, the predominant site for these tumors has been the submandibular glands (Ellis and Auclair 1996; Osaki et al. 1990). These are extremely rare lesions with no known frequency of occurrence.

Malignant Mixed Tumors

Carcinoma ex-pleomorphic adenoma, carcinosarcoma, and metastasizing mixed tumor have all been regarded as subtypes of malignant mixed tumors. The most common among these is the carcinoma ex-pleomorphic adenoma. On the other hand, the carcinosarcoma is a true malignant mixed tumor. However, the carcinosarcoma and the metastasizing mixed tumor, which is semantically an inexactness, are extremely rare (Ellis and Auclair 1996).

Carcinoma Ex-pleomorphic Adenoma

Carcinoma ex-pleomorphic adenoma, sometimes termed "carcinoma ex-mixed tumor," is a malignant epithelial neoplasm that demonstrates evidence of arising primarily from or in a benign pleomorphic adenoma in one of the major salivary glands (Roijer et al. 2002). Thus, diagnosis necessitates that the sample contains benign tumor as well as carcinomatous elements (LiVolsi and Perzin 1977). AFIP files have indicated that carcinoma ex-pleomorphic adenoma encompasses 8.8% of all mixed tumors and 4.6% of all malignant salivary gland tumors, making it the sixth most common malignant salivary gland tumor (Ellis and Auclair 1996). The most common clinical symptoms have been that of a painless mass, although one-third of patients have been noted to present with facial paralysis (Ellis and Auclair 1996). Similar to other major salivary gland tumors, tumor stage, grade, and degree of invasion determine prognosis (Brandwein et al. 2002).

Salivary Carcinosarcoma

Salivary carcinosarcoma has also been regarded and termed as a bona fide malignant mixed tumor. Consequently, these neoplasms contain elements that are both carcinoma and sarcomatous in nature. Either or both components are expressed in metastatic lesions. Although carcinosarcomas may develop on their own, others arise in association with or within benign mixed tumors. The majority of tumors occur in the major salivary glands, where they have presented clinically with swelling, pain, nerve palsy, and/or ulceration. These tumors are extremely unusual, with only a few cases being acknowledged by the AFIP (Ellis and Auclair 1996). Carcinosarcoma is an aggressive, high-grade malignancy with a survival of 3.6 years (Stephen et al. 1986).

Metastasizing Mixed Tumor

Metastasizing mixed tumor is an uncommon histological benign salivary gland neoplasm that enigmatically metastasizes. Reportedly, long intervals occur between the diagnosis of a primary "benign" tumor and the metastases. The histological attributes are essentially those that epitomize pleomorphic adenoma (Ellis and Auclair 1996). The majority of these lesions occur in the major salivary glands as a single, well-defined mass. Interestingly, metastases or recurrences may occur up to 26 years after excision of the primary neoplasm (Schneider et al. 1977).

Rare Carcinomas

Primary Squamous Cell Carcinoma

Primary squamous cell carcinoma is a rare neoplasm of salivary glands. This neoplasm occurs in the parotid gland approximately nine times more frequently than in the submandibular gland, with a partiality toward males (Ellis and Auclair 1996; Gaughan, Olsen, and Lewis 1992; Spitz and Batsakis 1984; Sterman et al. 1990). Patients generally present with an asymptomatic mass in the parotid region. However, with progression symptoms may comprise pain and/or facial nerve palsy (Shemen, Huvos, and Spiro 1987). Identification of these lesions requires segregating this primary carcinoma from metastatic disease originating from other head and neck or oral occurrences (Ellis and Auclair 1996). The diagnosis of primary disease probably cannot be made in minor salivary glands because of the size of the glands and proximity to mucosa that is vulnerable to develop squamous or epidermoid carcinoma (Ellis and Auclair 1996). Existing literature suggests that preceding exposure to ionizing radiation increases the risk for developing primary salivary squamous carcinoma; however, the sample size used in these studies was meager (Schneider et al. 1977; Shemen, Huvos, and Spiro 1987; Spitz and Batsakis 1984). The frequency of this primary salivary squamous carcinoma has ranged from 0.9% to 4.7% (Ellis and Auclair 1996). AFIP series have indicated that over a 10-year interval primary squamous cell carcinoma encompassed 2.7% of all tumors, 5.4% of malignant tumors, and 2.5% of parotid neoplasms and 2.8% of submandibular tumors, with an average age of 64 years (Ellis and Auclair 1996). Primary salivary gland squamous carcinoma is graded similar to extrasalivary squamous or epidermoid carcinomas, utilizing degree (low, intermediate, and high) of differentiation (Speight and Barrett 2002). The prognosis for these primary salivary gland cancers is dire, with an 18% 10-year survival rate (Shemen, Huvos, and Spiro 1987).

Epithelial-Myoepithelial Carcinoma

Epithelial-myoepithelial carcinoma, also designated by some as adenomyoepithelioma, clear cell adenoma, tubular solid adenoma, monomorphic clear cell tumor, glycogen-rich adenoma, glycogen-rich adenocarcinoma, clear cell carcinoma, and salivary duct carcinoma, is an uncommon, low-grade epithelial neoplasm composed of variable proportions of ductal and large, clear-staining, differentiated myoepithelial cells. These neoplasms embrace ~1% of all epithelial salivary gland tumors (Batsakis, el-Naggar, and Luna 1992; Ellis and

Auclair 1996). Epithelial-myoepithelial carcinomas are principally limited to the parotid glands. The lesions commonly present as localized painless swellings, although larger lesions may be associated with pain or compromise of the facial muscle tone (Collina et al. 1991; Daley et al. 1984). The best current data indicates that the mean age of patients with these lesions is ~60 years, with a gender bias of 60% toward females (Ellis and Auclair 1996). Although these tumors have a propensity to metastasize to parotid and cervical lymph nodes, and may on rare occasion give rise to distant metastasis and death, these tumors are generally regarded as low-grade carcinomas with a high frequency of recurrence (Batsakis, el-Naggar, and Luna 1992; Collina et al. 1991; Noel and Brozna 1992; Simpson et al. 1991).

Anaplastic Small Cell Carcinoma

Anaplastic small cell carcinoma is regarded by many as a neuroendocrine carcinoma (Gnepp and Wick 1990; Perez-Ordonez et al. 1998). These tumors often appear with the cells arranged as sheets, strands, and nests. The cells possess oval, hyperchromatic nuclei and limited cytoplasm and generally have a high mitotic index.

Undifferentiated Carcinomas

Undifferentiated carcinomas of salivary glands is a group of rare, malignant epithelial neoplasms that lack the specific light-microscopic morphologic features of other types of salivary gland carcinomas. These carcinomas are histologically similar to undifferentiated carcinomas that arise in other organs and tissues. Accordingly, metastatic carcinoma is a principal matter in the differential diagnosis of these tumors (Ellis and Auclair 1996).

Small Cell Undifferentiated Carcinoma

Small cell undifferentiated carcinomas have also been termed "extrapulmonary oat cell carcinomas." These primary malignant tumors are comprised of undifferentiated cells that do not exhibit neuroendocrine differentiation. As such these lesions have been regarded as the undifferentiated equivalent of the anaplastic small cell carcinoma. Small cell carcinoma has represented ~1.8% of all major salivary gland malignancies in the AFIP series. The tumors have a mean patient age of 56 years, with half of the cases presenting as an asymptomatic parotid mass of only a few months' duration (Ellis and Auclair 1996; Perez-Ordonez et al. 1998). These are high-grade neoplasms with an estimated survival rate at 2 and 5 years of 70% and 46%, respectively (Gnepp, Corio, and Brannon 1986).

Large Cell Undifferentiated Carcinoma

Large cell undifferentiated carcinoma is a malignant neoplasm that lacks any features of differentiation. However, in some instances poorly formed duct-like structures have been described. Rapid growth of a parotid swelling is a common clinical presentation (Gaughan, Olsen, and Lewis 1992). These tumors are high-grade lesions that commonly metastasize. Tumors that are T3 or greater have been noted to have a dire prognosis (Batsakis and Luna 1991). These neoplasms make up only ~1% of all epithelial salivary gland tumors, with the vast majority of cases occurring in the parotid glands of elderly patients (Batsakis and Luna 1991; Ellis and Auclair 1996; Hui et al. 1990).

Lymphoepithelial Carcinoma

Lymphoepithelial carcinoma, which is also known as undifferentiated carcinoma with lymphoid stroma and carcinoma ex-lymphoepithelial lesion, is an undifferentiated tumor coupled with a dense lymphoid stroma; notably these lesions have been linked with Epstein-Barr virus infection (Leung et al. 1995). Moreover, an unusually high incidence of these tumors has been identified most often in the parotid glands and to a lesser extent in the submandibular gland of Eskimo and Inuit populations (Bosch, Kudryk, and Johnson 1988; Ellis and Auclair 1996). Pain is a common presenting symptom; however, in 20% of patients facial nerve involvement has been recorded (Borg et al. 1993). Cervical lymph node metastasis has been a common finding at initial presentation, and 20% of patients develop distant metastases within a 3-year period (Borg et al. 1993; Bosch, Kudryk, and Johnson 1988).

Myoepithelial Carcinoma

Myoepithelial carcinoma is a very rare, malignant salivary gland neoplasm that almost entirely manifests myoepithelial differentiation. This tumor represents the malignant complement of benign myoepithelioma (Ellis and Auclair 1996). The majority of patients, mean age 55 years, present with a painless mass generally within the parotid gland (66%) (Ellis and Auclair 1996). The tumors are often intermediate-grade or high-grade carcinomas (Ellis and Auclair 1996; Savera et al. 2000). Interestingly, the histological grade of these neoplasms does not appear to correlate in a good way with clinical behavior, in that some tumors manifesting with a low-grade histologic pattern may behave in an aggressive manner (Savera et al. 2000).

Adenosquamous Carcinoma

Adenosquamous carcinoma is an extremely uncommon malignant neoplasm that emerges concurrently from surface mucosa and salivary gland ductal epithelium. These tumors possess histopathological characteristics of squamous cell carcinoma and of adenocarcinoma. Analysis of the few cases reported seems to indicate that this is an extremely aggressive malignancy with a dismal prognosis (Ellis and Auclair 1996).

Non-epithelial Neoplasms
Lymphomas and Benign Lymphoepithelial Lesion

Lymphomas of the major salivary glands are typically non-Hodgkin's lymphomas. AFIP reviews have indicated that non-Hodgkin's lymphoma constitutes 16.3% of all malignant tumors that arise in the major salivary glands. Moreover, non-Hodgkin's lymphoma of the parotid gland comprises 80% of all cases (Ellis and Auclair 1996).

Patients with benign lymphoepithelial lesion and with Sjogren's syndrome are considered at an increased risk for development of non-Hodgkin's lymphoma (Abbondanzo 2001; Ihrler et al. 2000). Benign lymphoepithelial lesion is clinically distinguished by bilateral enlargement of the salivary and lacrimal glands. In affected glands the lesion is composed of distinctive myoepithelial islands bounded by lymphocytes, which possess germinal centers (Ellis and Auclair 1996). Immunophenotypically and genotypically, the lymphocytic component consists of polyclonal B-lymphocytes and T-lymphocytes. The B-cell lymphocytic component has been noted to result in clonal expansion and progress to a non-Hodgkin's lymphoma. The majority of the non-Hodgkin's lymphomas arising within benign lymphoepithelial lesions are marginal zone lymphomas of mucosa-associated lymphoid tissue (MALT) (Abbondanzo 2001; Ihrler et al. 2000). MALT lymphomas of the salivary glands, similar to their complement in other sites, are clinically indolent lesions (Ellis and Auclair 1996; Harris 1991).

Notable is that primary non-MALT lymphomas of the salivary glands have been described and have a prognosis comparable to nodal lymphomas (Salhany and Pietra 1993). In contrast to non-Hodgkin's lymphoma, Hodgkin's lymphoma of the major salivary glands is most unusual. However, if present the majority of tumors arise in the parotid gland and manifest as either nodular-sclerosing or lymphocyte-predominant variants (Ellis and Auclair 1996; Gleeson, Bennett, and Cawson 1986).

Mesenchymal Neoplasms

Mesenchymal neoplasms make up 2–5% of all neoplasms that occur within the major salivary glands (Seifert and Oehne 1986). The most common varieties of benign mesenchymal salivary gland neoplasms include hemangiomas, lipomas, and lymphangiomas.

Malignant Mesenchymal Salivary Gland Tumors

Malignant mesenchymal salivary gland tumors include malignant schwannomas, hemangiopericytomas, malignant fibrous histiocytomas, rhabdomyosarcomas, and fibrosarcomas, as well as others, and account for ~1.5% of all malignant tumors of the major salivary glands (Luna et al. 1991; Seifert and Oehne 1986). Primary salivary gland sarcomas behave like soft tissue sarcomas in other locations; however, prognosis is governed by cell of origin, histological grade, tumor size, and stage (Auclair et al. 1986; Luna et al. 1991; Weiss and Goldblum 2001). The necessity of establishing a primary salivary gland origin by excluding the likelihood of metastasis and direct extension from other adjacent locations cannot be overemphasized. Furthermore, the consideration of salivary gland carcinosarcoma should be contemplated (Ellis and Auclair 1996).

Malignant Secondary Neoplasms

Malignant neoplasms from primary sites outside the salivary glands may involve the major salivary glands by: (a) direct invasion from cancers that lie adjacent to the salivary glands; (b) hematogenous metastases from distant primary tumors; and (c) lymphatic metastases to lymph nodes within the salivary gland (Ellis and Auclair 1996). It has been estimated that ~80% of metastases to the major salivary glands are from primary tumors somewhere else in the head and neck. The parotid gland is the site for most metastases, followed by the submandibular gland (Seifert et al. 1986). The majority of metastases to the major salivary glands are squamous cell carcinomas and melanomas. More rarely, carcinomas from the lung, kidney, and breast, have been recognized presumably reaching these sites by a hematogenous route (Batsakis and Bautina 1990; Seifert, Hennings, and Caselitz 1986). The peak incidence for metastatic tumors in the salivary glands is reported to be in the seventh decade of life (Ellis and Auclair 1996).

Grading and Staging of Salivary Gland Tumors

MOLECULAR SYSTEMATICS OF SALIVARY GLAND NEOPLASMS

One of the earliest attempts to use molecular systematics was to identify genes with altered expression in salivary adenoid cystic carcinoma (ACC). These studies observed expression of genes indicative of myoepithelial differentiation, including those whose protein products are components of basement membranes and extracellular matrix (Frierson et al. 2002). Other genes that were highly ranked for their expression in ACC were those encoding the transcription factors SOX4 and AP-2γ. Additional genes, which were highly expressed in ACC compared to the other carcinomas, included casein kinase 1, epsilon, and frizzled-7, which are members of the Wnt/β-catenin signaling pathway. More recent studies have indicated that the combination of copy number and gene expression profiling provides an improved strategy for gene identification in salivary gland ACCs (Kasamatsu et al. 2005).

To further relate gene expression profiles with progression and perineural invasion (PNI), laser capture microdissection (LCM) and high-throughput cDNA microarray analyses have been performed to monitor in vivo gene expression profiles of salivary ACC and to correlate the profile with PNI. These studies showed 53 genes as being two-fold or more differentially expressed in PNI cancer cell groups as compared to non-PNI cancer cell controls. Out of the 53 genes found consistently differentially expressed, 38 were up-regulated and 15 down-regulated. These findings substantiated many genes previously reported for ACC (Frierson et al. 2002; Patel et al. 2006), but also revealed several novel genes that appeared to be associated with initiation and progression of PNI, included among which were MCAM (CD146), AREG, MGEA6, CARD12, PMP22, TRAG-3, MMP-7, NTF-4, APOC1, MAGEA2, MAGEA4, MAGEA6, and MAGEA9 (Chen et al. 2007).

Initial attempts to use gene profiling to classify salivary gland neoplasms have shown differences between ACCs and other types of malignant tumors. Hierarchical clustering analysis revealed that the latter group, including salivary duct carcinoma (SDC), mucoepidermoid carcinoma (MEC), and acinic cell carcinoma (ACI), share overlapping gene expression patterns. Thirteen known genes were differentially expressed in MEC and ACI, 37 in SDC, and 59 in ACCs. Highly expressed genes included the genes for immunoglobulin J chain and chemokine HCC-1 in MEC, transcriptional factor IIF and SON DNA-binding protein in ACI, and von Hippel Lindau gene (VHL) in SDC. Underexpressed genes included the genes for the D13S824E locus in MEC, SKAP 55 protein in ACI, and KIAA0074 and prostate carcinoma tumor antigen in SDC. Interestingly, a distinctively different pattern within the ACIs was noted based on their site of origin. According to the heat map of clustering within ACI cases, 11 known genes were found to discriminate between ACI cases from major salivary gland (ACI-major) and ACI from minor salivary gland (ACI-minor). In particular, the expression of keratin 5 and keratin 13 was markedly lower in ACI-major than in ACI-minor (Maruya et al. 2004).

In a like fashion gene expression profiles have been studied in a variety of salivary gland carcinomas, including MEC, ACI, and SDC. These studies showed a total of 162 deregulated genes. However, only 5 genes were overexpressed in all carcinomas, including fibronectin 1 (FN1), tissue metalloproteinase inhibitor 1 (TIMP1), biglycan (BGN), tenascin-C (HXB), and insulin-like growth factor binding protein 5 (IGFBP5), whereas 16

Table 7.2. Grading of salivary gland tumors.

Low-grade
  Acinic cell carcinoma
  Basal cell adenocarcinoma
  Clear cell carcinoma
  Cystadenocarcinoma
  Epithelial-myoepithelial carcinoma
  Mucinous adenocarcinoma
  Polymorphous low-grade adenocarcinoma
Low-grade, intermediate-grade, and high-grade
  Adenocarcinoma, NOS
  Mucoepidermoid carcinoma*
  Squamous cell carcinoma
Intermediate-grade and high-grade
  Myoepithelial carcinoma
High-grade
  Anaplastic small cell carcinoma
  Carcinosarcoma
  Large cell undifferentiated carcinoma
  Small cell undifferentiated carcinoma
  Salivary duct carcinoma

*Some investigators consider mucoepidermoid carcinoma to be of only two grades: low-grade and high-grade (Spiro et al. 1978).

genes were underexpressed. Interestingly, diversity in gene expression between the carcinoma types was identified by hierarchical clustering. Each carcinoma entity was clustered together, but MEC, SDC, and ACI were separated from each other. Significance analysis of microarrays identified 27 genes expressed differently between the groups. In MEC, overexpressed genes included those of cell proliferation (IL-6 and SFN) and cell adhesion (SEMA3F and COL6A3), whereas many underexpressed genes were related to DNA modification (NTHL1 and RBBP4). Apoptosis-related genes CASP10 and MMP11 were overexpressed in SDC, in accordance with the typical tumor necrosis seen in this entity. An intermediate filament protein of basal epithelial cells, cytokeratin 14 (KRT14) was clearly differently expressed among the three types of carcinoma (Leivo et al. 2005).

Although molecular genomic and proteomic profiles are beginning to impact our consideration of many neoplasms, except for breast, the surgical pathologists are still guided in large part by histological grade and evidence of invasion, particularly when evaluating salivary gland tumors. Histological grading of salivary gland carcinomas along with clinical staging are the two most important considerations in determining the treatment and prognosis. Interestingly, clinical stage appears to be a more important prognostic indicator than histological grade (Ellis and Auclair 1996; Speight and Barrett 2002).

Generally, grading is used for mucoepidermoid carcinomas, adenocarcinomas, NOS, adenoid cystic carcinomas, and squamous cell carcinomas (Ellis and Auclair 1996; Speight and Barrett 2002), whereas other salivary gland carcinomas are generally collectively categorized according to histologic grade (Ellis and Auclair 1996; Goode, Auclair, and Ellis 1998; Guzzo et al. 2002; Spiro et al. 1978; Stephen et al. 1986) (Table 7.2).

Staging of Salivary Gland Tumors

Tumors of the major salivary glands are staged according to size, extraparenchymal extension, lymph node involvement (in parotid tumors, whether or not the facial nerve is involved), and presence of metastases (Fu et al. 1977; Kuhel et al. 1992; Levitt et al. 1981; Spiro, Huvos, and Strong 1975). Tumors arising in the minor salivary glands are staged according to the anatomic site of origin (e.g., oral cavity and sinuses).

The American Joint Committee on Cancer (AJCC) has designated staging by TNM classification (2002) (www.cancerstaging.net) (Table 7.3).

Table 7.3. Staging of salivary gland tumors.

TNM Definitions

Major Salivary Glands

Primary Tumor (T)
TX: Primary tumor cannot be assessed
T0: No evidence of primary tumor
T1: Tumor ≤2 cm in greatest dimension without extraparenchymal extension*
T2: Tumor >2 cm but ≤4 cm in greatest dimension without extraparenchymal extension*
T3: Tumor >4 cm and/or tumor having extraparenchymal extension*
T4a: Tumor invades skin, mandible, ear canal, and/or facial nerve
T4b: Tumor invades skull base and/or pterygoid plates and/or encases carotid artery

*Extraparenchymal extension is clinical or macroscopic evidence of invasion of soft tissues. Microscopic evidence alone does not constitute extraparenchymal extension for classification purposes.

Regional Lymph Nodes (N)
NX: Regional lymph nodes cannot be assessed
N0: No regional lymph node metastasis
N1: Metastasis in a single ipsilateral lymph node, ≤3 cm in greatest dimension
N2: Metastasis in a single ipsilateral lymph node, >3 cm but ≤6 cm in greatest dimension, or in multiple ipsilateral lymph
    nodes, ≤6 cm in greatest dimension, or in bilateral or contralateral lymph nodes, ≤6 cm in greatest dimension
N2a: Metastasis in a single ipsilateral lymph node >3 cm but ≤6 cm in greatest dimension
N2b: Metastasis in multiple ipsilateral lymph nodes, ≤6 cm in greatest dimension
N2c: Metastasis in bilateral or contralateral lymph nodes, ≤6 cm in greatest dimension
N3: Metastasis in a lymph node >6 cm in greatest dimension

Distant Metastasis (M)
MX: Distant metastasis cannot be assessed
M0: No distant metastasis
M1: Distant metastasis

Table 7.3. *Continued*

TNM Definitions

AJCC stage groupings

Stage I	T1, N0, M0
Stage II	T2, N0, M0
Stage III	T3, N0, M0
Stage III	T1, N1, M0
Stage III	T2, N1, M0
Stage III	T3, N1, M0
Stage IVA	T4a, N0, M0
Stage IVA	T4a, N1, M0
Stage IVA	T1, N2, M0
Stage IVA	T2, N2, M0
Stage IVA	T3, N2, M0
Stage IVA	T4a, N2, M0
Stage IVB	T4b, any N, M0
Stage IVB	Any T, N3, M0
Stage IVC	Any T, Any N, M1

Residual Tumor (R)
RX-Presence of residual tumor cannot be assessed
R0-No residual tumor
R1-Microscopic residual tumor
R2-Macroscopic residual tumor

Minor Salivary Glands
Lip and Oral Cavity

Primary Tumor (T)
TX: Primary tumor cannot be assessed
T0: No evidence of primary tumor
Tis: Carcinoma in situ
T1: Tumor 2 cm or less in greatest dimension
T2: Tumor more than 2 cm but ≤4 cm in greatest dimension
T3: Tumor >4 cm in greatest dimension
T4: (Lip) Tumor invades through cortical bone, inferior alveolar nerve, floor of mouth, or skin of face, i.e., chin or nose*
T4a: (Oral cavity) Tumor invades through cortical bone, into deep (extrinsic) muscle of tongue (genioglossus, palatoglossus, and styloglossus), maxillary sinus, or skin of face
T4b: Tumor involves masticator space, pterygoid plates, or skull base and/or encases internal carotid artery

*Superficial erosion alone of bone/tooth socket by gingival primary is not sufficient to classify as T4.

Regional Lymph Nodes (N)
NX: Regional lymph nodes cannot be assessed
N0: No regional lymph node metastasis
N1: Metastasis in a single ipsilateral lymph node, ≤3 cm in greatest dimension
N2: Metastasis in a single ipsilateral lymph node, >3 cm but ≤6 cm in greatest dimension, or in multiple ipsilateral lymph nodes, ≤6 cm in greatest dimension, or in bilateral or contralateral lymph nodes, ≤6 cm in greatest dimension
N2a: Metastasis in a single ipsilateral lymph node >3 cm but ≤6 cm in greatest dimension
N2b: Metastasis in multiple ipsilateral lymph nodes, ≤6 cm in greatest dimension
N2c: Metastasis in bilateral or contralateral lymph nodes, ≤6 cm in greatest dimension
N3: Metastasis in a lymph node >6 cm in greatest dimension

Table 7.3. *Continued*

TNM Definitions

Distant Metastasis (M)
MX: Distant metastasis cannot be assessed
M0: No distant metastasis
M1: Distant metastasis

AJCC Stage Groupings

Stage 0	Tis, N0, M0
Stage I	T1, N0, M0
Stage II	T2, N0, M0
Stage III	T3, N0, M0
Stage III	T1, N1, M0
Stage III	T2, N1, M0
Stage III	T3, N1, M0
Stage IVA	T4a, N0, M0
Stage IVA	T4a, N1, M0
Stage IVA	T1, N2, M0
Stage IVA	T2, N2, M0
Stage IVA	T3, N2, M0
Stage IVA	T4a, N2, M0
Stage IVB	T4b, any N, M0
Stage IVB	Any T, N3, M0
Stage IVC	Any T, Any N, M1

Histologic Grade (G)
GX-Grade cannot be assessed
G1-Well differentiated
G2-Moderately differentiated
G3-Poorly differentiated

Residual Tumor (R)
RX-Presence of residual tumor cannot be assessed
R0-No residual tumor
R1-Microscopic residual tumor
R2-Macroscopic residual tumor
Nasopharynx/Oropharynx

Primary Tumor (T)
TX: Primary tumor cannot be assessed
T0: No evidence of primary tumor
Tis: Carcinoma in situ

Nasopharynx
T1: Tumor confined to the nasopharynx
T2: Tumor extends to soft tissues
T2a: Tumor extends to oropharynx and/or nasal cavity without parapharyngeal extension
T2b: Any tumor with parapharyngeal extension
T3: Tumor involves bony structures and/or paranasal sinuses
T4: Tumor with intracranial extension and/or involvement of cranial nerves, infratemporal fossa, hypopharynx, orbit, or masticator space

Oropharynx
T1: Tumor 2 cm or less in greatest dimension
T2: Tumor more than 2 cm but ≤4 cm in greatest dimension

Table 7.3. *Continued*

TNM Definitions

T3: Tumor >4 cm in greatest dimension
T4a: Tumor invades the larynx, deep/extrinsic muscle of tongue, medial pterygoid, hard palate, or mandible
T4b: Tumor invades lateral pterygoid muscle, pterygoid plates, lateral nasopharynx, or skull base or encases carotid artery

Regional Lymph Nodes (N)
Nasopharynx
NX: Regional lymph nodes cannot be assessed
N0: No regional lymph node metastasis
N1: Unilateral metastasis in lymph node(s), 6 cm or less, above the supraclavicular fossa
N2: Bilateral metastasis in lymph node(s), 6 cm or less, above the supraclavicular fossa
N3: Metastasis in lymph node(s) 6 cm or greater and/or to supraclavicular fossa
N3a: Greater than 6 cm in dimension
N3b: Extension to the supraclavicular fossa

Oropharynx/Hypopharynx
NX: Regional lymph nodes cannot be assessed
N0: No regional lymph node metastasis
N1: Metastasis in a single ipsilateral lymph node, ≤3 cm in greatest dimension
N2: Metastasis in a single ipsilateral lymph node, >3 cm but ≤6 cm in greatest dimension, or in multiple ipsilateral lymph nodes, ≤6 cm in greatest dimension, or in bilateral or contralateral lymph nodes, ≤6 cm in greatest dimension
N2a: Metastasis in a single ipsilateral lymph node >3 cm but ≤6 cm in greatest dimension
N2b: Metastasis in multiple ipsilateral lymph nodes, ≤6 cm in greatest dimension
N2c: Metastasis in bilateral or contralateral lymph nodes, ≤6 cm in greatest dimension
N3: Metastasis in a lymph node >6 cm in greatest dimension

Distant Metastasis (M)
MX: Distant metastasis cannot be assessed
M0: No distant metastasis
M1: Distant metastasis

AJCC Stage Groupings
Nasopharynx

Stage 0	Tis, N0, M0
Stage I	T1, N0, M0
Stage IIa	T2a, N0, M0
Stage IIb	T1, N1, M0
Stage IIb	T2, N1, M0
Stage IIb	T2a, N1, M0
Stage IIb	T2b, N0, M0
Stage IIb	T2b, N1, M0
Stage III	T1, N2, M0
Stage III	T2a, N2, M0
Stage III	T2b, N2, M0
Stage III	T3, N0, M0
Stage III	T3, N1, M0
Stage III	T3, N2, M0
Stage IVA	T4, N0, M0
Stage IVA	T4, N1, M0
Stage IVA	T4, N2, M0
Stage IVB	Any T, N3, M0
Stage IVC	Any T, Any N, M1

Table 7.3. *Continued*

TNM Definitions

Oropharynx/Hypopharynx

Stage 0	Tis, N0, M0
Stage I	T1, N0, M0
Stage II	T2, N0, M0
Stage III	T3, N0, M0
Stage III	T1, N1, M0
Stage III	T2, N1, M0
Stage III	T3, N1, M0
Stage IVA	T4a, N0, M0
Stage IVA	T4a, N1, M0
Stage IVA	T1, N2, M0
Stage IVA	T2, N2, M0
Stage IVA	T3, N2, M0
Stage IVA	T4a, N2, M0
Stage IVB	T4b, Any N, M0
Stage IVB	Any T, N3, M0
Stage IVC	Any T, Any N, M1

Histologic Grade (G)
GX-Grade cannot be assessed
G1-Well differentiated
G2-Moderately differentiated
G3-Poorly differentiated

Residual Tumor (R)
RX-Presence of residual tumor cannot be assessed
R0-No residual tumor
R1-Microscopic residual tumor
R2-Macroscopic residual tumor

Nasal Cavity and Paranasal Sinuses—Maxillary Sinus

Primary Tumor (T)
TX: Primary tumor cannot be assessed
T0: No evidence of primary tumor
Tis: Carcinoma in situ
T1: Tumor confined to the maxillary sinus with no erosion or destruction of bone
T2: Tumor causing bone erosion or destruction including extension into the hard palate and/or middle nasal meatus, except extension to the posterior wall of the maxillary sinus and ptygeroid plates
T3: Invades any of the following: bone of the posterior wall of the maxillary sinus, subcutaneous tissues, floor of medial wall of orbit, ptyergoid fossa, ethmoid sinuses
T4a: Tumor invades anterior orbital contents, skin of cheek, pterygoid plates, infratemporal fossa, cribiform plate, sphenoid or frontal sinuses
T4b: Tumor invades any of the following: orbital apex, dura, brain, middle cranial fossa, cranial nerves other than maxillary division of the trigeminal nerve V_2, nasopharynx, or clivus

Nasal Cavity and Ethmoid Sinus

Primary Tumor (T)
TX: Primary tumor cannot be assessed
T0: No evidence of primary tumor
Tis: Carcinoma in situ
T1: Tumor restricted to any one subsite, with or without bony invasion

Table 7.3. *Continued*

TNM Definitions

T2: Tumor invading two subsites in a single region or extending to involve an adjacent region within the nasoethmoidal complex, with or without bony invasion

T3: Extends to invade the medial wall or floor of the orbit, maxillary sinus, palate, or cribiform plate

T4a: Tumor invades any of the following: anterior orbital contents, skin of nose, or cheek, minimal extension to anterior cranial fossa, ptygeroid plates, sphenoid or frontal sinuses

T4b: Tumor invades any of the following: orbital apex, dura, brain, middle cranial fossa, cranial nerves other than V_2, nasopharynx, or clivus

Regional Lymph Nodes (N)

NX: Regional lymph nodes cannot be assessed

N0: No regional lymph node metastasis

N1: Metastasis in a single ipsilateral lymph node, ≤3 cm in greatest dimension

N2: Metastasis in a single ipsilateral lymph node, >3 cm but ≤6 cm in greatest dimension, or in multiple ipsilateral lymph nodes, ≤6 cm in greatest dimension, or in bilateral or contralateral lymph nodes, ≤6 cm in greatest dimension

N2a: Metastasis in a single ipsilateral lymph node >3 cm but ≤6 cm in greatest dimension

N2b: Metastasis in multiple ipsilateral lymph nodes, ≤6 cm in greatest dimension

N2c: Metastasis in bilateral or contralateral lymph nodes, ≤6 cm in greatest dimension

N3: Metastasis in a lymph node >6 cm in greatest dimension

Distant Metastasis (M)

MX: Distant metastasis cannot be assessed

M0: No distant metastasis

M1: Distant metastasis

AJCC Stage Groupings

Stage 0	Tis, N0, M0
Stage I	T1, N0, M0
Stage II	T2, N0, M0
Stage III	T3, N0, M0
Stage III	T1, N1, M0
Stage III	T2, N1, M0
Stage III	T3, N1, M0
Stage IVA	T4a, N0, M0
Stage IVA	T4a, N1, M0
Stage IVA	T1, N2, M0
Stage IVA	T2, N2, M0
Stage IVA	T3, N2, M0
Stage IVA	T4a, N2, M0
Stage IVB	Any T, N3, M0
Stage IVB	T4b, Any N, M0
Stage IVC	Any T, Any N, M1

Histologic Grade (G)

GX-Grade cannot be assessed

G1-Well differentiated

G2-Moderately differentiated

G3-Poorly differentiated

Residual Tumor (R)

RX-Presence of residual tumor cannot be assessed

R0-No residual tumor

R1-Microscopic residual tumor

R2-Macroscopic residual tumor

Summary

- The classification of salivary gland tumors takes into account their cellular derivation from epithelial, mesenchymal, or lymphoid origins.
- The rarity of some of these tumors, some of which display a wide spectrum of morphological patterns within the same tumor, as well as the existence of hybrid tumors, results in a difficult task of differentiating benign from malignant tumors.
- For the most part, salivary gland tumors exist as benign or malignant neoplasms, with anticipated biologic behavior.
- The pleomorphic adenoma distinguishes itself as a benign tumor that may take on malignant characteristics and behavior.
- Some low-grade salivary gland malignancies represent highly curable neoplasms.
- Gene expression profiles may be used to predict biologic behavior of salivary gland malignancies. This notwithstanding, histologic grading and clinical staging remain the two most important considerations in determining the treatment of these neoplasms and their prognosis.
- Major salivary gland staging occurs according to size, extraparenchymal extension, lymph node involvement, the presence of metastases, and whether the facial nerve is involved, as may occur in parotid tumors.

References

Abbondanzo SL. 2001. Extranodal marginal-zone B-cell lymphoma of the salivary gland. *Ann Diagn Pathol* 5(4):246–254.

Allison DB, Cui X, Page GP, Sabripour M. 2006. Microarray data analysis: From disarray to consolidation and consensus. *Nat Rev Genet* 7(1):55–65.

American Joint Committee on Cancer. 2002. Major salivary glands (parotid, submandibular, and sublingual). In: AJCC Cancer Staging Manual (6th ed.). New York: Springer, pp. 53–58.

Auclair PL, Ellis GL, Gnepp DR (eds.). 1991. Surgical Pathology of Salivary Glands (1st ed.). Philadelphia: W.B. Saunders, p. 129.

Auclair PL, Goode RK, Ellis GL. 1992. Mucoepidermoid carcinoma of intraoral salivary glands: Evaluation and application of grading criteria in 143 cases. *Cancer* 69(8):2021–2030.

Auclair PL, Langloss JM, Weiss SW, Corio RL. 1986. Sarcomas and sarcomatoid neoplasms of the major salivary gland regions: A clinicopathologic and immunohistochemical study of 67 cases and review of the literature. *Cancer* 58(6):1305–1315.

Batsakis JG. 1979. Tumors of the Head and Neck: Clinical and Pathological Considerations. Baltimore: Williams & Wilkins, p. 9.

Batsakis JG, Bautina E. 1990. Metastases to major salivary glands. *Ann Otol Rhinol Laryngol* 99(6 Pt 1):501–503.

Batsakis JG, el-Naggar AK, Luna MA. 1992. Epithelial-myoepithelial carcinoma of salivary glands. *Ann Otol Rhinol Laryngol* 101(6):540–542.

Batsakis JG, Frankenthaler R. 1992. Embryoma (sialoblastoma) of salivary glands. *Ann Otol Rhinol Laryngol* 101(11):958–960.

Batsakis JG, Luna MA. 1991. Undifferentiated carcinomas of salivary glands. *Ann Otol Rhinol Laryngol* 100(1):82–84.

Batsakis JG, Luna MA, el-Naggar A. 1990. Histopathologic grading of salivary gland neoplasms: III. Adenoid cystic carcinomas. *Ann Otol Rhinol Laryngol* 99(12):1007–1009.

Borg MF, Benjamin CS, Morton RP, Llewellyn HR. 1993. Malignant lympho-epithelial lesion of the salivary gland: A case report and review of the literature. *Australas Radiol* 37(3):288–291.

Bosch JD, Kudryk WH, Johnson GH. 1988. The malignant lymphoepithelial lesion of the salivary glands. *J Otolaryngol* 17(4):187–190.

Brandwein MS, Ferlito A, Bradley PJ, Hille JJ, Rinaldo A. 2002. Diagnosis and classification of salivary neoplasms: Pathologic challenges and relevance to clinical outcomes. *Acta Otolaryngol* 122(7):758–764.

Brandwein MS, Ivanov K, Wallace DI, Hille JJ, Wang B, Fahmy A, Bodian C, Urken ML, Gnepp DR, Huvos A et al. 2001. Mucoepidermoid carcinoma: A clinicopathologic study of 80 patients with special reference to histological grading. *Am J Surg Pathol* 25(7):835–845.

Brookstone MS, Huvos AG. 1992. Central salivary gland tumors of the maxilla and mandible: A clinicopathologic study of 11 cases with an analysis of the literature. *J Oral Maxillofac Surg* 50(3):229–236.

Buyse M, Loi S, van't Veer L, Viale G, Delorenzi M, Glas AM, d'Assignies MS, Bergh J, Lidereau R, Ellis P et al. 2006. Validation and clinical utility of a 70-gene prognostic signature for women with node-negative breast cancer. *J Natl Cancer Inst* 98(17):1183–1192.

Chen W, Zhang HL, Shao XJ, Jiang YG, Zhao XG, Gao X, Li JH, Yang J, Zhang YF, Liu BL et al. 2007. Gene expression profile of salivary adenoid cystic carcinoma associated with perineural invasion. *Tohoku J Exp Med* 212(3):319–334.

Collina G, Gale N, Visona A, Betts CM, Cenacchi V, Eusebi V. 1991. Epithelial-myoepithelial carcinoma of the parotid gland: A clinico-pathologic and immunohistochemical study of seven cases. *Tumori* 77(3):257–263.

Daley TD, Wysocki GP, Smout MS, Slinger RP. 1984. Epithelial-myoepithelial carcinoma of salivary glands. *Oral Surg Oral Med Oral Pathol* 57(5):512–519.

Delgado R, Klimstra D, Albores-Saavedra J. 1996. Low grade salivary duct carcinoma: A distinctive variant with a low-grade histology and a predominant intraductal growth pattern. *Cancer* 78(5):958–967.

Ellis GL, Auclair PL. 1996. Tumors of the Salivary Glands (3rd ed.). Washington, DC: Armed Forces Institute of Pathology.

Evans HL, Luna MA. 2000. Polymorphous low-grade adenocarcinoma: A study of 40 cases with long-term follow up and an evaluation of the importance of papillary areas. *Am J Surg Pathol* 24(10):1319–1328.

Evans RW, Cruickshank AH. 1970. Epithelial Tumors of Salivary Glands. Philadelphia: W.B. Saunders, p. 19.

Eveson JW, Cawson RA. 1985. Salivary gland tumours: A review of 2410 cases with particular reference to histological types, site, age and sex distribution. *J Pathol* 146(1):51–58.

Foote FW Jr, Frazell EL. 1954. Tumors of Major Salivary Glands. Washington, DC: Armed Forces Institute of Pathology, p. 8.

Friedrich RE, Bleckmann V. 2003. Adenoid cystic carcinoma of salivary and lacrimal gland origin: Localization, classification, clinical pathological correlation, treatment results and long-term follow-up control in 84 patients. *Anticancer Res* 23(2A):931–940.

Frierson HF, Jr., El-Naggar AK, Welsh JB, Sapinoso LM, Su AI, Cheng J, Saku T, Moskaluk CA, Hampton GM. 2002. Large scale molecular analysis identifies genes with altered expression in salivary adenoid cystic carcinoma. *Am J Pathol* 161(4):1315–1323.

Fu KK, Leibel SA, Levine ML, Friedlander LM, Boles R, Phillips TL. 1977. Carcinoma of the major and minor salivary glands: Analysis of treatment results and sites and causes of failures. *Cancer* 40(6):2882–2890.

Gaughan RK, Olsen KD, Lewis JE. 1992. Primary squamous cell carcinoma of the parotid gland. *Arch Otolaryngol Head Neck Surg* 118(8):798–801.

Gleeson MJ, Bennett MH, Cawson RA. 1986. Lymphomas of salivary glands. *Cancer* 58(3):699–704.

Gnepp DR. 1983. Sebaceous neoplasms of salivary gland origin: A review. *Pathol Annu* 18 Pt 1:71–102.

Gnepp DR, Brannon R. 1984. Sebaceous neoplasms of salivary gland origin: Report of 21 cases. *Cancer* 53(10):2155–2170.

Gnepp DR, Corio RL, Brannon RB. 1986. Small cell carcinoma of the major salivary glands. *Cancer* 58(3):705–714.

Gnepp DR, Wick MR. 1990. Small cell carcinoma of the major salivary glands: An immunohistochemical study. *Cancer* 66(1):185–192.

Goode RK, Auclair PL, Ellis GL. 1998. Mucoepidermoid carcinoma of the major salivary glands: Clinical and histopathologic analysis of 234 cases with evaluation of grading criteria. *Cancer* 82(7):1217–1224.

Guzzo M, Andreola S, Sirizzotti G, Cantu G. 2002. Mucoepidermoid carcinoma of the salivary glands: Clinicopathologic review of 108 patients treated at the National Cancer Institute of Milan. *Ann Surg Oncol* 9(7):688–695.

Hamper K, Lazar F, Dietel M, Caselitz J, Berger J, Arps H, Falkmer U, Auer G, Seifert G. 1990. Prognostic factors for adenoid cystic carcinoma of the head and neck: A retrospective evaluation of 96 cases. *J Oral Pathol Med* 19(3):101–107.

Harris NL. 1991. Extranodal lymphoid infiltrates and mucosa-associated lymphoid tissue (MALT): A unifying concept. *Am J Surg Pathol* 15(9):879–884.

Hui KK, Luna MA, Batsakis JG, Ordonez NG, Weber R. 1990. Undifferentiated carcinomas of the major salivary glands. *Oral Surg Oral Med Oral Pathol* 69(1):76–83.

Ihrler S, Baretton GB, Menauer F, Blasenbreu-Vogt S, Lohrs U. 2000. Sjogren's syndrome and MALT lymphomas of salivary glands: A DNA-cytometric and interphase-cytogenetic study. *Mod Pathol* 13(1):4–12.

Ioannidis JP. 2007. Is molecular profiling ready for use in clinical decision making? *Oncologist* 12(3):301–311.

Kasamatsu A, Endo Y, Uzawa K, Nakashima D, Koike H, Hashitani S, Numata T, Urade M, Tanzawa H. 2005. Identification of candidate genes associated with salivary adenoid cystic carcinomas using combined comparative genomic hybridization and oligonucleotide microarray analyses. *Int J Biochem Cell Biol* 37(9):1869–1880.

Kuhel W, Goepfert H, Luna M, Wendt C, Wolf P. 1992. Adenoid cystic carcinoma of the palate. *Arch Otolaryngol Head Neck Surg* 118(3):243–247.

Leivo I, Jee KJ, Heikinheimo K, Laine M, Ollila J, Nagy B, Knuutila S. 2005. Characterization of gene expression in major types of salivary gland carcinomas with epithelial differentiation. *Cancer Genet Cytogenet* 156(2):104–113.

Leung SY, Chung LP, Yuen ST, Ho CM, Wong MP, Chan SY. 1995. Lymphoepithelial carcinoma of the salivary gland: In situ detection of Epstein-Barr virus. *J Clin Pathol* 48(11):1022–1027.

Levitt SH, McHugh RB, Gomez-Marin O, Hyams VJ, Soule EH, Strong EW, Sellers AH, Woods JE, Guillamondegui OM. 1981. Clinical staging system for cancer of the salivary gland: A retrospective study. *Cancer* 47(11):2712–2724.

LiVolsi VA, Perzin KH. 1977. Malignant mixed tumors arising in salivary glands. I. Carcinomas arising in benign mixed tumors: A clinicopathologic study. *Cancer* 39(5):2209–2230.

Luna MA, Tortoledo ME, Ordonez NG, Frankenthaler RA, Batsakis JG. 1991. Primary sarcomas of the major salivary glands. *Arch Otolaryngol Head Neck Surg* 117(3):302–306.

Maruya S, Kim HW, Weber RS, Lee JJ, Kies M, Luna MA, Batsakis JG, El-Naggar AK. 2004. Gene expression screening of salivary gland neoplasms: Molecular markers of potential histogenetic and clinical significance. *J Mol Diagn* 6(3):180–190.

Matsuba HM, Mauney M, Simpson JR, Thawley SE, Pikul FJ. 1988. Adenocarcinomas of major and minor salivary gland origin: A histopathologic review of treatment failure patterns. *Laryngoscope* 98(7):784–788.

Muller S, Barnes L. 1996. Basal cell adenocarcinoma of the salivary glands. Report of seven cases and review of the literature. *Cancer* 78(12):2471–2477.

Noel S, Brozna JP. 1992. Epithelial-myoepithelial carcinoma of salivary gland with metastasis to lung: Report of a case and review of the literature. *Head Neck* 14(5):401–406.

Osaki T, Hirota J, Ohno A, Tatemoto Y. 1990. Mucinous adenocarcinoma of the submandibular gland. *Cancer* 66(8):1796–1801.

Patel KJ, Pambuccian SE, Ondrey FG, Adams GL, Gaffney PM. 2006. Genes associated with early development, apoptosis and cell cycle regulation define a gene expression profile of adenoid cystic carcinoma. *Oral Oncol* 42(10):994–1004.

Perez-Ordonez B, Caruana SM, Huvos AG, Shah JP. 1998. Small cell neuroendocrine carcinoma of the nasal cavity and paranasal sinuses. *Hum Pathol* 29(8):826–832.

Perzin KH, Gullane P, Clairmont AC. 1978. Adenoid cystic carcinomas arising in salivary glands: A correlation of histologic features and clinical course. *Cancer* 42(1):265–282.

Roijer E, Nordkvist A, Strom AK, Ryd W, Behrendt M, Bullerdiek J, Mark J, Stenman G. 2002. Translocation, deletion/amplification, and expression of HMGIC and MDM2 in a carcinoma ex pleomorphic adenoma. *Am J Pathol* 160(2):433–440.

Salhany KE, Pietra GG. 1993. Extranodal lymphoid disorders. *Am J Clin Pathol* 99(4):472–485.

Savera AT, Sloman A, Huvos AG, Klimstra DS. 2000. Myoepithelial carcinoma of the salivary glands: A clinicopathologic study of 25 patients. *Am J Surg Pathol* 24(6):761–774.

Schneider AB, Favus MJ, Stachura ME, Arnold MJ, Frohman LA. 1977. Salivary gland neoplasms as a late consequence of head and neck irradiation. *Ann Intern Med* 87(2):160–164.

Seifert G, Donath K. 1996. Hybrid tumours of salivary glands: Definition and classification of five rare cases. *Eur J Cancer B Oral Oncol* 32B(4):251–259.

Seifert G, Hennings K, Caselitz J. 1986. Metastatic tumors to the parotid and submandibular glands—analysis and differential diagnosis of 108 cases. *Pathol Res Pract* 181(6):684–692.

Seifert G, Miehlke A, Haubrich J, Chilla R. 1986. Diseases of the Salivary Glands: Pathology-Diagnosis-Treatment-Facial Nerve Surgery. Stuttgart, Gev.: George Thieme Verlag.

Seifert G, Oehne H. 1986. Mesenchymal (non-epithelial) salivary gland tumors: Analysis of 167 tumor cases of the salivary gland register. *Laryngol Rhinol Otol* (Stuttg) 65(9):485–491.

Shemen LJ, Huvos AG, Spiro RH. 1987. Squamous cell carcinoma of salivary gland origin. *Head Neck Surg* 9(4):235–240.

Simpson RH, Clarke TJ, Sarsfield PT, Gluckman PG. 1991. Epithelial-myoepithelial carcinoma of salivary glands. *J Clin Pathol* 44(5):419–423.

Speight PM, Barrett AW. 2002. Salivary gland tumours. *Oral Dis* 8(5):229–240.

Spiro RH, Huvos AG, Berk R, Strong EW. 1978. Mucoepidermoid carcinoma of salivary gland origin: A clinicopathologic study of 367 cases. *Am J Surg* 136(4):461–468.

Spiro RH, Huvos AG, Strong EW. 1975. Cancer of the parotid gland: A clinicopathologic study of 288 primary cases. *Am J Surg* 130(4):452–459.

Spitz MR, Batsakis JG. 1984. Major salivary gland carcinoma: Descriptive epidemiology and survival of 498 patients. *Arch Otolaryngol* 110(1):45–49.

Stephen J, Batsakis JG, Luna MA, von der Heyden U, Byers RM. 1986. True malignant mixed tumors (carcinosarcoma) of salivary glands. *Oral Surg Oral Med Oral Pathol* 61(6):597–602.

Sterman BM, Kraus DH, Sebek BA, Tucker HM. 1990. Primary squamous cell carcinoma of the parotid gland. *Laryngoscope* 100(2 Pt 1):146–148.

Sugimoto T, Wakizono S, Uemura T, Tsuneyoshi M, Enjoji M. 1993. Malignant oncocytoma of the parotid gland: A case report with an immunohistochemical and ultrastructural study. *J Laryngol Otol* 107(1):69–74.

Thackray AC, Sobin LH. 1972. Histological Typing of Salivary Gland Tumors. Geneva: World Health Organization.

Thackray AC, Lucas RB. 1974. Tumors of Major Salivary Glands (2nd series ed.). Washington, DC: Armed Forces Institute of Pathology.

Weiss SW, Goldblum JR. 2001. Weiss's Soft Tissue Tumors (4th ed.). St. Louis: Mosby.

Chapter 8
Tumors of the Parotid Gland

Outline

Introduction

This chapter will discuss the diagnosis and management of parotid tumors arising from epithelial cells, that is, salivary derived parotid tumors. Non-epithelial tumors will be discussed in chapter 11. Although the commonest tumor is the benign pleomorphic adenoma, there is currently much controversy in the literature over the surgical management of this tumor regarding the place of extracapsular dissection vs. the traditional parotidectomy, which will be discussed at length. Changing approaches to neck dissection and adjuvant radiotherapy in malignant parotid tumors will also be highlighted.

Etiology and Epidemiology

The etiology of salivary gland tumors is largely unknown. There is an increase in salivary tumors from exposure to radiation documented from Hiroshima and Nagasaki (Saku, Hayashi, Takahara et al. 1997). An increase in poorly differentiated carcinoma of the parotid, which may be associated with Epstein-Barr virus, is reported in Inuit people.

It is thought that Warthin's tumors arise from salivary duct remnants enclaved in lymph nodes during embryologic development and that irritation from tobacco smoke may cause these ducts to proliferate (Lamelas, Terry, and Alfonso 1987). At the present time data does not show any connection between cell phone use and increased risk of parotid tumors (Lonn, Alholm, and Christensen et al. 2006). There is a reported increase in other solid tumors, particularly breast cancer, in conjunction with salivary malignancies (In der Maur, Klokman, and van Leeuwen et al. 2005).

Salivary gland tumors are rare: 1.5–2 per 100,000 in the United States, and they comprise approximately 3% of head and neck malignancies. Eighty percent of all salivary tumors are located in the parotid gland and of these tumors approximately 80% will be benign. The "rule of 80s" also states that 80% of parotid tumors are located in the superficial lobe and that 80% of these will be pleomorphic adenomas (PAs). This chapter will discuss the epithelial derived salivary tumors of the parotid.

Diagnosis

The diagnosis of a tumor of the parotid gland will be dependent upon the history, clinical examination, imaging, and fine needle aspiration biopsy (FNAB). In most cases the history will be of a painless slow-growing lump that the patient had been aware of for some months or even years, and that was noticed initially when shaving, washing, or applying makeup. Occasionally the patient will report a rapidly growing mass, but this is not always a malignancy, as a long-standing retromandibular tumor that can no longer be accommodated in this space may have "popped out" and become prominent. Pain in a parotid mass is usually an ominous sign and can be an indication of adenoid cystic carcinoma. A history of facial nerve weakness, numbness of the ear or facial skin, or enlarged nodes in the neck are signs of malignancy.

Clinical examination will begin with the cervical nodes and palpation of the parotid. The facial nerve and muscles of facial expression are tested and intraoral examination of the soft palate and lateral pharynx is done to exclude deep lobe tumors extending into the parapharyngeal space. Most parotid tumors will present as smooth, sometimes lobulated, firm or hard nontender masses in the superficial lobe. Most are discrete and mobile. Fixation to the skin, ulceration, or deep muscle fixation are signs of malignancy. Facial nerve palsy and associated hard lymph nodes are also signs of parotid cancer. However, only 2.6–22% of parotid cancers will have VII nerve palsy (Ord 1995). Overall, 30% of malignancies are diagnosed on clinical features with palpable cervical nodes, facial nerve palsy, deep fixation, and rapid enlargement being significant signs (Wong 2001). The majority of cancers present clinically as benign tumors.

The differential diagnosis of a parotid tumor includes lesions arising outside the parotid as well as intra-parotid masses. Skin lesions such as sebaceous or dermoid cysts are usually distinguished by their superficial origin in the overlying skin. Neoplasms of the masseter and masseteric hypertrophy will become fixed and more prominent on clenching the jaws. Condylar masses usually move with jaw opening and jaw lesions are usually bony hard to palpation. Intra-parotid masses that mimic parotid tumors include enlarged parotid nodes, and, as these may be metastatic, clinical examination of the parotid mass should always include the ear and the scalp for skin cancers. Parotid cysts may be difficult to distinguish from common parotid tumors such as PAs and low-grade mucoepidermoid carcinoma, which can present as fluctuant cysts. Tumors arising in the parotid tail may be mistaken for submandibular or neck masses (Figure 8.1), while those arising in the accessory gland may be thought to arise in the cheek itself (Figure 8.2).

In imaging the parotid, technetium scans may confirm a diagnosis of Warthin's tumor or oncocytoma but are largely of historical interest. The same is true for sialography, which is no longer used for tumors. Ultrasound can distinguish cystic from solid masses and may be helpful to guide

FNAB; however, CT scanning or MR are the imaging modalities of choice if the clinician feels the information gained is worth the financial cost. Little is added to the diagnosis when imaging tumors in the superficial lobes; however, imaging deep lobe tumors, particularly those with parapharyngeal extension, gives the surgeon useful information. Recent papers have claimed that high-resolution MR using a surface coil may allow imaging of the facial nerve and its relationship to the tumor (Takahashi et al. 2005). Other methods of predicting facial nerve position include use of anatomic lines drawn on the images, such as the facial nerve line, which connects the lateral surface of the posterior belly of the digastric muscle with the lateral surface of the cortical bone of the ascending ramus of the mandible, and which has been assessed as 88% accurate in determining the location of the tumor in relation to the nerve (Ariyoshi and Shimahara 1998). Another proposed guideline is the Utrecht line connecting the most

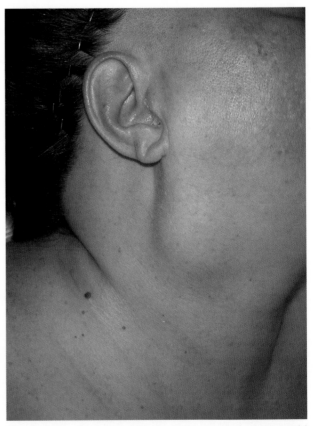

Figure 8.1a. A woman with Warthin's tumor in the parotid tail presenting as a neck mass.

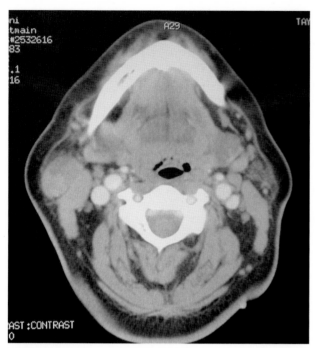

Figure 8.1b. CT scan confirms the mass is in the parotid tail.

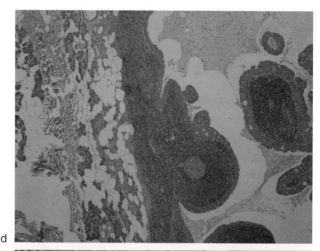

d

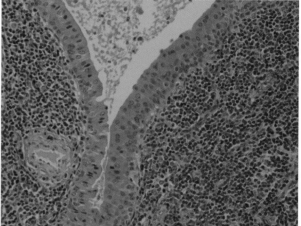

e

Figures 8.1d and 8.1e. Low- and high-power microscopic views of specimen, which was a Warthin's tumor.

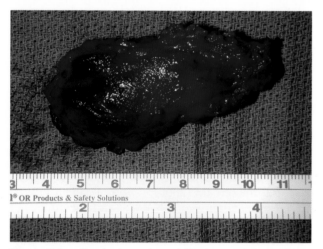

Figure 8.1c. Surgical specimen following partial parotidectomy of parotid tail with tumor.

dorsal point visible of C1 or C2 vertebra to the retromandibular vein (RMV) (de Ru, Van Bentham, and Hordijk 2002). Magnetic resonance imaging may be helpful in distinguishing benign PAs from malignant tumors, by post-contrast enhancement, a higher T2 signal, and lack of invasion (Figure 8.2). However, Fee and Tran (2003) suggest that neither MR nor ultrasound is accurate enough to

be routinely used in the workup of parotid masses and that careful history and examination are sufficient for most cases. This conclusion was echoed by de Ru, Maartens, and Van Bentham et al. (2007), who concluded that MRI and palpation are almost equally accurate for assessing tumor location and both are superior to ultrasound. They recommend the use of FNAB as an accurate method of assessing whether a tumor is malignant, and MR only for tumors in the deep lobe or malignant tumors. PET scan and fused PET/CT have so far not been shown to reliably differentiate between benign and malignant parotid tumors (Rubello, Nanni, and Castellucci et al. 2005).

FNAB may be utilized to give a preoperative cytologic diagnosis. Open biopsy is contraindicated, as it will cause spillage and seeding of

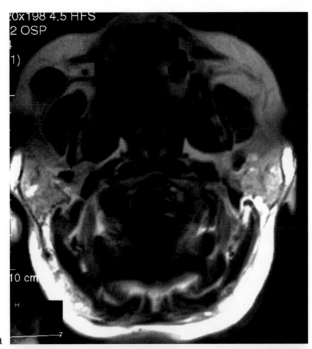

a

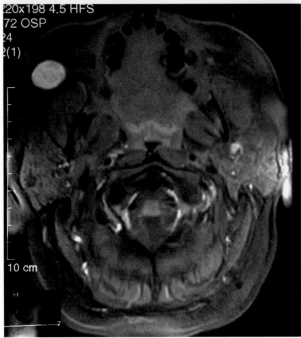

b

Figures 8.2a and 8.2b. MR T1 and T2 weighted images of a cystic pleomorphic adenoma deep in the cheek is a diagnostic challenge as to whether this is a minor salivary gland tumor or an accessory parotid tumor.

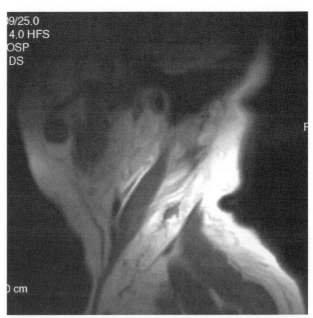

Figure 8.2c. Clinically this lesion appears to be inferior to the parotid duct, as seen in the sagittal view, which would make an accessory lobe tumor unlikely.

benign PAs and lead to increased recurrence (Figure 8.3). Although FNAB will not usually change the proposed treatment plan of parotidectomy, a malignant diagnosis may allow better presurgical counseling for possible facial nerve sacrifice. In addition, when extracapsular dissection or limited superficial parotidectomy is contemplated (see below), it is best to have confirmation of the benign nature of the tumor (O'Brien 2003). There is still controversy whether FNAB is mandatory as part of the diagnostic workup for a presumed parotid tumor. Although Schroder, Eckel, and Rasche et al. (2000) report a sensitivity of 93.1%, specificity of 99.2%, and accuracy of 98.2%, other papers have shown lower figures, sensitivity 81.5% and specificity 97.5% (Longuet et al. 2001).

Zbaren, Schar, and Hotz et al. (2001) recommended FNAB as a valuable adjunct to preoperative diagnosis, reporting 86% accuracy, 64% sensitivity, and 95% specificity. However, in a study of 6,249 participant responses from the database of the College of American Pathologists Interlaboratory Comparison Program in Nongynecologic Cytology, the sensitivity and specificity for interpreting salivary tumors as benign or malignant was 73% and 91%. Benign cases with the commonest false positive rates were monomorphic

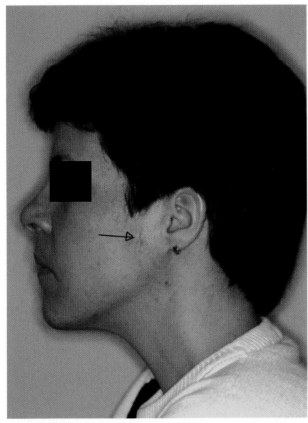

Figure 8.3a. A 45-year-old woman with parotid pleomorphic adenoma biopsied through the cheek. The arrow points to the biopsy scar.

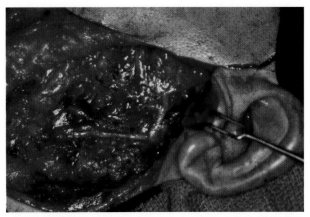

Figure 8.3c. Superficial parotidectomy with complete nerve dissection.

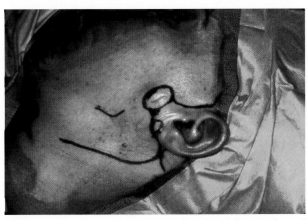

Figure 8.3b. The surgical incision is delineated and includes a 1 cm skin paddle surrounding the biopsy scar.

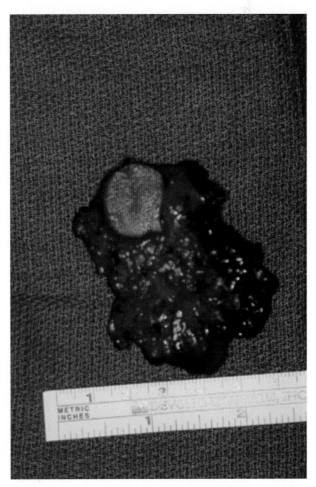

Figure 8.3d. Surgical specimen of parotid with overlying skin.

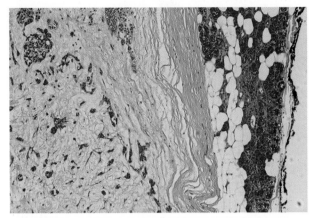

Figure 8.3e. Histopathology confirms diagnosis of pleomorphic adenoma. Note marked pseudocapsule of collagenous tissue. The patient is disease free 10+ years post-surgery.

adenoma (53%) and intra-parotid lymph node (36%). Malignant salivary gland tumors with the highest false negative rate were acinic cell carcinoma (49%), low-grade mucoepidermoid carcinoma (43%), and adenoid cystic carcinoma (33%). It was felt the data confirmed the difficulty inherent in FNAB of salivary glands (Hughes, Volk, and Wilbur 2005). A paper from the Memorial Sloan Kettering Cancer Center concluded that an FNAB result positive for a malignant neoplastic process is generally predictive of the final histologic diagnosis, whereas the predictive value of a negative FNAB is low (Cohen, Patel, and Lin et al. 2004).

Surgical Management

The basic surgical procedure is the superficial parotidectomy in which the superficial lobe of the parotid is removed, preserving the facial nerve unless it is directly infiltrated by the tumor. The author's usual incision is the modified Blair or "lazy S." The skin flap is elevated in a plane through the subcutaneous fat superficial to the parotid capsule (Figure 8.4). Recently the use of a face lift incision has been advocated to improve esthetic results of the scar (Honig 2005; Meningaud, Bertolus, and Bertrand 2006). These authors have also combined face lift incisions with a separate SMAS (superficial musculoaponeurotic system) dissection to eliminate hollowing and reduce Frey's syndrome. Concerns regarding access to anteriorly sited tumors when using a face lift approach for

parotidectomy do not appear to be borne out in anatomic studies (Nouraei, Al-Yaghchi, and Ahmed et al. 2006) (Figures 8.5 and 8.6).

Once the skin flap is elevated, the sternocleidomastoid muscle (SCM) is identified with the overlying greater auricular nerve, whose branch to the earlobe may be preserved if it does not compromise tumor resection (Figure 8.4e). The anterior border of the SCM is dissected free of the posterior parotid gland, which is retracted anteriorly. Deeper dissection at the superior end of the SCM will allow identification of the posterior belly of the digastric muscle. The facial nerve trunk lies 4 mm superior to the digastric and at the same depth and is an important landmark. Next, attention is turned to the preauricular region with sharp and blunt dissection down the cartilage of the external auditory meatus to the bony portion of the meatus. A strip of parotid tissue remains, which separates the cervical from the preauricular dissection, and this tissue is carefully dissected away to the depth of the digastric muscle. Some troublesome bleeding has to be controlled with bipolar diathermy under direct vision superficial to where the facial nerve will be identified. The facial nerve trunk can be confirmed with a nerve stimulator and the nerve branches are dissected out peripherally to mobilize and remove the superficial parotid. It is usually best to dissect either the frontal or mandibular branches first, depending on the site of the tumor, and then proceed stepwise inferiorly or superiorly dissecting the branches in order and staying superficial to the nerves.

If the tumor directly overlies the facial nerve trunk, making it impossible to access safely, then the peripheral branches can be identified and followed backward as a retrograde parotidectomy, although this is more tedious. The mandibular branch of the facial nerve, where it crosses the anterior facial vein or the buccal branch with its close relationship to the parotid duct (Pogrel, Schmidt, and Ammar 1996), can be found initially. Despite a 66% incidence of weakness 1 week post-parotidectomy, normal facial nerve function was present in 99% of 136 retrograde parotidectomies in one series (O'Regan et al. 2007).

In tumors of the deep lobe it is usually necessary to undertake a total parotidectomy. The superficial parotidectomy is performed, preserving the facial nerve and dissecting the superficial lobe from superiorly so that it remains attached to the deep lobe inferiorly and at the tail. Most deep lobe

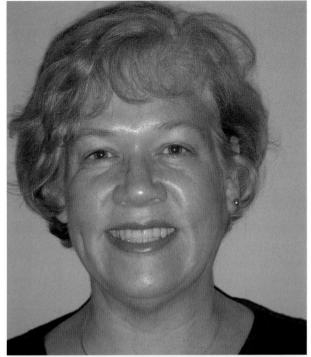

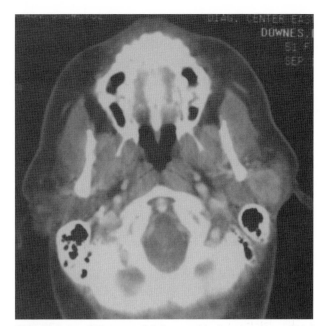

Figure 8.4c. CT scan of left parotid showing superficial lobe tumor.

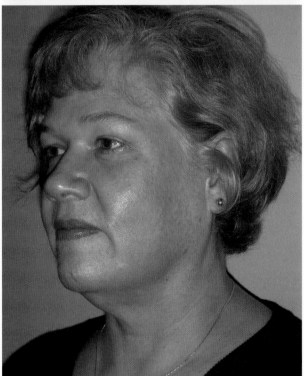

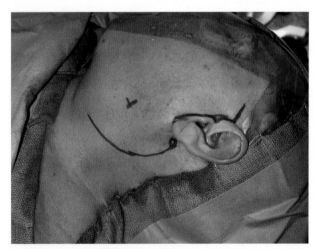

Figures 8.4a and 8.4b. Patient with pleomorphic adenoma of the left parotid gland preoperatively.

Figure 8.4d. Modified Blair incision.

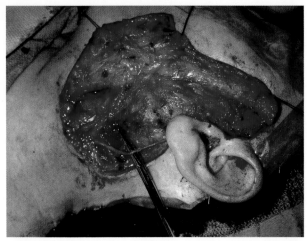

Figure 8.4e. Skin flap raised, the instrument indicates the sensory branch of the greater auricular nerve to the ear, which was preserved in this case.

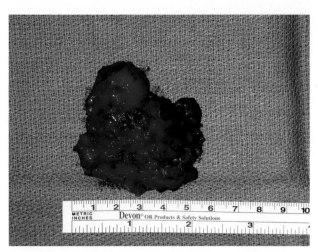

Figure 8.4g. The surgical specimen is seen with the tumor superiorly with no good surrounding "cuff" of tissue.

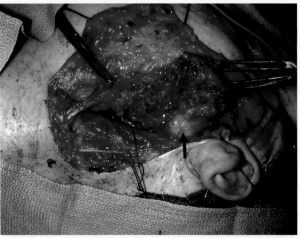

Figure 8.4f. The parotidectomy has been commenced from inferiorly and the superficial lobe is being retracted superiorly. The arrow indicates the deep surface of the tumor, which was adjacent to the nerve bifurcation (seen inferior to the tumor) and has no normal parotid tissue covering the tumor capsule.

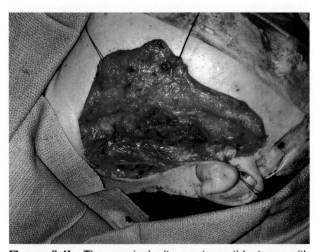

Figure 8.4h. The surgical site post-parotidectomy with complete dissection of the facial nerve.

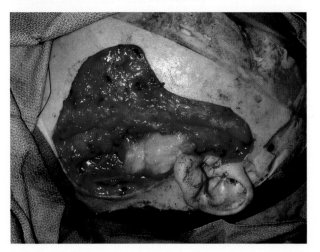

Figure 8.4i. A free abdominal fat graft is placed to reduce "hollowing," which was a concern of the patient.

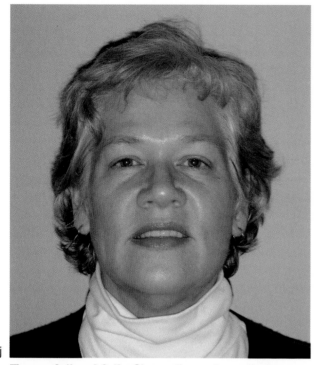

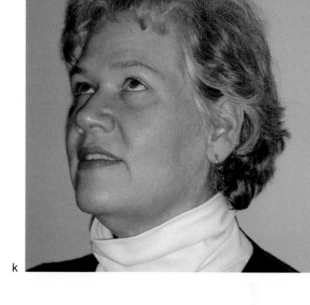

j

k

Figures 8.4j and 8.4k. Six months postoperatively.

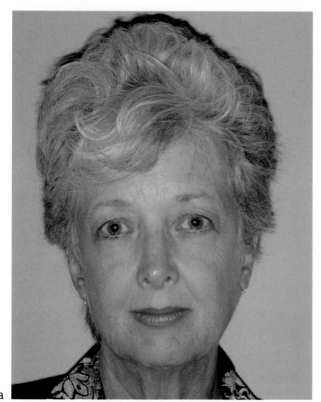

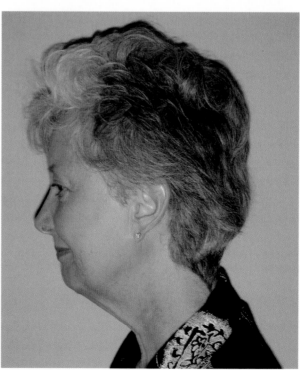

a

b

Figures 8.5a and 8.5b. Preoperative facial views of patient with left parotid pleomorphic adenoma. Patient requests bilateral face lift at the same time as parotidectomy.

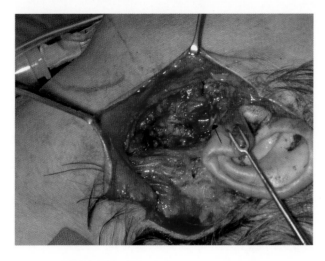

Figure 8.5c. Surgical access through face lift incision running into occipital hair line. Arrow shows facial nerve trunk being dissected.

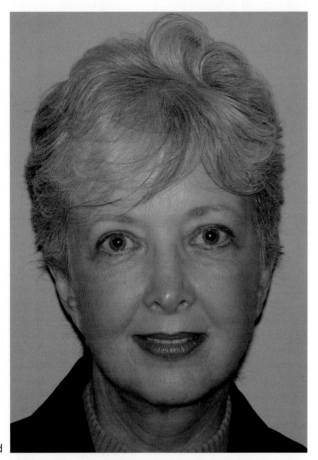

d

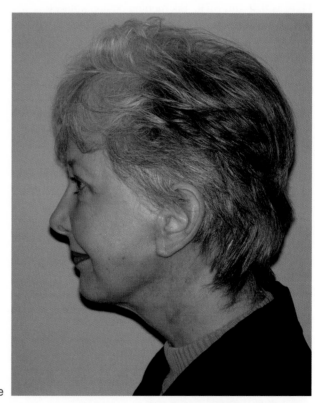

e

Figures 8.5d and 8.5e. Six months postoperatively. Notice absence of neck incision. (Aesthetic portions of this case undertaken by Dr. A. Pazoki, DDS, MD.)

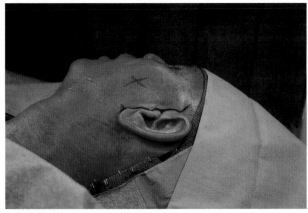

Figure 8.6a. Preauricular portion of omega face lift incision for parotidectomy for benign cystic lesion in the retromandibular portion of the superficial lobe of the left parotid gland.

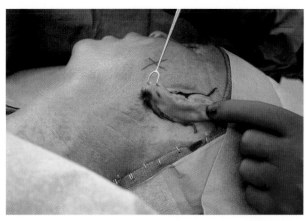

Figure 8.6b. Post-auricular portion of omega incision runs in the post-auricular sulcus.

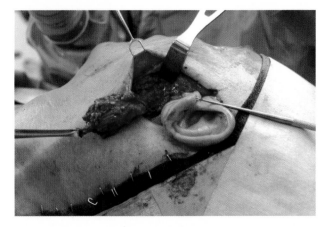

Figure 8.6c. A partial parotidectomy of the retroauricular portion of the superficial lobe is almost completed. The specimen is pedicled to the remains of the parotid tail.

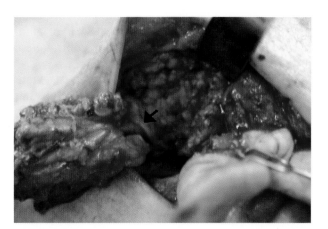

Figure 8.6d. Close-up of the dissection. Arrow points to the mandibulo-cervical trunk, which was the only branch of the facial nerve that was dissected, as it crosses superficial to the retromandibular vein.

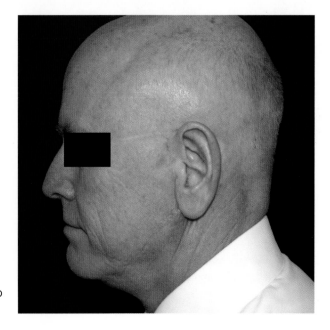

Figure 8.6e. The patient 3 months postoperatively with no visible scar.

181

tumors will be retromandibular and lie inferior to the trunk of the nerve. The space inferiorly is larger and by gentle retraction of the nerve trunk and blunt dissection around the tumor it can usually be delivered into the neck. In larger tumors the neoplasm may be impacted between the mandible and the mastoid with no means of mobilizing it without either dislocating the mandible forward or a subsigmoid or "C" osteotomy to give more space. As contemporary surgery has evolved, more emphasis has been placed on reducing morbidity. Deep lobe tumors may be removed without removing the superficial lobe but leaving it attached anteriorly and then replacing it after excising the deep lobe tumor (Coleela et al. 2007). This technique preserves facial contour and 84% of glandular function compared to the contralateral parotid.

In those tumors with parapharyngeal extension, blind finger enucleation may lead to capsular rupture or cause brisk hemorrhage. In order to visualize and safely remove these tumors an osteotomy of the mandible with or without lip split is utilized (Kolokythas, Fernandes, and Ord 2007) (Figures 8.7 and 8.8).

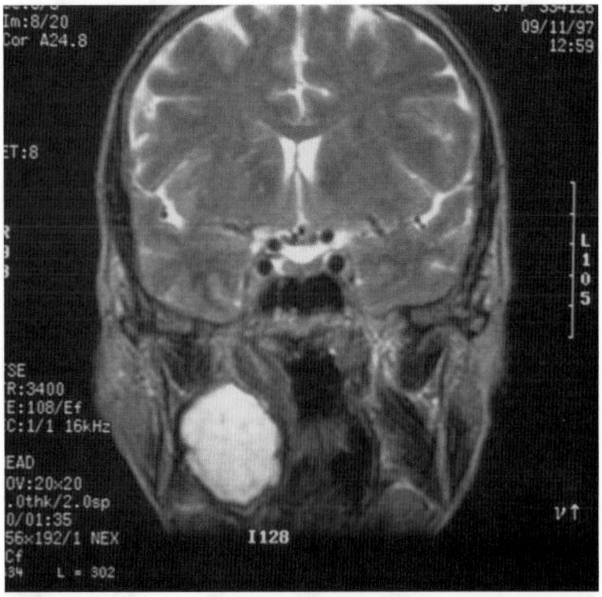

There is currently a controversy among surgeons regarding superficial parotidectomy or extracapsular dissection. This important topic will be discussed below in the section on pleomorphic adenomas.

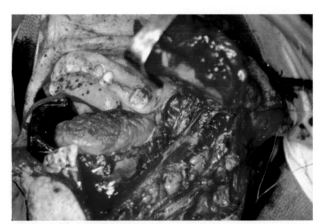

Figure 8.7b. Standard lip split incision for mandibulotomy.

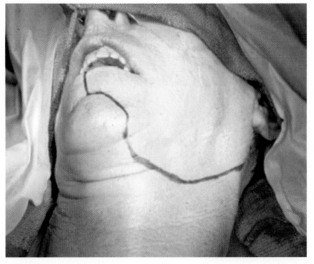

Figure 8.7a. MR shows parapharyngeal pleomorphic adenoma.

Figure 8.7c. Mandible is retracted out of the field and the pleomorphic adenoma is dissected preserving the overlying lingual nerve.

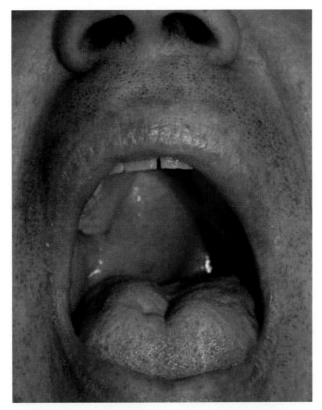

Figure 8.8a. Deep lobe parotid tumor with parapharyngeal extension presenting as a palatal mass.

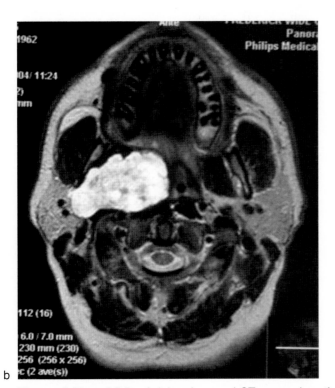 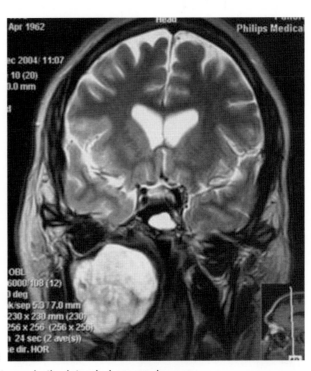

Figures 8.8b and 8.8c. Axial and coronal CT scans show the tumor in the lateral pharyngeal space.

183

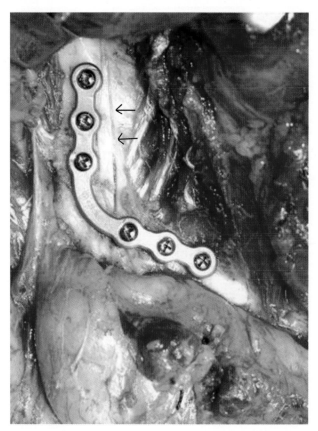

Figure 8.8d. The mandible is accessed via a cervical incision from mastoid to chin without lip split. Subsigmoid osteotomy cut marked with saw through buccal cortex only (arrows) and plate has been applied prior to completing the osteotomy.

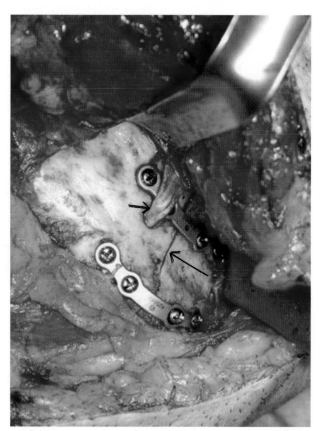

Figure 8.8e. Osteotomy marked with a saw through the buccal cortex (long arrow) anterior to the mental nerve (short arrow). Two miniplates applied prior to completing the osteotomy.

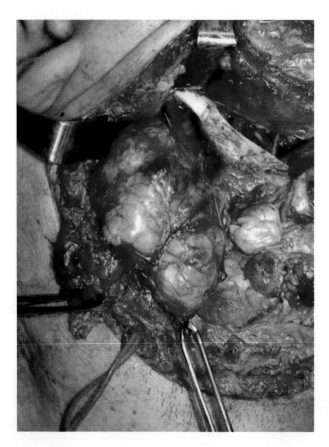

Figure 8.8f. The plates are removed, the double osteotomy is completed, and the osteotomized hemimandible is retracted upward and rotated to expose the lateral pharyngeal space, and the tumor is being delivered under direct vision.

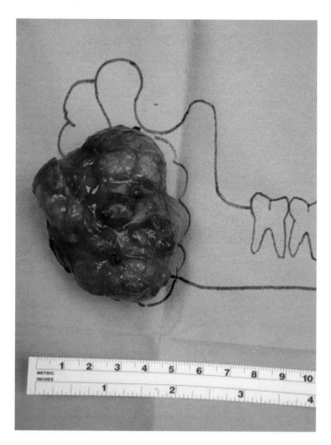

Figure 8.8g. The final specimen, which was PA, seen in relation to the mandible.

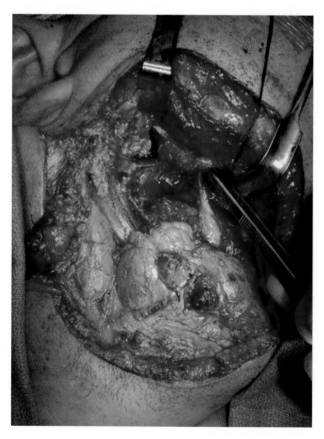

Figure 8.8h. The post-resection tumor bed. The plates are reapplied to reconstruct the original position of the mandible and occlusion.

185

BENIGN TUMORS

Pleomorphic Adenomas

The PA is the commonest benign salivary gland tumor and the commonest salivary tumor overall, although it is comparatively rare in young children. It is slow growing and can reach giant proportions if neglected, and there is a 2–4% malignant change. PAs will recur if the tumor is inadequately removed. Although PAs have a pseudo-capsule of compressed fibrous tissue, the buds and pseudopodia from the tumor involve the capsule so that simple enucleation will leave tumor remnants and lead to multifocal recurrence. The concept of whether the capsule is incomplete and whether pseudopodia of the tumor involves the parotid tissue is currently being questioned, and with it the need for complete superficial parotidectomy. Although parotidectomy is designed to remove PAs with a cuff or margin of normal tissue to prevent recurrence, the tumor's proximity to the facial nerve frequently means that the dissection at some points leaves no tissue around the capsule. In a recent histologic analysis of the capsular form in PAs, 81% showed capsular exposure following parotidectomy or submandibular gland excision (Webb and Eveson 2001) (Figure 8.4f). This paper also showed 57% bosselations, 33% enveloping of the capsule, with 42% microinvasion and 12% "tumor buds" in the capsule; and large >25 mm hypocellular tumors had thinner capsules, possibly easier to rupture at surgery. The article suggested that a minimum of 1 mm of normal tissue around PAs was required as a margin. However, in an article reviewing 475 PAs of the superficial lobe of the parotid, 380 treated by extracapsular dissection and 95 by superficial parotidectomy, there was no difference in recurrence rate or permanent facial nerve palsy (McGurk et al. 1996). These surgeons postulated that tumor buds or micro-invasion into the capsule had little significance and that extracapsular dissection could be done safely. In 1999 a series of 59 partial parotidectomies with selective nerve dissection for benign and low-grade malignant tumors reported a zero incidence of permanent facial nerve paralysis or paresis and zero recurrence (Witt 1999). Although Witt in a later paper confirmed that capsular exposure occurred in virtually all types of parotid surgery, and could find no difference in recurrence, capsular rupture, tumor-facial nerve interface, and permanent facial palsy between total parotidectomy, superficial parotidectomy, and extracapsular dissection, he recommended against minimum margin resection in extracapsular dissection (Witt 2002). Further evidence for extracapsular dissection is provided by a series of 83 cases in which the overall recurrence rate was 6%, but 17.6% when the tumor itself was at the margins; however, cases with margins of <1 mm had a recurrence of only 1.8% (Ghosh et al. 2003). Ghosh et al. also reported that intraoperative capsular rupture and microscopic invasion of the capsule had no influence on recurrence, suggesting that a fraction of a millimeter of normal tissue was an adequate margin and that only tumors that actually involved the margin were at risk for recurrence. These authors recommend that preservation of vital structures is a more important consideration than preserving a cuff of normal tissue.

In contrast, Piekarski, Nejc, and Szymczak et al. (2004) found a recurrence rate of 8.2% and an unacceptable rate of complications with extracapsular dissection and did not recommend the technique as too "technically demanding." In a separate publication with 213 patients who were operated for pleomorphic adenoma of the parotid, 5 of 9 primary tumors (56%) that recurred were found to have pseudopodia extending outside the capsule on histologic review. This was statistically higher than the examined cases that did not recur (8%), and the authors concluded that pseudopodia extending outside the capsule was a significant risk for recurrence (Henriksson et al. 1998). Interestingly, in the same study only 2 of 28 cases that ruptured during surgical removal recurred (7.1%), which was not significantly different than the 4.1% recurrence rate for the tumors that had no rupture. A further cautionary note is raised by the histologic analysis of Zbaren and Stauffer (2007), in which 160 of 218 (73%) of PAs were found to have adverse capsular characteristics, 33% with an incomplete capsule and 13% with satellite nodules. These were most frequently seen in the stroma rich myxoid subtype. Similar findings with stroma rich PAs showing 71% of focal absence of a capsule and 33% of satellite nodules have been reported with recommendations against local dissection (Stennert et al. 2004.)

It does not appear that extracapsular dissection is just a "euphemism for enucleation" as some have claimed, as recurrence rates are comparable to parotidectomy and most papers show lower morbidity. The exact margin required for complete removal of PA remains controversial. A criticism of extracapsular dissection has been that even if this technique is suitable for a presumed benign PA, what should the surgeon do if the final histopathologic diagnosis turns out to be malignant? In a review of 662 clinically benign parotid tumors, 503 treated by extracapsular dissection and 159 by superficial parotidectomy, 5% were malignant and there was no difference in 5- or 10-year survival or recurrence rates between the malignant tumors in the two surgical groups, although morbidity was significantly lower in the extracapsular dissection group (McGurk, Thomas, and Renehan 2003).

A superficial lobe parotid tumor clinically benign and diagnosed as a PA on FNAB may also be treated with a limited superficial parotidectomy (without complete dissection of the facial nerve) and may not require a complete superficial parotidectomy for cure (O'Brien 2003). This is probably most commonly undertaken for tumors in the parotid tail (Figure 8.9).

Deep lobe PAs are usually larger and frequently will have less surrounding parotid tissue, especially deeply, where they abut the prevertebral muscles of the neck. However, the inability to obtain a surrounding cuff of parotid does not seem

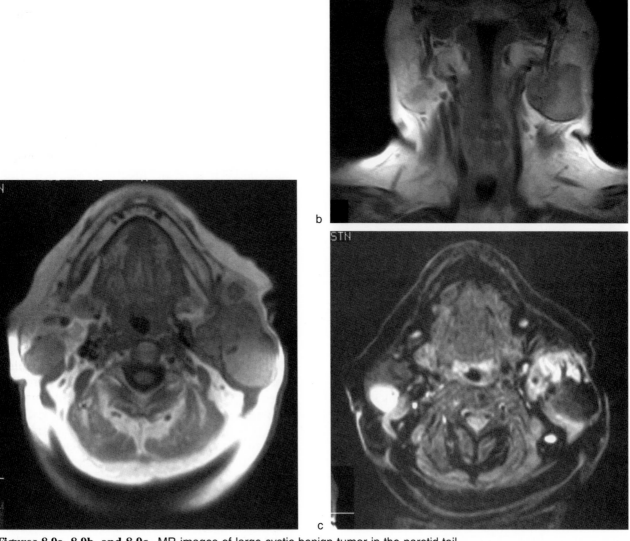

Figures 8.9a, 8.9b, and 8.9c. MR images of large cystic benign tumor in the parotid tail.

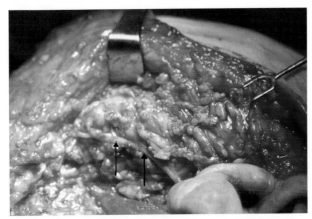

Figure 8.9d. Following partial parotidectomy the two arrows point to the dissected cervico-mandibular branch of the facial nerve, the parotid tail tumor having been resected inferior to this nerve branch. The upper branches of the facial nerve have not been dissected in this case.

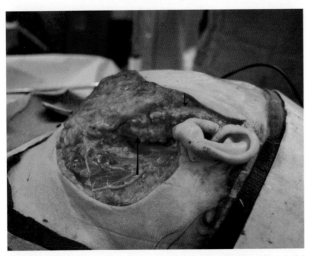

Figure 8.9e. The long arrow points to the resected parotid tail region, while the shorter arrow points to the remaining superficial parotid lobe preserved intact.

to lead to increased recurrence. Harney, Murphy, and Hone et al. (2003) found that the capsules of deep lobe tumors were significantly thicker and that there was less extracapsular extension of tumor in the deep lobe tumors (58% vs. 79%), which may explain this phenomenon.

If the capsule of the tumor is ruptured during surgery, then recurrence is not inevitable and perhaps liberal irrigation with sterile water followed by normal saline may be tumoricidal (Webb and Eveson 2001). When recurrence occurs it is frequently multinodular (Figure 8.10) and requires

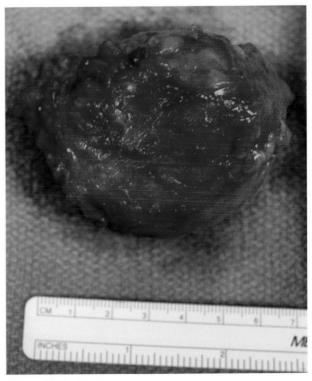

Figure 8.9f. Surgical specimen.

more radical en bloc surgery with excision of the previous scar, muscle, overlying skin, and facial nerve if they are involved. Maxwell, Hall, and Freeman (2004) in a retrospective study of 35 patients treated with surgery alone found a locoregional control of 77% with a malignant transformation of 5.7%. In a separate study of 42 cases of multinodular recurrence (6 with prior radiation), there were 2 patients with malignant transformation who died of distant metastases. Twelve patients had subtotal parotidectomy, 25 total parotidectomy, 5 subtotal petrosectomy; 14 had facial nerve resection. Seven patients of 36 who were followed developed further recurrences (19.4%), all of whom had only undergone subtotal parotidectomy (Leonetti et al. 2005). In a further series of 33 patients, 73% multifocal, 9% with malignant transformation, treated surgically, 6 (18%) recurred at an average of 9 years, and 23% of patients with initial enucleation and 14% with initial superficial parotidectomy had permanent partial facial nerve injury (Zbaren Tschumi et al. 2006). Renehan, Gleave, and McGurk (1996) reviewed 144 cases of recurrent PAs and suggested a role for radiation in multinodular cases. A recent paper of 34 cases of

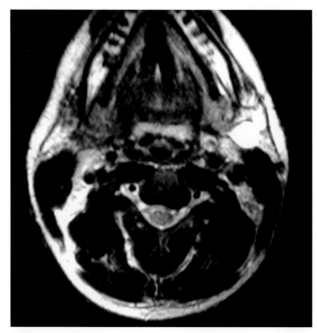

Figure 8.10a. Two large nodules of recurrent pleomorphic adenoma exist in the left parotid gland.

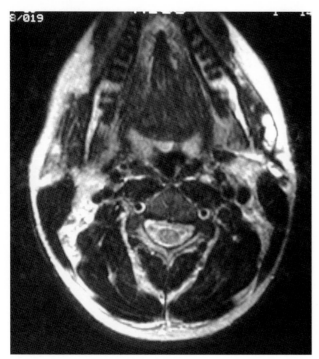

Figure 8.10b. Two smaller nodules are seen in the parotid tail.

recurrent PAs with radiation therapy post–gross resection shows a 20-year actuarial control rate of 94% (Chen et al. 2006)

Warthin's Tumor

This is the second commonest benign tumor of the parotid. If it is diagnosed when small and asymptomatic it may not require treatment in an old or infirmed patient. There is a 12% incidence of multiple ipsilateral or bilateral tumors. There appears to be a link to heavy smoking and bilateral Warthin's tumors (Klussman, Wittekindt, and Preuss et al. 2006). Eight percent of these tumors occur in extra-parotid cervical lymph nodes and may be found at the time of parotidectomy or serendipidously in neck dissection specimens. Treatment is as for PA. Warthin's tumors have a tendency to occur in the parotid tail, where the majority of parotid lymph nodes occur, so partial parotidectomy is often all that is required.

MALIGNANT TUMORS

Principles of Management of Parotid Carcinoma

There is no universally agreed method for managing parotid cancer; however, prognosis and management are related to two variables: the histologic classification/grade of the tumor and the staging. In reviewing 2,465 patients with carcinoma of parotid and submandibular glands, Wahlberg, Anderson, and Bjorklund et al. (2002) found 10-year survival of 88% for acinic cell carcinoma, 80% for mucoepidermoid carcinoma (MEC), and 74% for adenoid cystic carcinoma (ACC), but only 55% for adenocarcinoma unspecified and 44% for undifferentiated carcinoma. It should be noted that 5-year survival figures for ACC will give an artificially high value, as late local recurrence and distant metastasis continue over a 20+ year period (Chen, Garcia, Bucci et al. 2006; Lima, Tavares, Dias et al. 2005; Longuet, Nallet, Guedon et al. 2001). Harbo, Bungaard, and Pederson et al. (2002) also found acinic cell carcinoma to have the best 10-year survival, but in their Cox hazard regression analysis found T stage, N stage, M stage, and histologic differentiation to be significant in predicting prognosis and recommended the use of both staging and histologic diagnosis to assess prognosis. In other series significant factors include extraglandular extension, aggressive histology, and nodal disease (Bhattacharyya and Fried 2005), histologic grade, T stage, N stage, and facial nerve dysfunction (Lima et al. 2005), and N stage and perineural involvement (Hocwald, Korkmaz, and Yoo et al. 2001).

The only other predictor of adverse prognosis reported in several series was advancing age (Bhattacharyya and Fried 2005; Lima et al. 2005; Kirkbridge, Liu, and O'Sullivan et al. 2001).

The reported survival related to stage varies between authors, which may reflect differences in therapy as well as different patterns of histopathology. Luukkaa, Klemi, and Leivo et al. (2005) found

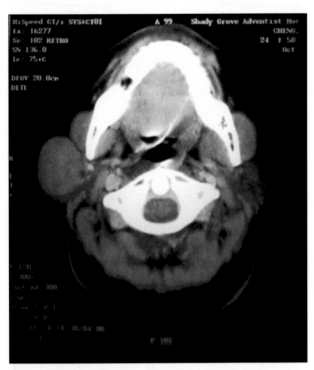

Figure 8.11a. CT scan of large superficial lobe tumor in 22-year-old woman.

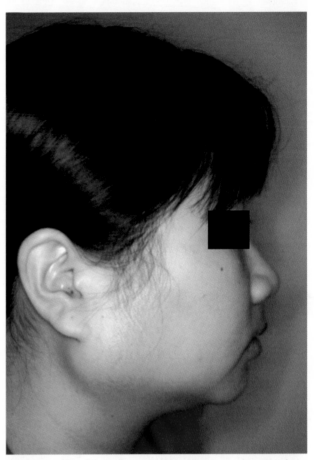

Figure 8.11b. Clinical appearance; the tumor has no signs of malignancy.

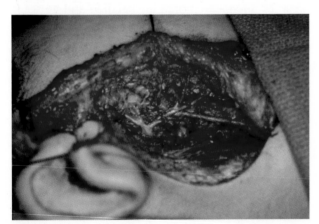

Figure 8.11c. Complete parotidectomy. The facial nerve was not involved.

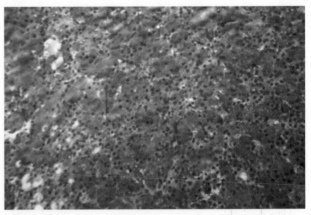

Figure 8.11d. Histopathology of acinic cell carcinoma. The patient is alive and well 8+ years postoperatively.

5-year survival Stage I–IV 78%, 25%, 21%, and 23%, while Lima et al. (2005) found 10-year disease-specific survival Stage I–IV 97%, 81%, 56%, and 20%.

In considering management, Kaplan and Johns (1986) divide parotid cancers into 4 groups to recommend treatment. Group I T1-2 low-grade tumors are treated by parotidectomy with preservation of the facial nerve (Figures 8.11 and 8.12). Group II T1-2 high-grade are treated with parotidectomy plus first echelon node removal and postoperative radiation therapy (RT) (Figure 8.13). Group III T3 tumors, any positive nodes and recurrent tumor not in Group IV, are treated with radical parotidectomy with sacrifice of the facial nerve if necessary and radical neck dissection plus RT. Group IV includes T4 and tumors with significant local extension; they are treated by radical paroti-

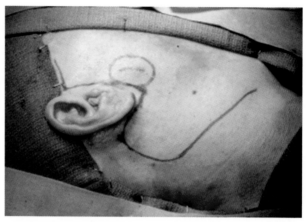

Figure 8.12b. Operative image shows Blair incision incorporating 1 cm skin margin surrounding the biopsy.

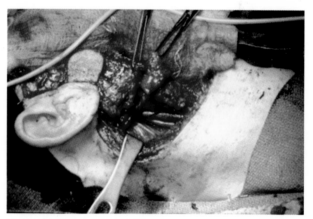

Figure 8.12c. The level II nodes (first echelon nodes) will be taken in continuity in this case.

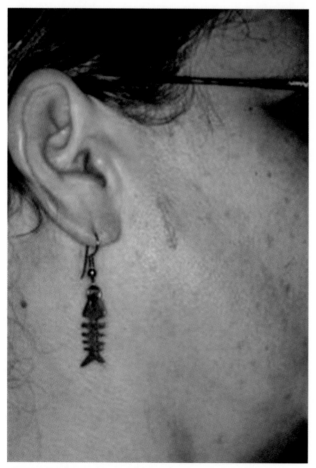

Figure 8.12a. Patient who had a "skin cyst" biopsied; it was histologically a low-grade mucoepidermoid carcinoma of the parotid. Note preauricular biopsy scar.

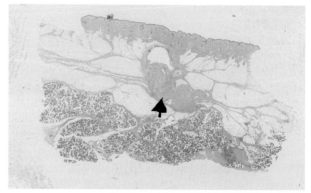

Figure 8.12d. Histology shows a focus of mucoepidermoid carcinoma (arrow) in the biopsy scar between the skin and parotid, demonstrating the importance of excising "seeded" skin.

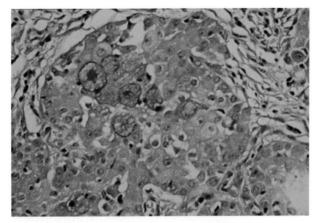

Figure 8.12e. Mucicarmine stain confirms intracellular mucus.

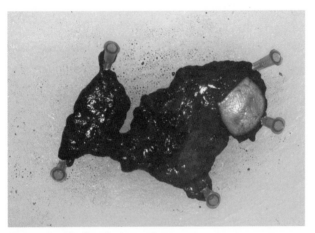

Figure 8.12f. Surgical specimen.

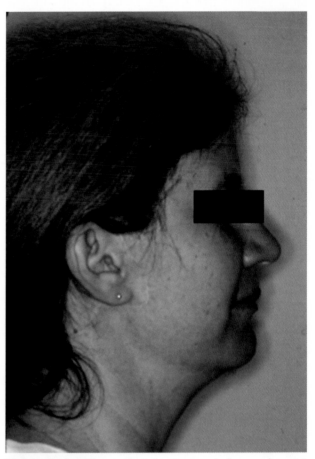

Figure 8.12g. The patient is alive and disease-free 14 years postoperatively.

dectomy plus skin, muscle, and bone as indicated with radical neck dissection and postoperative RT (see chapter 11, Figure 11.16).

Controversy exists in the exact indications for RT, neck dissection, and facial nerve sacrifice. The majority of recent papers do show that RT is indicated for advanced parotid carcinoma and confers a survival benefit (Bhattacharyya and Fried 2005) or longer disease-free survival (Hocwald, Korkmaz, and Yoo et al. 2001). However, there is a move toward suggesting RT for earlier stage disease. Zbaren, Nuyens, and Caversaccio et al. (2006) retrospectively analyzed T1-2 carcinomas with and without postoperative RT and found local recurrence rates of 3% and 33%, respectively, and actuarial and disease-free survival of 93% and 92% with and 83% and 70% without RT. In an earlier publication from the same unit RT was suggested

not just for high-grade tumors but low-grade T2-4 (Zbaren, Schupbach, and Nuyens et al. 2003). So perhaps RT is indicated for earlier stage disease than was previously recommended. The latest data regarding fast neutron therapy in the management of advanced salivary cancer with gross residual disease shows a 6-year local-regional control of 59%, and 100% with no evidence of gross residual disease (Douglas et al. 2003.) Benefits of chemotherapy have not been clearly demonstrated for parotid cancer.

Similarly, although lymph node dissection was recommended for positive nodes and high-grade tumors, there is an increasing interest in the N0 neck. Occult metastasis rates of 22–45% led Stennert, Kisner, and Jungehuelsing et al. (2003) and Zbaren, Schupbach, and Nuyens et al. (2003) to recommend an elective neck dissection in the

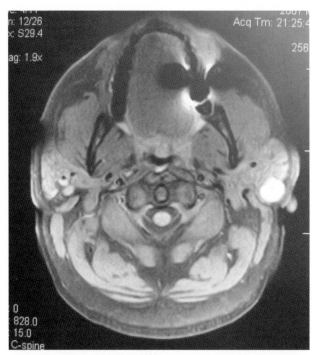

Figure 8.13a. MR of parotid tumor that radiologically was diagnosed as a pleomorphic adenoma, but fine needle aspiration biopsy showed adenoid cystic carcinoma.

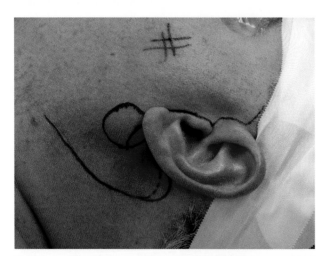

Figure 8.13b. In view of the cytologic diagnosis, proposed treatment includes resection of overlying skin (which clinically was felt to be tethered) and level II cervical nodes.

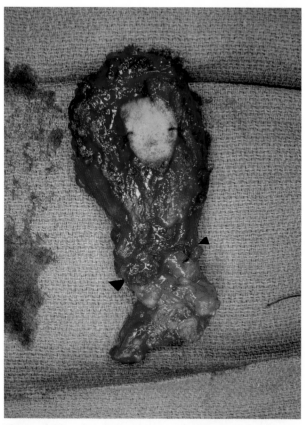

Figure 8.13c. Surgical specimen shows parotid with skin. The arrows show where level II nodes and fat are in continuity with the parotid tail. Final diagnosis was cellular pleomorphic adenoma with the FNAB diagnosis being a false positive.

N0 neck for parotid cancer (Figure 8.14). Elective neck dissection for high-grade tumors and >T2 low-grade tumors should encompass levels I–III and upper V (Teymoortash and Werner 2002). In comparing elective neck dissection for the N0 neck against observation, Zbaren et al. (2005) found an actuarial and disease-free survival of 80% and 86% for the elective neck dissection patients vs. 83% and 69% for the observation group in a retrospective study.

Regarding the facial nerve, Spiro and Spiro (2003) recommend preservation unless the nerve is adherent to/embedded in the tumor. They feel that close margins to the nerve can be treated successfully by RT. This view is supported by the work of Carinci, Farina, and Pelucchi et al. (2001), who found that sacrifice of the nerve was not always able to improve survival rate. In a series of 107 patients with parotid cancer, 91 had normal nerve function preoperatively and facial nerve preservation was possible in 79 patients. The 5-year disease-free rate and 5- and 10-year survival rates were 65%, 83%, and 54% in the preserved nerve cohort and 56%, 62%, and 42% in the patients with nerve sacrifice. The authors felt that

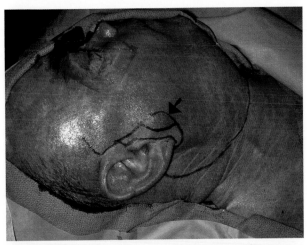

Figure 8.14a. High-grade parotid malignancy with skin fixation and N0 neck. Incision modified to include skin excision (arrow), and cervical incision extended to allow supra-omohyoid neck dissection.

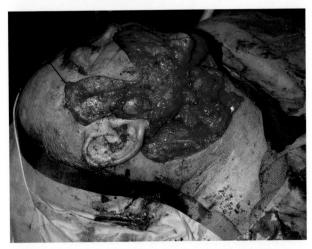

Figure 8.14b. The skin flaps developed with the skin overlying the tumor left on the parotid gland.

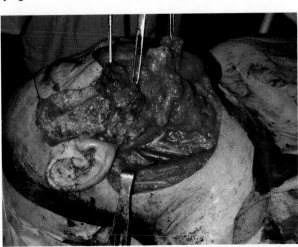

Figure 8.14c. The selective neck dissection is complete with the specimen in continuity with the parotid gland. The facial nerve trunk has been exposed and the superficial parotidectomy is being performed.

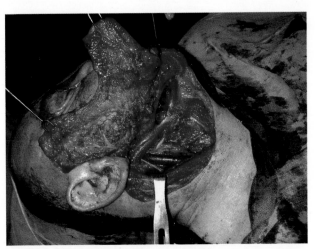

Figure 8.14d. The surgical site following parotidectomy and selective neck dissection.

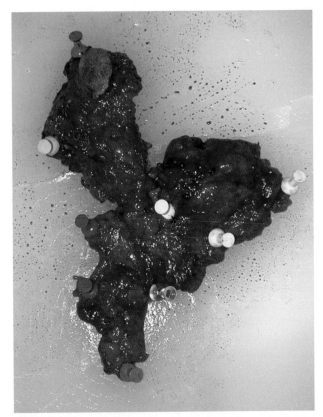

Figure 8.14e. The surgical specimen with the parotid superiorly and level I nodes pinned out with white pins.

preservation of the facial nerve by careful dissection gave favorable oncologic results (Guntinas-Lichius, Klussman, and Schroeder et al. 2004). Finally, a disease-free survival in patients with normal, partially, and completely impaired facial nerve function preoperatively of 69%, 37%, and 13% despite the use of facial nerve sacrifice and postoperative RT indicates what a poor prognosis invasion of the nerve confers (Terhaard, Lubsen, and Tan et al. 2006).

In specific histologic tumor types variable results for different treatments have been reported. Mucoepidermoid carcinoma is the commonest salivary malignancy and most cases are fortunately low or intermediate grade. A series of 89 cases at the Mayo Clinic, 69 T1-2, 85 N0, and 83 low/intermediate grade, were treated by parotidectomy with "appropriate" neck dissection and only 7 had RT. Kaplan-Meier estimated cancer-specific survival rates at 5, 15, and 25 years were 98.9%, 97.4%, and 97.4% (Boahene, Olsen, and Lewis et al. 2004). Using a point grading system for histopathologic features in a series of 234 mucoepidermoid carcinomas of the major salivary glands, cystic component <20%, 4 or more mitotic figures per 10 high power fields, neural involvement, necrosis, and anaplasia were found to have prognostic significance for parotid MEC (Goode, Auclair, and Ellis 1998). Intermediate-grade MEC tends to behave more like low-grade MEC, while high-grade MEC behaves aggressively with local recurrence and regional and distant metastases in the majority of cases. Other low-grade tumors such as acinic cell carcinoma, epimyoepithelial carcinoma, and low-grade adenocarcinoma all can be treated like low-grade MEC. Polymorphous low-grade adenocarcinoma is rare in the major glands, being seen mostly in the minor salivary glands of the oral cavity.

On the other hand, results for high-grade tumors such as primary squamous carcinoma of the parotid are poor; in one published series two-thirds were treated with radical surgery and RT and one-third with RT alone, but 5-year actuarial survival and disease-free survival was 31% and 33%, respectively (Lee, Kim, and Parks et al. 2001). Malignant change in PAs is most commonly seen as carcinoma ex-pleomorphic adenoma, and prognosis will depend on the histologic type of malignancy and whether the malignancy has spread outside the capsule. In carcinoma ex-pleomorphic adenoma the use of postoperative RT improved 5-year local control from 49% to 75%

and improved survival in patients without cervical metastasis (Chen, Garcia, and Bucci et al. 2007). Two other forms of malignant PA occur, both rare: the "true" malignant mixed tumor or carcinosarcoma where malignant change is seen in both the epithelial and myoepithelial component of the PA, and the benign metastasizing PA, which as its name suggests retains a benign histologic appearance despite the presence of metastases.

It is hard to interpret survival figures in some series, as ACC is very slow growing and 5-year survival is less meaningful in this neoplasm as survival continues to fall on 20-year follow-up. Thus in series with short follow-up ACC will erroneously be thought to have a good prognosis. Typical long-term survival figures are 84.3% 2 year, 75.9% 5 year, 50.49% 10 year, and 20.11% after 20 years (Issing, Hemmanouil, and Wilkens et al. 2002). The type of histologic appearance, solid vs. cylindrical, and the presence of perineural invasion are important prognostic factors. Even with documented lung metastases patients can live 5+ years, the average survival between the appearance of lung metastases and death being 32.3 months in one series (van der Waal et al. 2002). Wide field adjuvant RT post–radical surgery is usually recommended for ACC.

The histologic grade of the tumor must be taken into account as well as TNM staging when interpreting survival results in reported series. Every parotid cancer will be unique and the decision for what is the correct surgery will be made on an individual basis for each patient.

Summary

- 80% of parotid tumors are benign and most commonly pleomorphic adenomas.
- Less than one-third of malignant tumors will have obvious clinical signs of malignancy, for example, facial nerve palsy, ulceration, fixation, or lymphadenopathy.
- Routine use of CT or MR imaging does not appear justified and should be used selectively for malignant neoplasms and deep lobe tumors.
- Preoperative open biopsy is contraindicated and FNAB is the modality of choice for preoperative cytologic diagnosis.

- Although superficial parotidectomy remains the basic surgical procedure, there is currently much debate regarding the roles of partial parotidectomy and extracapsular dissection in the management of PA. The role of the capsule and the acceptable margin for PA remain undefined.
- Recurrent PAs will frequently require en bloc resection due to their infiltrative and multinodular nature. Cure in this situation is probably achieved in approximately two-thirds of cases.
- Management of malignant parotid tumors will depend on both the histologic diagnosis and the staging of the tumor.
- Radiation therapy may be more helpful in earlier stage disease and lower-grade tumors than previously advocated.
- Selective neck dissection for the N0 neck may be justified in early stage disease given the high reported rate of occult nodes.
- The facial nerve should be preserved in parotid cancer unless it is directly infiltrated by the tumor.

References

Ariyoshi Y, Shimahara M. 1998. Determining whether a parotid tumor is in the superficial or deep lobe using magnetic resonance imaging. *J Oral Maxillofac Surg* 56:23–27.

Bhattacharyya N, Fried MP. 2005. Determinants of survival in parotid gland carcinoma: A population based study. *Am J Otolaryngol* 26(1):39–44.

Boahene DK, Olsen KD, Lewis JE et al. 2004. Mucoepidermoid carcinoma of the parotid gland: The Mayo Clinic experience. *Arch Otolaryngol Head Neck Surg* 130(7):849–856.

Carinci F, Farina A, Pelucchi S et al. 2001. Parotid gland carcinoma: Surgical strategy based on local risk factors. *J Craniofac Surg* 12(5):434–437.

Chen AM, Garcia J, Bucci MK et al. 2007. The role of postoperative radiation therapy in carcinoma ex pleomorphic adenoma of the parotid gland. *Int J Radiat Oncol Biol Phys* 67(1):138–143.

Chen AM, Garcia J, Bucci MK, Quivey JM, Eisle DW. 2006. Recurrent pleomorphic adenoma of the parotid gland: Long term outcome of patients treated with radiation therapy. *Int J Radiol Biol Phys* 66(4):1031–1035.

Cohen EG, Patel SG, Lin O et al. 2004. Fine needle aspiration biopsy of salivary gland lesions in a selected patient population. *Arch Otolaryngol Head Neck Surg* 130(6):773–778.

Coleela C, Giudice A, Rambali PF, Cuccurullo V. 2007. Parotid function after selective deep lobe parotidectomy. *Brit J Oral Maxillofacial Surg* 45:108–111.

de Ru JA, Maartens SVL, Van Bentham PPG et al. 2007. Do magnetic resonance imaging and ultrasound add anything to the preoperative workup of parotid tumors? *J Oral Maxillofac Surg* 65:945–952.

de Ru JA, Van Bentham PPG, Hordijk GJ. 2002. The location of parotid gland tumors in relation to the facial nerve on magnetic resonance images and computed tomography scans. *J Oral Maxillofac Surg* 60:992–996.

Douglas JG, Koh WJ, Austin-Seymour M, Laramore GE. 2003. Treatment of salivary gland neoplasms with fast neutron radiotherapy. *Arch Otolaryngol Head Neck Surg* 129:944–948.

Fee WE Jr, Tran LE. 2003. Evaluation of a patient with a parotid tumor. *Arch Otolaryngol Head Neck Surg* 129:937–938.

Ghosh S, Panarese A, Bull PD, Lee JA. 2003. Marginally excised parotid pleomorphic adenomas: Risk factors for recurrence and management. A 12.5 year mean follow up study of histologically marginal excisions. *Clin Otolaryngol* 28:262–266.

Goode RK, Auclair PL, Ellis GL. 1998. Mucoepidermoid carcinoma of the major salivary glands: Clinical and histopathologic analysis of 234 cases with evaluation of grading criteria. *Cancer* 82(7):1217–1224.

Guntinas-Lichius O, Klussman JP, Schroeder U et al. 2004. Primary parotid malignant surgery in patients with normal preoperative facial nerve function: Outcome and long-term postoperative facial nerve function. *Laryngoscope* 114(5):949–956.

Harbo G, Bungaard T, Pedersen D et al. 2002. Prognostic indicators for malignant tumors of the parotid gland. *Clin Otolaryngol Allied Sci* 27(6):512–516.

Harney MS, Murphy C, Hone S et al. 2003. A histological comparison of deep and superficial lobe pleomorphic adenomas of the parotid gland. *Head Neck* 25(8):649–653.

Henriksson G, Westrin KM, Carlsoo B, Silversward C. 1998. Recurrent primary pleomorphic adenomas of salivary gland origin: Intrasurgical rupture, histopathologic features, and pseudopodia. *Cancer* 82(4):617–620.

Hocwald E, Korkmaz H, Yoo GH et al. 2001. Prognostic factors in major salivary gland cancer. *Laryngoscope* 111(8):1434–1439.

Honig JF. 2005. Omega incision face lift approach and SMAS rotation advancement in parotidectomy for the prevention of contour deficiency and conspicuous scars affecting the neck. *Int J Oral Maxillofac Surg* 34(6):612–618.

Hughes JH, Volk EE, Wilbur DC. 2005. Pitfalls in salivary gland fine-needle aspiration cytology: Lessons from the College of American Pathologists Interlaboratory Comparison Program in Nongynecologic Cytology. *Arch Pathol Lab Med* 129(1):26–31.

In der Maur CD, Klokman WJ, van Leeuwen FE et al. 2005. Increased risk of breast cancer development after diagnosis of salivary gland cancer. *European Journal of Cancer* 41(9):1311–1315.

Issing PR, Hemmanouil I, Wilkens L et al. 2002. Long term results in adenoid cystic carcinoma. (Article in German.) *Laryngorhinootologie* 81(2):98–105.

Kaplan MJ, Johns ME. 1986. Salivary gland cancer. *Clin Oncology* 5:525–547.

Kirkbridge P, Liu FF, O'Sullivan B et al. 2001. Outcome of curative management of malignant tumors of the parotid gland. *J Otolaryngol* 30(5):271–279.

Klussman PJ, Wittekindt C, Preuss FS et al. 2006. High risk for bilateral Warthin's tumors in heavy smokers—review of 185 cases. *Acta Otolaryngol* 126(11):1213–1217.

Kolokythas A, Fernandes RP, Ord RA. 2007. A non-lip-splitting-double mandibular osteotomy technique for resection of tumors in the parapharyngeal and pterygo-mandibular spaces. *J Oral Maxillofac Surg* 65(3):66–69.

Lamelas J, Terry JH, Alfonso AE. 1987. Warthin's tumor: Multicentricity and increasing incidence in women. *Am J Surg* 154:347–351.

Lee S, Kim GE, Parks CS et al. 2001. Primary squamous cell carcinoma of the parotid gland. *Am J Otolaryngol* 22(6):400–406.

Leonetti JP, Marzo SJ, Petrzelli GJ, Herr B. 2005. Recurrent pleomorphic adenoma of the parotid gland. *Otolaryngol Head Neck Surg* 133(3):319–322.

Lima RA, Tavares MR, Dias FL, Kligerman J, Nascimento MF, Barbosa MM, Cernea CR, Soares JR, Santos IC, Salviano S. 2005. Clinical prognostic factors in malignant parotid gland tumors. *Otolaryngol Head Neck Surg* 133(5):702–708.

Longuet M, Nallet E, Guedon C et al. 2001. Diagnostic value of needle biopsy and frozen section histological examination in the surgery of primary parotid tumors. *Rev Laryngolo Otol Rhinol* 122(1):51–55.

Lonn S, Alholm A, Christensen HC et al. 2006. Mobile phone use and risk of parotid gland tumor. *Am J Epidemiol* 164(7):637–643.

Luukkaa H, Klemi P, Leivo I et al. 2005. Salivary gland cancer in Finland 1991–96. *Acta Otolaryngol* 125(2):207–214.

Maxwell EL, Hall FT, Freeman JL. 2004. Recurrent pleomorphic adenoma of the parotid gland. *J Otolaryngol* 33(3):181–184.

McGurk M, Renehan A, Gleave EN, Hancock BD. 1996. Clinical significance of the tumor capsule in the treatment of parotid pleomorphic adenomas. *Br J Surg* 83(12):1747–1749.

McGurk M, Thomas BL, Renehan AG. 2003. Extracapsular dissection for clinically benign parotid lumps: Reduced morbidity without oncological compromise. *Br J Cancer* 89(9):1610–1613.

Meningaud JP, Bertolus C, Bertrand JC. 2006. Parotidectomy: Assessment of a surgical technique including face-lift incision and SMAS advancement. *J Craniomaxillofac Surg* 34(10):34–37.

Nouraei SA, Al-Yaghchi C, Ahmed J et al. 2006. An anatomical comparison of Blair and facelift incisions for parotid surgery. *Clin Otolaryngol* 31(6):531–534.

O'Brien CJ. 2003. Current management of benign parotid tumors—the role of limited superficial parotidectomy. *Head Neck* 25:946–952.

Ord RA. 1995. Surgical management of parotid tumors. *Oral and Maxillofac Surg Clin of North America* 7(3):529–564.

O'Regan BO, Bharadwaj G, Bhopal S, Cook V. 2007. Facial nerve morbidity after retrograde nerve dissection in parotid surgery for benign disease: A 10-year prospective observational study of 136 cases. *Brit J Oral Maxillofac Surg* 45(2):101–107.

Piekarski J, Nejc D, Szymczak W et al. 2004. Results of extracapsular dissection of pleomorphic adenoma of the parotid gland. *J Oral Maxillofac Surg* 62(10):1198–1202.

Pogrel MA, Schmidt B, Ammar A. 1996. The relationship of the buccal branch of the facial nerve to the parotid duct. *J Oral Maxillofac Surg* 54(1):71–73.

Renehan A, Gleave EN, McGurk M. 1996. An analysis of the treatment of 114 patients with recurrent pleomorphic adenoma of the parotid gland. *Am J Surg* 172:710–714.

Rubello D, Nanni C, Castellucci P et al. 2005. Does 18F-FDG PET/CT play a role in the differential diagnosis of parotid masses. *Panminerva Med* 47(3):187–189.

Saku T, Hayashi Y, Takahara O et al. 1997. Salivary tumors among atom bomb survivors, 1950–1987. *Cancer* 79(8):1465–1475.

Schroder U, Eckel HE, Rasche V et al. 2000. Value of fine needle puncture cytology in neoplasms of the parotid gland. *HNO* 48(6):421–429.

Spiro JD, Spiro RH. 2003. Cancer of the parotid gland: Role of 7th nerve preservation. *World J Surg* 27(7):863–867.

Stennert E, Kisner D, Jungehuelsing M et al. 2003. High incidence of lymph node metastasis in major salivary gland cancer. *Arch Otolaryngol Head Neck Surg* 129(7):720–723.

Stennert E, Wittekindt C, Klussman JP, Guntinas-Lichas O. 2004. New aspects in parotid surgery. *Otolaryngol Pol* 58(1):109–114.

Takahashi N, Okamoto K, Ohkubo M, Kawana M. 2005. High-resolution magnetic resonance of the extracranial facial nerve and parotid duct: Demonstration of the branches of the intraparotid facial nerve and its relation to parotid tumors by MRI with a surface coil. *Clin Radiology* 60(3):349–354.

Terhaard C, Lubsen H, Tan B et al. 2006. Facial nerve function in carcinoma of the parotid gland. *Eur J Cancer* 42(16):2744–2750.

Teymoortash A, Werner JA. 2002. Value of neck dissection in patients with cancer of the parotid gland and a clinical N0 neck. *Onkologie* 25(2):122–126.

van der Waal JE, Becking AG, Snow GB, van der Waal I. 2002. Distant metastases of adenoid cystic carcinoma of the salivary glands and the value of diagnostic examinations during follow up. *Head Neck* 24(8):779–783.

Wahlberg P, Anderson H, Bjorklund A et al. 2002. Carcinoma of the parotid and submandibular glands—a study of survival in 2,465 patients. *Oral Oncol* 38(7):706–713.

Webb AJ, Eveson JW. 2001. Pleomorphic adenomas of the major salivary glands: A study of the capsular form in relation to surgical management. *Clin Otolaryngol* 26:134–142.

Witt RL. 1999. Facial nerve function after partial superficial parotidectomy: An 11 year review 1987–1997. *Otolaryngol Head Neck Surg* 121(3):210–213.

Witt RL. 2002. The significance of the margin in parotid surgery for pleomorphic adenoma. *Laryngoscope* 112(12):2141–2154.

Wong DS. 2001. Signs and symptoms of malignant parotid tumors: An objective assessment. *J R Coll Surg Edinb* 46(2):91–95.

Zbaren P, Nuyens M, Caversaccio M et al. 2006. Postoperative radiation for T1 and T2 primary parotid carcinoma: Is it useful? *Otolaryngol Head Neck Surg* 135(1):140–143.

Zbaren P, Schar C, Hotz MA et al. 2001. Value of fine-needle aspiration cytology of parotid gland masses. *Laryngoscope* 111(11 part 1):1989–2002.

Zbaren P, Schupbach J, Nuyens M et al. 2003. Carcinoma of the parotid gland. *Am J Surg* 186(1):57–62.

Zbaren P, Schupbach J, Nuyens M, Stauffer E. 2005. Elective neck dissection versus observation in primary parotid cancer. *Otolaryngol Head Neck Surg* 132(3):387–391.

Zbaren P, Stauffer E. 2007. Pleomorphic adenoma of the parotid gland: Histopathologic analysis of the capsular characteristics of 218 tumors. *Head Neck* 29:751–757.

Zbaren P, Tschumi I, Nuyens M, Stauffer E. 2006. Recurrent pleomorphic adenoma of the parotid gland. *Am J Surg* 192(2):203–207.

Chapter 9
Tumors of the Submandibular and Sublingual Glands

Outline

Introduction

This chapter will discuss the diagnosis and management of epithelial derived tumors of the submandibular and sublingual glands. These tumors are much less common than tumors of the parotid gland and a long series of cases from which to apply evidence-based medicine treatment protocols is lacking, particularly with regard to the sublingual gland neoplasms. Current approaches are highlighted, although the diversity of histologic types, paucity of cases, and lack of long-term follow-up results in many of these cases being treated empirically based on oncologic principles derived from other tumors and sites in the head and neck region.

Epidemiology and Etiology

The etiology of tumors of the submandibular and sublingual glands is the same as discussed in relation to salivary gland tumors of the parotid gland (see chapter 8). At a molecular level in a study that examined PCNA, Ki-67, and p53 in pleomorphic adenomas (PAs), mucoepidermoid carcinomas (MECs), and adenoid cystic carcinomas (ACCs), PCNA, Ki-67, and p53 expression for PA and ACC in the submandibular gland was similar to that reported for tumors of the parotid gland and minor salivary glands. However, there was a higher expression of these markers in MEC of the submandibular gland (Alves, Pires, and DeAlemeda et al. 2004). This may indicate that MEC of the submandibular gland is potentially more aggressive.

Approximately 10–15% of all salivary gland tumors will occur in the submandibular gland, and only 0.5–1% in the sublingual gland, so these tumors are very rare. In the submandibular gland approximately 50% of these tumors are benign. Series vary in their percentages, from 657 of 1,235 tumors (53%) benign (Auclair, Ellis, and Gnepp et al. 1991), 55% benign (Oudidi, El-Alami, and Boulaich et al. 2006), which included nonepidermoid cancers, to 39.2% benign (Rapidis et al. 2004). Pleomorphic adenoma is the commonest benign tumor in the submandibular gland, while ACC predominates for malignant tumors. In examining malignant tumors, Bhattacharyya (2004) analyzed 370 cases from the Surveillance, Epidemiology, and End Results (SEER) database, finding ACC 42.2% and MEC 22.2%, while the Rapidis et al. (2004) literature review of 356 cases showed ACC 45.3%, adenocarcinoma 14.3%, MEC 12.9%, and carcinoma ex-pleomorphic adenoma 11.2%, and Auclair, Ellis, and Gnepp et al. (1991) found ACC 24% and MEC 19% of 578 cases.

Although sublingual gland tumors are extremely rare they are important to recognize, as they have an extremely high rate of malignancy. In a review of approximately 4,000 patients with salivary tumors collected over a 55-year period, only 18 (0.5%) had sublingual gland tumors, all of which were malignant (Spiro 1995). There are very few other large series of sublingual gland tumors in the literature. Yu, Gao, and Wang et al. (2007) reported 30 cases collected over a 50-year period, all of which were malignant. In one of the author's personal series (Ord) of 9 sublingual gland tumors collected over a 16-year period at the University of Maryland, there were no benign tumors. Adenoid cystic carcinoma appears to be the commonest histologic type, followed by MEC: ACC 50%, MEC 28% (Spiro 1995), ACC 56.7% (Yu, Gao, and Wang et al. 2007), and ACC 66%, MEC 33% (Perez, Pires, and Alves et al. 2005).

Diagnosis

SUBMANDIBULAR GLAND TUMORS

Most submandibular gland tumors present with a slow-growing, painless mass inferior to the man-

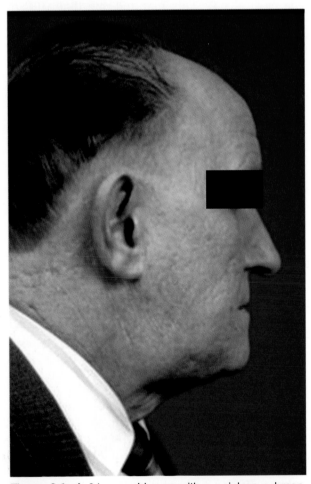

Figure 9.1. A 64-year-old man with a painless submandibular mass.

dible (Figure 9.1). In a series of 87 submandibular gland carcinomas, 94% presented with a palpable mass and 39% with pain (Kaszuba, Zafero, and Rosenthal et al. 2007). As tumors of the gland are rare and inflammatory swelling secondary to sialolithiasis is seen more often, they may not be initially diagnosed and can present with late disease. In one series 50% of all referred patients with submandibular gland tumors had already had their submandibular gland removed on the presumption that the involved process was benign (Camilleri et al. 1998). The average tumor size in 370 cases of cancer of the submandibular gland was 2.9 cm (Bhattacharyya 2004). Inflammatory disease, however, is often painful and usually characterized by exacerbations and resolutions of the swelling in relation to eating. In a series of 258 submandibular gland excisions, 119 (46%) had sialolithiasis, 88 (34%) sialadenitis, and 51 (20%) tumors (Preuss, Klussmann, and Wittekindt et al. 2007).

Examination usually reveals a smooth, firm to hard mass in the submandibular triangle that is most commonly discrete and mobile. Fixation of the mass to the skin or underlying mylohyoid muscle is a sign of malignancy with advanced extracapsular infiltration (Figure 9.2). Neural involvement of the mandibular branch of the facial nerve with ipsilateral lower lip palsy, the lingual nerve with ipsilateral anesthesia/paresthesia of the tongue, or the hypoglossal nerve with ipsilateral palsy of the tongue muscles are also signs of cancer. Associated hard cervical nodes due to regional metastasis may also be present in malignant tumors.

The differential diagnosis of a solitary mass in the submandibular triangle with no overt signs of malignancy will include lymphadenopathy, plunging ranula, vascular malformation, and branchial cysts. It may be difficult to differentiate a lymph node from the enlarged gland on clinical examination alone. If the mass is bimanually palpable from within the floor of the mouth it is more likely to be a submandibular gland mass, and if it can be "rolled" over the lower border of the mandible on palpation it is a lymph node. The plunging ranula is usually soft-cystic in consistency but can become firm if chronically encysted. Vascular lesions are also soft and may "pit" on firm pressure or have thrills and murmurs. Branchial cysts lie more posterior and are partially

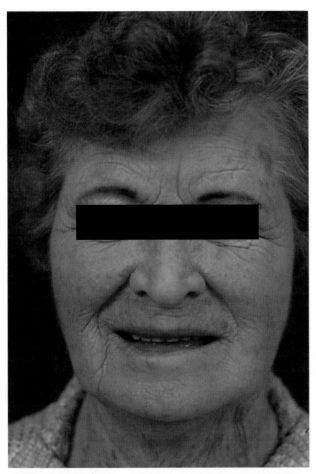

Figure 9.2a. Elderly lady with hard submandibular mass (adenoid cystic carcinoma on fine needle aspiration biopsy) who presented with a palsy of the marginal mandibular branch of the facial nerve.

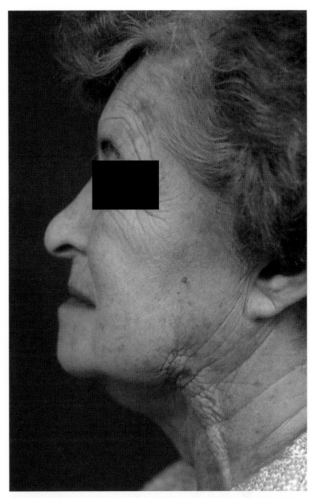

Figure 9.2b. Lateral facial view shows skin fixation and tethering.

beneath the anterior border of the sternocleido-mastoid muscle.

Imaging techniques to delineate submandibular gland lesions include ultrasound, CT, and MR. As the submandibular gland is superficial in the neck high-resolution ultrasound can distinguish intraglandular from extraglandular masses and can differentiate benign tumors from those that are malignant (Alyas, Lewis, and Williams et al. 2005). CT scanning may be useful in detecting early cortical erosion of the mandible and identifying cervical nodes in malignant cases (Figure 9.3). In a study to identify whether a submandibular mass was intra- or extraglandular, the accuracy of contrast enhanced CT was 87%, CT sialography 85%, and MR 91% (Chikui, Shimizu, and Goto et al. 2004).

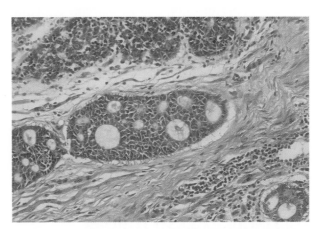

Figure 9.2c. Histopathology of adenoid cystic carcinoma of submandibular gland.

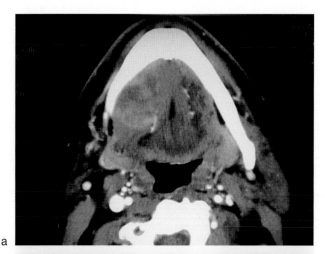

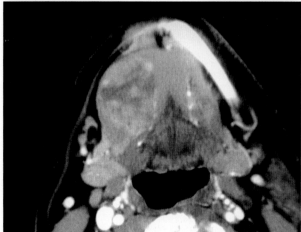

a

b

Figures 9.3a and 9.3b. CT scans showing submandibular mass with differing regions of radiolucency and opacity. Histopathology showed pleomorphic adenoma.

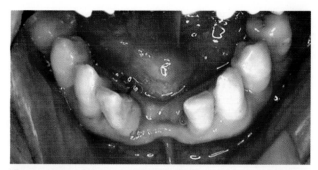

Figure 9.4a. Adenocarcinoma of right sublingual gland.

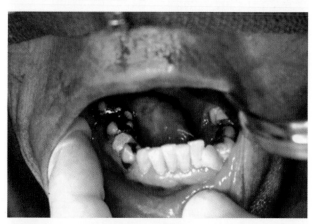

Figure 9.4b. Polymorphous low-grade adenocarcinoma of the sublingual gland. Re-published with permission from Blanchaert RG, Ord RA, Kumar D. 1998. Polymorphous low-grade adenocarcinoma of the sublingual gland. *Int J Oral Maxillofac Surg* 27:115–117.

These authors did not find displacement of the facial vein and its relationship to the mass a helpful guide.

Open biopsy of the submandibular gland mass is contraindicated for similar reasons that were discussed in relation to the parotid (see chapter 8). Fine needle aspiration biopsy (FNAB) is the method of choice for these tumors, one literature review finding an overall accuracy of greater than 80% in skilled hands, which is comparable with the accuracy of frozen section (Pogrel 1995).

SUBLINGUAL GLAND TUMORS

Tumors of the sublingual gland present as a mass in the floor of the mouth, usually painless and

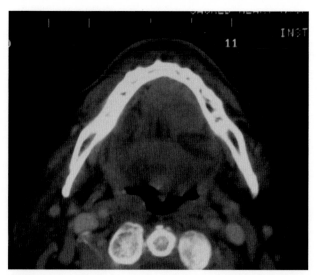

Figure 9.5. CT scan of large malignant sublingual gland tumor.

slow-growing. They may be large enough to impair tongue movement with speech difficulty or to prevent wearing a lower denture (Figure 9.4). Occasionally they may cause obstruction of Wharton's duct either due to pressure or malignant infiltration and present with a submandibular swelling. Virtually 100% of these tumors are malignant and involvement of the lingual nerve or hypoglossal nerve with ipsilateral anesthesia or weakness of the tongue may be seen. Examination by palpation reveals a firm to hard mass that may be tender and fixed to the lingual periosteum. Infiltration of the tongue muscles with slurring of speech or dysphagia can occur.

The only other entity on the differential diagnosis is a ranula, which can resemble a cystic tumor.

Imaging is usually by CT or MR. CT scans will be more accurate for early cortical bone invasion (Figure 9.5). In MR imaging T1 weighted signal intensity of carcinomas in and near the sublingual gland is lower than the gland, whereas T2 weighted signal intensity of carcinomas exceeds that of the gland (Sumi et al. 1999).

In the sublingual gland histologic diagnosis is accomplished by incisional biopsy through the overlying oral mucosa.

Management

SUBMANDIBULAR GLAND TUMORS

As in all salivary gland tumors surgery is the primary modality of treatment. When the diagnosis is established preoperatively as benign PA by FNAB, then an extracapsular excision of the submandibular gland is indicated (Figures 9.6 and 9.7). Pleomorphic adenomas should be treated in the same manner as for the parotid gland (see chapter 8). There is some evidence that the capsule of PAs in the submandibular gland is thinner than in the parotid (Webb and Eveson 2001), and it is important to maintain a margin of normal tissue around the tumor. If the entire gland and tumor is not removed but the PA merely enucleated, there is a higher risk of recurrence (Laskawi et al. 1995). In this dissection it is easy to maintain a little extra fat and connective tissue over areas where the PA may approach the surface of the gland (Figure 9.8). In a series of 15 PAs of the submandibular gland 20% were in the surface of the gland

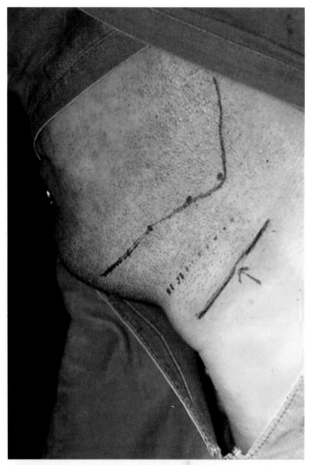

Figure 9.6a. The incision for submandibular gland tumor removal lays approximately 1–2 finger-breadths below the lower border of the mandible and is placed in a natural skin crease.

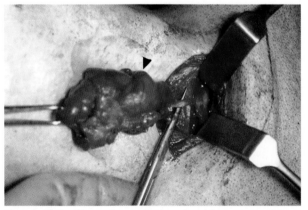

Figure 9.6b. The submandibular gland is separated from its duct, which is indicated by the sharp scissors. The arrow points to the tumor in the hilum.

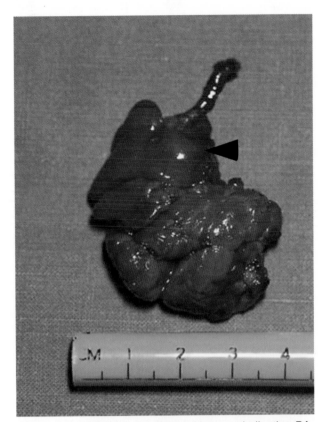

Figure 9.6c. Surgical specimen with arrow indicating PA.

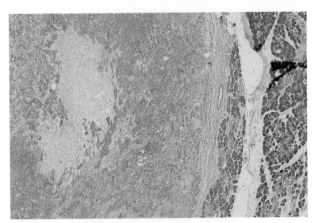

Figure 9.6d. Histopathology shows pleomorphic adenoma of submandibular gland.

(Laskawi et al. 1995) (Figure 9.9). The marginal mandibular branch of the facial nerve lies between the platysma superficially and the capsule of the submandibular gland (superficial layer of the deep cervical fascia) deeply and can be preserved either by dissecting it along its course and retracting it superiorly or by ligating and cutting the anterior

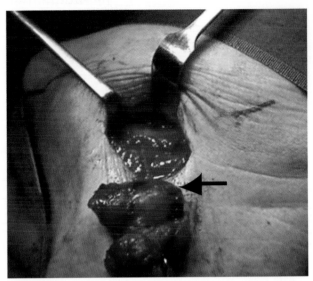

Figure 9.7. Another case of submandibular pleomorphic adenoma dissected to the duct. The larger tumor at the hilum is indicated by the arrow.

facial vein inferior to the nerve and using traction on the tied distal end of the vessel to retract the nerve out of the field (the Hayes Martin maneuver). The incidence of transient palsy of the marginal mandibular branch of the facial nerve is 7% in excising benign tumors and 21% in excising malignant tumors, with only 1 case (<1%) of permanent palsy in this series (Preuss, Klussmann, and Wittekindt et al. 2007). The facial artery is sacrificed if it passes through the gland itself, but if not its numerous small branches including the submental branch can be clipped and the main vessel preserved.

In recurrent PA the disease will frequently be multinodular as in the parotid, and as 45% of these cases involve the subcutaneous tissue under the previous operative scar, excision of the scar with a margin of the surrounding skin is recommended as part of the en bloc excision (Laskawi et al. 1995).

Where a definite diagnosis of a benign tumor is not established preoperatively or when a low-grade malignant tumor is diagnosed, an en bloc resection of level I is safest. If the final histologic diagnosis is benign no important structures have been sacrificed, only the gland and tumor plus fat with lymph nodes. If the tumor is a low-grade malignancy, then no further surgery is indicated. In the case of a high-grade tumor a selective or radical neck dissection can be completed at the same time (Figure 9.10).

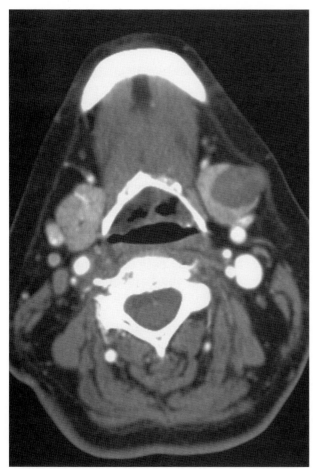

Figure 9.8a. Axial CT shows tumor projecting beyond the gland surface.

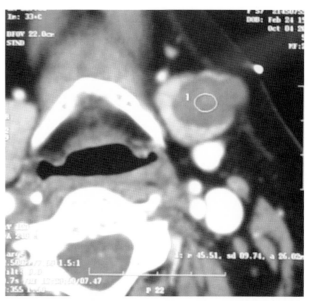

Figure 9.8c. High-power axial CT scan shows the tumor marked with a circle.

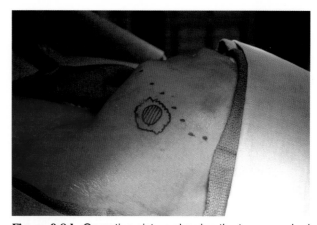

Figure 9.8d. Operative picture showing the tumor marked by palpation.

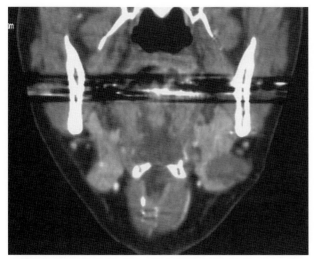

Figure 9.8b. Coronal CT confirms the surface involvement.

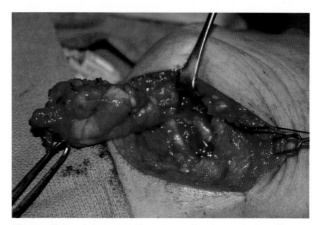

Figure 9.8e. Intraoperative view of extracapsular dissection preserving soft tissue over the tumor surface.

205

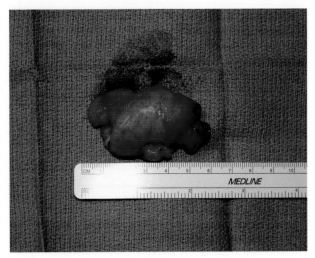

Figure 9.8f. Surgical specimen.

In undertaking the level I dissection the cervical skin flap is lifted in a subplatysmal plane and the marginal mandibular branch of the facial nerve is preserved. The anterior belly of the digastric muscle is identified and its fascia dissected free. The fascia is dissected off the mylohyoid muscle, freeing the fat and nodes from the digastric, mylohyoid, and inferior border of the mandible. The posterior edge of the mylohyoid muscle is retracted to identify the lingual nerve, which is preserved if it is uninvolved by cutting the branch to the gland and allowing the nerve to retract into the mouth. The duct is sectioned and the facial vein and artery tied off or dissected free as indicated to release the specimen. In low-grade N0 tumors a neck dissection is usually not indicated, but the excision can be extended to encompass lymph node levels II and III as a supraomohyoid neck dissection. If lymph nodes are clinically involved, then a type I modified radical neck dissection is required.

In high-grade tumors or advanced low-grade tumors with extracapsular infiltration and involvement of the skin, muscle, or mandible extended resections with incorporation of these structures will be necessary to obtain clear margins. These resections will be dictated by the size and extent of the tumor. In N0 cases selective neck dissection levels I-III or I-IV will be used and modified radical neck dissections for clinically positive necks. In the case of ACC, widespread infiltrative growth beyond the palpable tumor makes obtaining clear margins challenging. The propensity for perineural inva-

sion with ACC will necessitate sacrifice of involved nerves, for example, lingual, hypoglossal, and facial, tracing the nerves proximally using frozen section guidance to determine clearance. Unfortunately, "skip" metastases can occur along the nerve and a negative frozen section is no guarantee of success. ACC is more prone to metastasize hematogenously than through lymphatics such that a selective neck dissection is usually sufficient.

Postoperative radiation therapy is administered for high-grade tumors, positive margins, positive nodes, and perineural spread if re-resection is not possible. Chemotherapy has not been shown to improve survival in salivary gland cancer.

Prognosis will depend on the histologic grade and the stage of the tumor. Some authors (Anderson, Thrkildsen, and Ockelman et al. 1991) have found a crude 10-year survival of 50% with 10% local recurrence and 39% of cases having metastasized at the time of diagnosis. In the series reported by Rapidis et al. (2004), 8 of 14 patients died during follow-up with a survival rate of 38.5%, but 11 of 14 of these patients presented with stage III or IV disease. Bhattacharyya (2004) analyzed 370 cases of submandibular gland cancer from the SEER database and reported a 59.7% 5-year survival; however, this figure is high, as 42.2% of his cases were ACC with a mean survival of 99 months. In the same series the patients with squamous cell carcinoma had a mean survival of 52 months. Younger age, low-grade histology, and the use of radiation therapy were factors in improving survival. Weber, Byers, and Petit et al. (1990) found a 69% 5-year survival, with extracapsular infiltration and lymph node metastases indicating a poor prognosis. Stages TI-TIVA had a case-specific 5-year survival of 88% compared to 55% for T4B, and 5-year survival of 86% for negative nodes compared to 30% for positive nodes.

Most published series have found a survival benefit conferred by radiation therapy, with 75% of patients receiving adjuvant radiation in one study (Camilleri et al. 1998). Storey, Garden, and Morrison et al. (2001) report actuarial locoregional control of 88% at 5 and 10 years; however, the corresponding disease-free survival rates were 60% and 53% due to 36% of patients with locoregional control developing distant metastases.

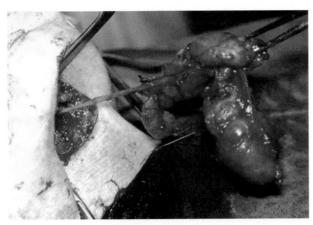

Figure 9.9a. Submandibular gland attached only by its duct. The pleomorphic adenoma is large and hangs beneath the gland attached only by the enveloping fascia of the capsule.

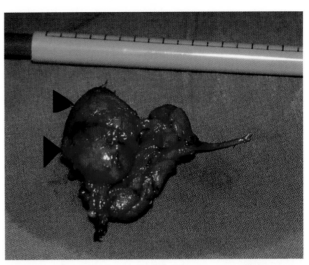

Figure 9.9b. Surgical specimen with arrows pointing to the large PA, which has no real attachment to the gland.

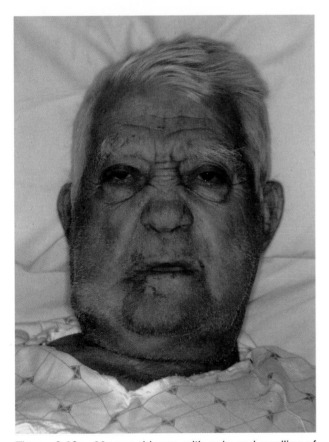

Figure 9.10a. 82-year-old man with pain and swelling of the right submandibular region.

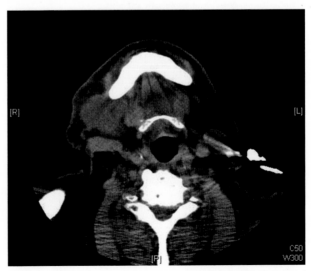

Figure 9.10b. CT scan confirms a submandibular gland mass diagnosed as malignant on fine needle aspiration biopsy.

207

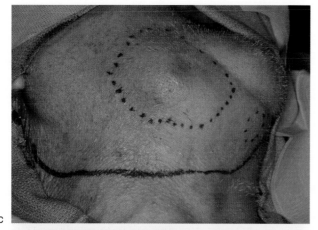

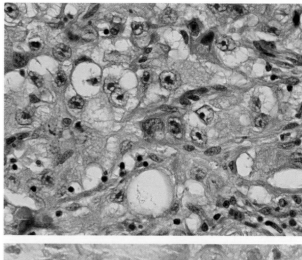

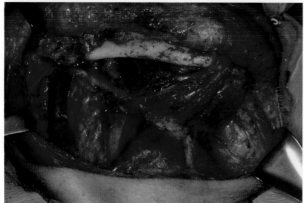

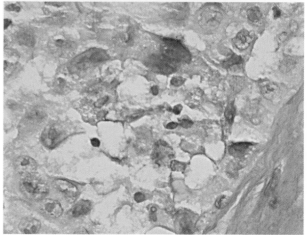

Figures 9.10c and 9.10d. Intraoperative figures showing level I excision combined with a selective neck dissection in view of high-grade cytology.

Figures 9.10f and 9.10g. Hematoxylin and eosin stain (f) and Alcian Blue stain (g) confirm a diagnosis of high-grade mucoepidermoid carcinoma.

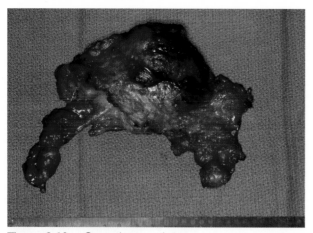

Figure 9.10e. Operative specimen.

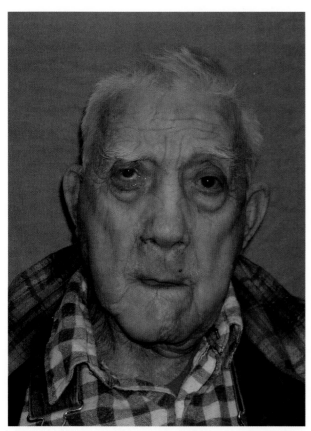

Figure 9.10h. One year postoperative view of the patient. He died 3 years postoperatively with distant metastases of the lung.

Nonetheless the median survival time for patients with locoregional control was 183 months compared to 19 months for those patients without locoregional control. In a similar study of adjuvant radiation therapy, cancer-specific survival was 79% and 57% at 5 and 10 years, with local control of 85% and 74%, respectively. Twenty percent of patients (all ACC) developed distant metastases (Sykes et al. 1999). A retrospective study of 87 patients that compared patients who received either initial enucleation of the gland (subcapsular dissection) with no evidence of residual primary or nodal disease followed by postoperative radiation therapy; or who had evidence of gross residual primary or nodal disease, grossly positive margins, or piecemeal removal following initial treatment who underwent definitive surgical resection followed by postoperative radiation therapy, found no difference in locoregional control, disease-specific survival, or overall survival (Kaszuba,

Zafero, and Rosenthal et al. 2007). This suggests patients without evidence of gross residual disease post-enucleation might be satisfactorily treated with radiation therapy without further surgery.

In a series of 22 patients with ACC of the submandibular gland, disease-free survival at 5 years of 57% and 10 years of 41% and overall survival of 70% and 37%, respectively, were found (Cohen, Damrose, and Huang et al. 2004). These authors concluded that early diagnosis, wide surgical intervention, and postoperative radiotherapy were associated with a favorable prognosis, while not surprisingly large tumor size, positive surgical margins, perineural invasion, and local recurrence were negative prognostic factors.

In comparing submandibular gland cancers to parotid cancer a poorer overall prognosis was associated with submandibular gland tumors (Hocwald, Korkmaz, and Yoo et al. 2001). In addition, the likelihood of developing distant metastasis is greater in the submandibular gland than the parotid (Schwenter et al. 2006); however, this may be due to the higher percentage of ACC. In one large series of 370 cases only 12 (3%) presented with distant metastases, but 24.9% were found to have positive regional nodes (Bhattacharyya 2004). Interestingly, in this retrospective review extraglandular extension and nodal positivity did not affect survival. Goode, Auclair, and Ellis (1998) in a study of 234 cases of MEC of the major salivary glands stated that MECs with equal histopathologic grade had a better prognosis when their tumors were in the parotid gland rather than in the submandibular gland. This finding was confirmed in a Swedish study of 2,465 major salivary gland tumors (Wahlberg, Anderson, and Bjorklund et al. 2002). High-grade MEC is also more common in the submandibular gland, with 32 of 82 cases (39%) occurring in this gland (Bhattacharyya 2004).

SUBLINGUAL GLAND TUMORS

Virtually all sublingual gland tumors will be malignant and as for all salivary tumors, primary surgery is the treatment of choice. Prognosis will be determined by the histologic grade and the stage of the tumor. In the very rare benign tumor or with small low-grade carcinomas a transoral wide local resection may be successfully performed (Blanchaert, Ord, and Kumar 1998). This will be easier to undertake in edentulous patients, and Wharton's

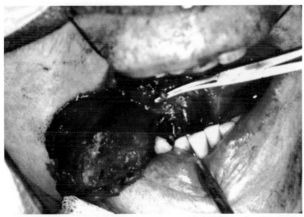

Figure 9.11. Delivering sublingual gland with low-grade malignant tumor via an intraoral wide local excision. Republished with permission from Blanchaert RG, Ord RA, Kumar D. 1998. Polymorphous low-grade adenocarcinoma of the sublingual gland. *Int J Oral Maxillofac Surg* 27:115–117.

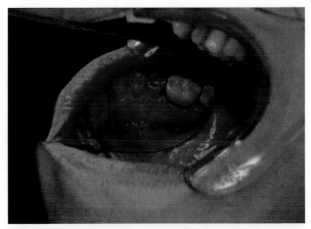

Figure 9.12a. Adenoid cystic carcinoma of sublingual gland closely approximated to the mandible (seen via an intraoral mirror photograph).

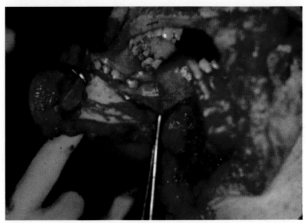

Figure 9.12b. Following lip split and mandibulotomy the periosteum is found to be uninvolved and is stripped from the mandible, which is preserved.

duct will require a sialodochoplasty procedure (Figure 9.11). In most cases due to grade, tumor size, the presence of teeth, and involvement of mandibular periosteum/bone a wider access will be required. If the periosteum is uninvolved and can be safely peeled from the lingual bone a standard "pull through" approach or a lip split with mandibulotomy can be used (Figure 9.12). The functional result of the lip split/mandibulotomy is better than the pull through (Devine, Rogers, and McNally et al. 2001). As both of these methods of access involve entering the neck, a supraomohyoid neck dissection is usually carried out in the N0 neck even for low-grade tumors (Figure 9.13).

When positive nodes are present, type I modified radical neck dissection is required. Both lingual and hypoglossal nerves can be involved by these tumors at an early stage, particularly the ACC. Sacrifice of the nerve with proximal tracing and frozen section guidance as described for the submandibular tumors may be needed. In tumors fixed to periosteum or where minimal cortical erosion is present, an oblique marginal mandibular resection angling the cut to take a greater height of the lingual plate will be utilized. The marginal mandibular resection can be performed with the pull through or mandibulotomy approach. Where the medullary bone is invaded a segmental mandibular resection with a composite en bloc resection of the floor of the mouth is safest and will provide excellent access (Figure 9.14). In these larger soft tissue resections a thin pliable flap such as the radial forearm flap probably gives the best results in maintaining tongue mobility. Where the mandible has been resected a fibular flap (Rinaldo, Shaha, and Pellitteri et al. 2004) or deep circumflex iliac artery (DCIA) flap is appropriate.

Adjuvant radiation therapy is indicated for positive nodes, perineural invasion, extracapsular nodal spread, positive margins, and high-grade histology. Prognosis for these tumors is difficult to assess, as the literature is mostly composed of case reports and small series. Spiro (1995) reported only 3 of 18 patients (16.6%) dying of their tumor with a median follow-up of 74 months. However, Yu, Gao, and Wang et al. (2007) reported distant

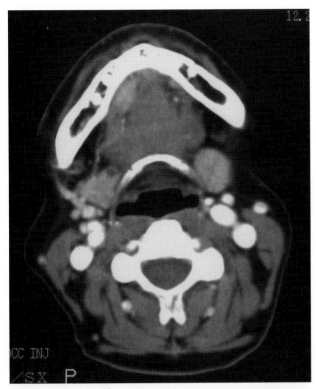

Figure 9.13a. CT scan shows low-grade mucoepidermoid carcinoma of the right sublingual gland.

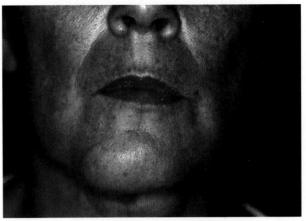

Figure 9.13c. Cosmetic result of lip split incision. Patient is alive and tumor-free 13 years postoperatively.

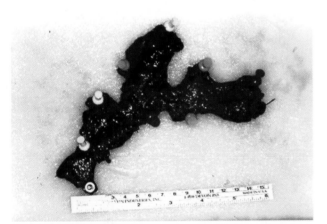

Figure 9.13b. This tumor was accessed via a lip split incision and mandibulotomy. Bilateral supraomohyoid neck dissections were undertaken, as can be seen in the surgical specimen.

metastases and local recurrence as the main cause of death with local recurrence rates of 30% and distant metastases 26.7%. In this series 56.7% of tumors were stage III.

It is reasonable to conclude that although 5-year survival from submandibular and sublingual gland cancer is reasonable, the high percentage of ACC found in these glands leads to a continuing decrease in survival at 10 years and beyond due to late local recurrence and distant metastases.

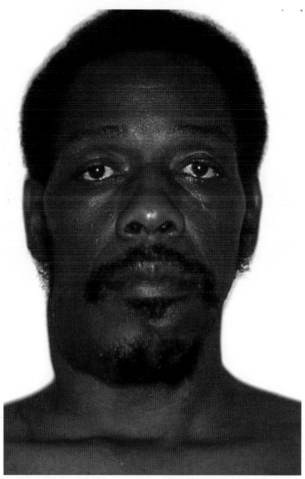

Figure 9.14a. 46-year-old African American man with left cervical lymphadenopathy.

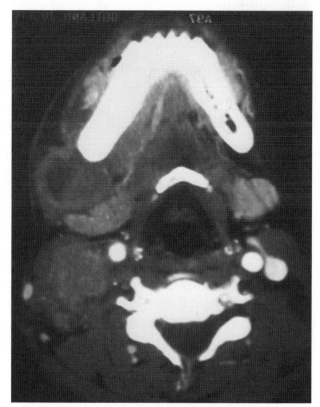

Figure 9.14c. CT scan confirms necrotic node.

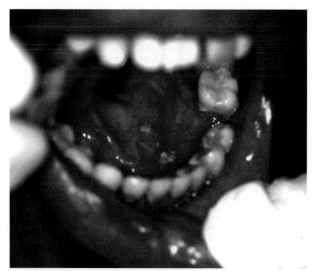

Figure 9.14b. Intraoral view of high-grade mucoepidermoid carcinoma fixed to the right mandible.

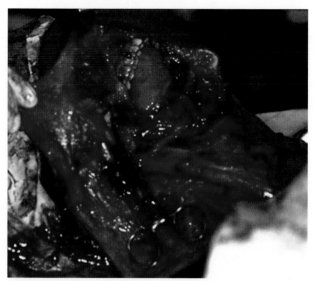

Figure 9.14d. A modified radical neck dissection and hemimandibulectomy with lip split was performed.

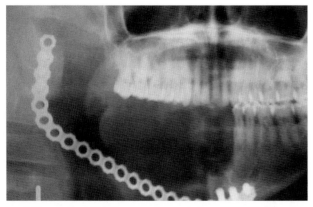

Figure 9.14e. Postoperative panoramic film showing the reconstruction plate.

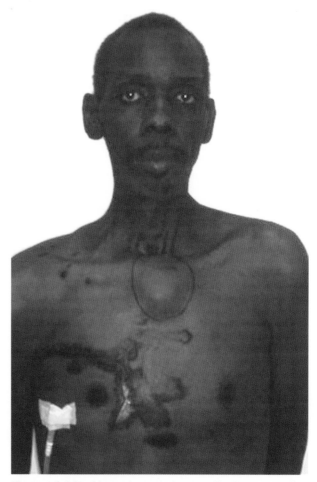

Figure 9.14g. Mass in anterior mediastinum eroding sternum and manubrium.

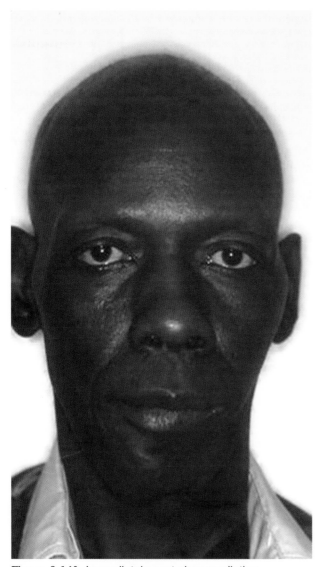

Figure 9.14f. Immediately post-chemoradiation.

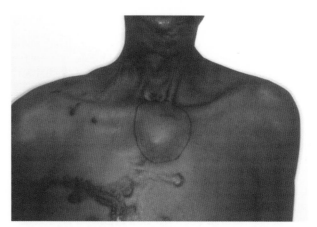

Figure 9.14h. Close-up view of manubrial mass. The patient died shortly thereafter due to lung metastases. Re-published with permission from Ord RA. 2000. Salivary gland disease. In: Fonseca R (ed.), Oral and Maxillofacial Surgery, Volume 5, Surgical Pathology. Philadelphia: W.B. Saunders Co., pp. 288–289 (Figures 10-21 a, b, c, d, e, f, g).

213

Summary

- Submandibular gland tumors comprise only 10% of salivary tumors.
- Most submandibular swellings are inflammatory in etiology.
- 50% of submandibular tumors will be malignant.
- Open biopsy should not be used for submandibular gland tumors. FNAB is the preoperative diagnostic method of choice.
- Sublingual gland tumors comprise <1% of salivary tumors.
- 90% of sublingual gland tumors are malignant.
- ACC followed by MEC are the commonest cancers in both the submandibular and sublingual glands.
- Surgical management is based on both histologic diagnosis and stage.

References

Alves FA, Pires FR, DeAlemeda OP et al. 2004. PCNA, Ki-67 and p53 expression in submandibular salivary gland tumors. *Int J Oral Maxillofac Surg* 33(6):593–597.

Alyas F, Lewis K, Williams M et al. 2005. Diseases of the submandibular gland as demonstrated using high resolution ultrasound. *Br J Radiol* 78(928):362–369.

Anderson LJ, Thrkildsen MH, Ockelman HH et al. 1991. Malignant epithelial tumors in the minor salivary glands, the submandibular gland and the sublingual gland. *Cancer* 68:2431–2437.

Auclair PL, Ellis GL, Gnepp DR et al. 1991. Salivary gland neoplasms: General considerations. In: Ellis GL, Auclair PL, Gnepp DR (eds.), Surgical Pathology of the Salivary Glands. Philadelphia: W.B. Saunders, pp. 144–145.

Bhattacharyya N. 2004. Survival and prognosis for cancer of the submandibular gland. *J Oral Maxillofac Surg* 62(4):427–430.

Blanchaert RH, Ord RA, Kumar D. 1998. Polymorphous low-grade adenocarcinoma of the sublingual gland. *Int J Oral Maxillofac Surg* 27:115–117.

Camilleri IG, Malata CM, McLean NR, Kelly CG. 1998. Malignant tumors of the submandibular salivary gland: A 15 year review. *Br J Plast Surg* 51(3):181–185.

Chikui T, Shimizu M, Goto TK et al. 2004. Interpretation of the origin of a submandibular mass by CT and MR imaging. *Oral Surg Oral Med Oral Pathol Radiol Endod* 98(6):721–729.

Cohen AN, Damrose EJ, Huang RY et al. 2004. Adenoid cystic carcinoma of the submandibular gland: A 35 year review. *Otolaryngol Head Neck Surg* 131(6):994–1000.

Devine JC, Rogers SN, McNally D et al. 2001. A comparison of aesthetic, functional and patient subjective outcomes following lip-split mandibulotomy and mandibular lingual releasing access procedures. *Int J Oral Maxillofac Surg* 30(3):199–204.

Goode RK, Auclair PL, Ellis GL. 1998. Mucoepidermoid carcinoma of the major salivary glands: Clinical and histopathologic analysis of 234 cases with evaluation of grading criteria. *Cancer* 82(7):1217–1224.

Hocwald E, Korkmaz H, Yoo GH et al. 2001. Prognostic factors in major salivary gland cancer. *Laryngoscope* 111(8):1434–1439.

Kaszuba SM, Zafero ME, Rosenthal DI et al. 2007. Effects of initial treatment on disease outcome for patients with submandibular gland carcinoma. *Arch Otolaryngol Head Neck Surg* 133(6):546–550.

Laskawi R, Ellies M, Arglebe C, Schott A. 1995. Surgical management of benign tumors of the submandibular gland: A follow up study. *J Oral Maxillofac Surg* 53(5):506–508.

Oudidi A, El-Alami MN, Boulaich M et al. 2006. Primary submandibular gland tumors: Experience based on 68 cases. *Rev Laryngol Otol Rhinol* (Bord) 127(3):187–190.

Perez DE, Pires FR, Alves FA et al. 2005. Sublingual gland tumors: Clinicopathologic study of six cases. *Oral Surg Oral Med Oral Pathol Radiol Endod* 100(4):449–453.

Pogrel MA. 1995. The diagnosis and management of tumors of the submandibular and sublingual glands. *Oral Maxillofac Clin North Amer* 7(3):565–571.

Preuss SF, Klussmann JP, Wittekindt C et al. 2007. Submandibular gland excision: 15 years of experience. *J Oral Maxillofac Surg* 65:953–957.

Rapidis AD, Stavrianos S, Lagogiannis G, Faratzis G. 2004. Tumors of the submandibular gland: Clinicopathologic analysis of 23 patients. *J Oral Maxillofac Surg* 62(10):1203–1208.

Rinaldo A, Shaha AR, Pellitteri PK et al. 2004. Management of malignant sublingual salivary gland tumors. *Oral Oncol* 40:2–5.

Schwenter I, Obrist P, Thumfart W, Sprinzi G. 2006. Distant metastasis of parotid tumors. *Acta Otolaryngol* 126(4):340–345.

Spiro RH. 1995. Treating tumors of the sublingual glands, including a useful technique for repair of the floor of mouth after resection. *Am J Surg* 170(5):457–460.

Storey MR, Garden AS, Morrison WH et al. 2001. Postoperative radiotherapy for malignant tumors of the submandibular gland. *Int J Radiat Oncol Phys* 51(4):952–958.

Sumi M, Izumi M, Yonetsu K, Nakamura T. 1999. Sublingual gland: MR features of normal and diseased states. *Am J Roentgenol* 172(3):717–722.

Sykes AJ, Slevin NJ, Birzgalis AR, Gupta NK. 1999. Submandibular gland carcinoma: An audit of local control and survival following adjuvant radiotherapy. *Oral Oncol* 35(2):187–190.

Wahlberg P, Anderson H, Bjorklund A et al. 2002. Carcinoma of the parotid and submandibular glands—a study of survival in 2,465 patients. *Oral Oncol* 38(7):706–713.

Webb AJ, Eveson JW. 2001. Pleomorphic adenomas of the major salivary glands: A study of the capsular form in relation to surgical management. *Clin Otolaryngol* 26: 134–142.

Weber RS, Byers RM, Petit B et al. 1990. Submandibular gland tumors. *Arch Otolaryngol Head Neck Surg* 116: 1055–1060.

Yu T, Gao GH, Wang XY et al. 2007. A retrospective clinicopathologic study of 30 cases of sublingual gland malignant tumors (in Chinese). *Hua Xi Kou Qiang Yi Xue Za Zhi* 25(1):64–66.

Chapter 10
Tumors of the Minor Salivary Glands

Outline

Introduction

The evaluation, diagnosis, and treatment of a patient with a mass occupying the territory of minor salivary gland tissue in the palate, buccal mucosa, or lips represent intellectually stimulating disciplines. This statement is clearly derived from the relative paucity of lesions in these anatomic areas. Salivary gland tumors in general are quite rare, accounting for only 0.2–6.6% of all human tumors (Chidzonga, Lopez-Perez, and Portilla-Alvarez 1995). Both geographic and racial factors may

explain the relative paucity of these tumors (Ansari 2007). The average annual incidence of salivary gland tumors per 100,000 population is 4.7 for benign tumors and 0.9 for malignant tumors (Ansari 2007). Both neoplastic and non-neoplastic entities are diagnosed in the salivary glands, including the minor salivary glands, thereby adding to the stimulating nature of the differential diagnosis, microscopic diagnosis, and treatment of minor salivary gland tumors. Data regarding the incidence of salivary gland tumors in general may be difficult to obtain. This is not only due to the rarity of these tumors but also to the previous non-routine nature of reporting of these diagnoses to hospital tumor registries and the occasional treatment of these lesions in office settings (Melrose 1994). It has been estimated that minor salivary gland tumors account for only 2–5% of all head and neck tumors, with malignant minor salivary gland tumors accounting for only 2–4% of all head and neck cancers (MacIntosh 1995). In 1985 Regezi et al. reported on 238 minor salivary gland tumors among 72,282 (0.33%) total oral biopsy specimens diagnosed over a 19-year period (Regezi et al. 1985). Similarly, Rivera-Bastidas, Ocanto, and Acevedo reported 62 minor salivary gland tumors from a total of 9,000 oral biopsies (0.7%) during a 24-year period (Rivera-Bastidas, Ocanto, and Acevedo 1996). Another review of 40,000 head and neck tumors over a 40-year period of time revealed 196 (0.5%) minor salivary gland tumors. Approximately 10% of all salivary gland tumors arise in the minor glands (Ord 1994). Of these minor salivary gland tumors, 70% occur in the oral cavity, 25% in the nasal cavity/sinuses/nasopharynx, and 3% occur in the larynx (MacIntosh 1995). Of the oral minor salivary gland tumors, at least 50% have been diagnosed in the palate, according to most large series (Eveson and Cawson 1985; Spiro 1986). In addition to relatively low numbers of minor salivary gland tumor diagnoses, there are controversies regarding the precise microscopic diagnosis of these tumors. In Waldron's review of 426 oral minor salivary gland tumors (Waldron, El-Mofty, and Gnepp 1988), each of these cases was reviewed by the three authors and complete concurrence of the microscopic diagnoses was reached in 346 cases (81.2%). In 49 cases, there were minor disagreements as to the diagnoses, mainly related to the subclassification of the tumors. Significant disagreement, regarding a benign vs. malignant diagnosis of the neoplasm, was noted in 21 cases (5%). Moreover, following the authors' review, their diagnoses were compared to those of the contributing pathologists. There was complete agreement in 374 cases (87.8%). These statistics exemplify the complex nature of intraoral minor salivary gland tumors, thereby questioning the exact incidence of these neoplasms as a whole as well as specific diagnoses in particular.

Minor salivary gland tumors occur not only as benign and malignant entities but also as a spectrum of cell types within these glands (Carlson 1998). The frequency of benign versus malignant tumors occurring throughout the minor glands in the oral cavity is one feature that distinguishes these tumors from their counterparts in the major glands. One series reported 15% of parotid gland tumors and 37% of submandibular gland tumors to be malignant (Eveson and Cawson 1985). In general terms, published series record that approximately 20–70% of minor salivary gland tumors are malignant (Epker and Henny 1969; Ord 1994) (Table 10.1). It seems that the center that reports the incidence of benign vs. malignant minor salivary gland tumors of the oral cavity is the primary bias in these reports. For example, tertiary care referral centers with a cancer initiative may preferentially receive patients on referral with malignant diagnoses. Spiro's report of his 35-year experience with salivary gland neoplasia at Memorial Sloan Kettering Cancer Center is a case in point. He reported on 2,807 patients, 607 of whom had minor salivary gland tumors. The frequency of malignant tumors in this report was 87%. The Armed Forces Institute of Pathology (AFIP) reported 2,945 cases of minor salivary gland tumors in 1991. By contrast, 49% of these cases were malignant. Numerous other series have reported similar figures, such that it has become reasonably well accepted that approximately 50% of minor salivary gland tumors of the oral cavity are benign and 50% are malignant.

Etiology of Minor Salivary Gland Tumors

Risk factors for salivary gland tumors have been studied extensively. Carcinoma of the major salivary glands, for example, has identified a relationship with prior radiation therapy and previous skin cancer (Spitz, Tilley, and Batsakis et al. 1984). Another study reported 31 patients who had both a newly diagnosed salivary gland tumor and a history of radiation therapy to the head and neck region (Katz and Preston-Martin 1984). Radiation therapy had been administered with a range of 11–66 years prior to the development of the salivary gland tumors. No course of radiation therapy was administered for a malignant condition, but rather for acne, hypertrophied tonsils, keloids, and other benign conditions. As such, it is reasonable to assume that a low dose of radiation therapy was administered. Only 3 cases of minor salivary gland tumors were identified among these 31 cases, including 2 adenoid cystic carcinomas and 1 mucoepidermoid carcinoma. One of the tumors was located in the palate and 2 were located in the cheek/retromolar region.

Benign and malignant salivary gland tumors have also been linked to exposure to ionizing radiation related to the atomic bombings in Hiroshima and Nagasaki during World War II. One hundred forty-five salivary gland tumors have been studied in survivors of these bombings (Saku, Hayashi, and Takahara et al. 1997). One hundred nineteen major gland tumors (27 malignant tumors, 82 benign tumors, 10 undetermined tumors) and 26 minor gland tumors (14 malignant tumors, 12 benign tumors) were identified. Among the 41 malignant tumors, the frequency of mucoepidermoid carcinoma was disproportionately high, and among the 94 benign tumors, the frequency of Warthin's tumor was high.

The association between first primary benign and malignant neoplasms of the salivary glands and the subsequent development of breast cancer has also been investigated (Abbey et al. 1984). This study identified a four-fold to five-fold increased risk of a second primary breast cancer subsequent to the first salivary gland tumor. Of note is that all of the primary salivary gland tumors were of the major glands, and 3 of the 4 patients described had benign salivary gland tumors. While no association between minor salivary gland neo-

Table 10.1. Incidence of minor salivary gland tumors

Authors	Year	Location	Number of Cases	Histology
Ansari	2007	Iran	18	Benign 11.1% Malignant 88.9%
AFIP (Auclair, Ellis, Gnepp et al.)	1991	USA	2,945	Benign 51% Malignant 49%
Chau, Radden	1986	Australia	98	Benign 62% Malignant 38%
Chidzonga, Lopez-Perez, Portilla-Alvarez	1995	Zimbabwe	282	Benign 80% Malignant 20%
Eveson, Cawson	1985	England	336	Benign 54% Malignant 46%
Isacsson, Shear	1983	Sweden	201	Benign 28% Malignant 72%
Ito, Ito, Vargas et al.	2005	Brazil	113	Benign 37% Malignant 63%
Jaber	2006	Libya	75	Benign 39% Malignant 61%
Lopes, Kowalski, Santos, Almeida	1999	Brazil	196	Benign 35% Malignant 65%
Potdar, Paymaster	1969	India	110	Benign 49% Malignant 51%
Regezi, Lloyd, Zarbo, McClatchey	1985	USA	238	Benign 65% Malignant 35%
Rivera-Bastidas, Ocanto, Acevedo	1996	Venezuela	62	Benign 55% Malignant 45%
Satko, Stanko, Longauerova	2000	Slovakia	31	Benign 48% Malignant 52%
Spiro	1986	USA	607	Benign 13% Malignant 87%
Stuteville, Corley	1967	USA	80	Benign 10% Malignant 90%
Toida, Shimokawa, Makita et al.	2005	Japan	82	Benign 67% Malignant 33%
Waldron, El-Mofty, Gnepp	1988	USA	426	Benign 58% Malignant 42%

plasia and breast cancer was established, the study nonetheless attempted to develop a relationship between the two. Moreover, the study investigated subsequent breast cancer in patients with a history of salivary gland neoplasia, rather than vice versa. As such, a risk factor for salivary gland tumor development would not be established in patients with breast cancer. In addition, minor salivary gland neoplasia was not represented in this cohort of patients. In the final analysis, there is some evidence to identify risk factors for the develop-ment of minor salivary gland tumors, yet not as much evidence as exists for the development of major salivary gland tumors.

Diagnosis of Minor Salivary Gland Tumors

The diagnosis of a minor salivary gland tumor begins with the establishment of a differential diagnosis. This differential diagnosis should be classified categorically and in order of decreasing likelihood (Carlson 1998). The evaluation of a lesion of the palate, lip, or buccal mucosa might suggest inflammatory, neoplastic, and non-neoplastic entities. Ultimately, the differential diagnosis is based on the patient's history, physical examination, and the anatomic location of the pathologic entity under scrutiny. Generally speaking, benign and malignant minor salivary gland tumors present as painless, slowly enlarging intraoral masses. When present, ulceration predicts a malignant diagnosis, although many minor salivary gland malignancies do not create ulceration of the oral mucosa. Pain is an ominous sign and is associated with perineural invasion, typically by adenoid cystic carcinoma. A painful enlargement of the minor salivary glands is malignant until proven otherwise. The presence or absence of pain therefore represents an important element of the patient's history. Special imaging studies may be obtained prior to performing the biopsy, if required at all, or they may be obtained after the establishment of a diagnosis based on incisional biopsy. Experience shows, however, that their purpose is to anatomically delineate the extent of the tumor rather than to assist in the establishment of the diagnosis. The experienced salivary gland surgeon may detect nuances on imaging studies that favor various diagnoses on the differential diagnosis. While fine needle aspiration biopsy is an essential part of the diagnosis of parotid neoplasms, it has no practical role in the diagnosis of minor salivary gland neoplasms. Rather, an incisional biopsy should be routinely performed, for example, when planning treatment of palatal tumors due to the diverse nature of possible histopathologic diagnoses, as well as the diverse nature of surgical treatment plans based on these diagnoses.

Other minor salivary gland tumor sites, such as the buccal mucosa and upper lip, require greater attention to the differential diagnosis in order to determine whether incisional or excisional biopsy best serves the needs of the patient. In many instances, the differential diagnosis may strongly support a benign neoplasm such that proceeding directly to excision is the most appropriate therapy. For example, a tumor in the upper lip that is freely moveable and associated with normal overlying mucosa indicates that an excisional biopsy may be performed in most instances due to the high likelihood of a benign tumor. A minor salivary gland tumor of the buccal mucosa, similar to the palate, has a diverse number of possibilities on the differential diagnosis such that an incisional biopsy should be considered to establish the diagnosis (Table 10.2). There are instances, however, where a freely moveable buccal mucosal tumor may be excised without preceding incisional biopsy, similar to the upper lip tumor previously described.

Treatment of Minor Salivary Gland Tumors

GENERAL PRINCIPLES OF SURGERY FOR MINOR SALIVARY GLAND TUMORS

The treatment of minor salivary gland tumors is distinctly surgical. The specific type of surgery is a function of the anatomic site of the tumor, the invasion of surrounding structures, and the histopathologic diagnosis, provided that an incisional biopsy has been performed. In general terms, a palatal minor salivary gland tumor requires an incisional biopsy so as to definitively establish the histopathologic diagnosis prior to the tumor surgery. This biopsy should be performed in the center of the mass so as to not seed the surrounding normal tissue (Freedman and Jones 1994). The decision as to whether to perform an incisional biopsy of buccal mucosal and lip masses thought to represent minor salivary gland tumors rests on the surgeon's intuition as to the benign vs. malignant nature of the mass. Smooth, freely moveable submucosal masses without fixation to the overlying mucosa are likely benign and may be treated with excisional biopsies without first performing an incisional biopsy due to the high likelihood of a benign process. By contrast, sizeable masses with mucosal fixation in these areas should probably be subjected to incisional biopsy so as to establish the diagnosis due to the concern for malignant disease. As with tumor surgery for other diagnoses, minor salivary gland tumor surgery requires a preoperative assessment of the anatomic barriers. Physical examination and imaging studies serve to delineate invasion of surrounding anatomic barriers by the tumor. In the palate, for example, it is important to determine whether the palatal bone has been invaded by the tumor. Benign tumors typically do not invade bone but may "cup it out." In such situations, it is not necessary to resect bone. Malignant tumors of the

Table 10.2. Incidence of benign and malignant minor salivary gland tumors at various sites.

Authors	Year	Palate	Lip	Buccal Mucosa
AFIP (Auclair, Ellis, Gnepp et al.)	1991	Benign 53% Malignant 47%	Benign 73% Malignant 27%	Benign 50% Malignant 50%
Chau, Radden	1986	Benign 67% Malignant 33%	Benign 77% Malignant 23%	Benign 64% Malignant 36%
Eveson, Cawson	1985	Benign 53% Malignant 47%	Benign 73% Malignant 27%	Benign 50% Malignant 50%
Isacsson, Shear	1983	Benign 78% Malignant 22%	Benign 71% Malignant 29%	Benign 89% Malignant 11%
Jaber	2006	Benign 58% Malignant 42%	Benign 46% Malignant 54%	Benign 46% Malignant 54%
Lopes, Kowalski, Santos, Almeida	1999	Benign 42% Malignant 58%	Benign 60% Malignant 40%	Benign 0% Malignant 100%
Potdar, Paymaster	1969	Benign 49% Malignant 51%	Benign 67% Malignant 33%	Benign 78% Malignant 22%
Regezi, Lloyd, Zarbo, McClatchey	1985	Benign 30% Malignant 70%	Benign 88% Malignant 12%	Benign 43% Malignant 57%
Rivera-Bastidas, Ocanto, Acevedo	1996	Benign 56% Malignant 44%	Benign 18% Malignant 82%	Benign 50% Malignant 50%
Spiro	1986	Benign 26% Malignant 84%	Benign 18% Malignant 82%	
Stuteville, Corley	1967	Benign 4% Malignant 96%	Benign 33% Malignant 67%	Benign 27% Malignant 73%
Toida, Shimokawa, Makita et al.	2005	Benign 69% Malignant 31%	Benign 67% Malignant 33%	Benign 60% Malignant 40%
Waldron, El-Mofty, Gnepp	1988	Benign 58% Malignant 42%	Benign 75% Malignant 25%	Benign 54% Malignant 46%

palate display variable involvement of the palatal bone. Imaging studies, particularly coronal bone windows, must be obtained so as to assess the involvement of the anatomic barrier of palatal bone. Minor salivary gland tumors of the upper lip and buccal mucosa exhibit different behavior regarding their invasion of the anatomic barrier of the surrounding mucosa. In general terms, it is appropriate to preserve the mucosa surrounding a benign minor salivary gland tumor of these sites, while a malignant tumor surgery in these sites requires sacrifice of the surrounding mucosa (Table 10.3).

Treatment of minor salivary gland tumors becomes predicated on the histopathologic diagnosis, which largely translates to the known biologic behavior of the neoplasm. Descriptive surgical terms may describe the sacrifice of surrounding soft and hard tissues as a matter of convenience (Carlson 1998). For example, surgical management of palatal tumors may be as straightforward as a periosteal sacrificing, bone sparing wide local excision with split thickness dissection of the soft palate. This specific surgical procedure is the main procedure performed for benign palatal tumors and also has a role to play in some low-grade malignancies (Carlson 1998). The bone-sparing, periosteally sacrificing wide local excision with full thickness sacrifice of the soft palate is reserved for deeply infiltrative low-grade malignancies of the palate. The most aggressive surgery for palatal minor salivary gland tumors is the maxillectomy, specifically reserved for the highly aggressive minor salivary gland malignancies of the palate.

SURGICAL TREATMENT OF BENIGN MINOR SALIVARY GLAND TUMORS

The treatment of benign tumors of the minor salivary glands centers on the pleomorphic adenoma, with a brief discussion of the surgery for the cana-

Table 10.3 Management of the anatomic barriers in minor salivary gland tumor surgery

Histology	Site		
	Palate	Lip	Buccal mucosa
Benign	– Mucosal sacrificing	– Mucosal sparing	– Mucosal sparing
	– Periosteal sacrificing	– Muscle sparing	– Muscle sparing
	– Bone sparing	– Skin sparing	– Skin sparing
Malignant	– Mucosal sacrificing	– Mucosal sacrificing	– Mucosal sacrificing
	– Periosteal sacrificing	– Muscle sacrificing	– Muscle sacrificing
	– Bone sacrificing (variable)	– Skin sparing (variable)	– Skin sparing (variable)

licular adenoma. The three most common minor salivary gland anatomic sites will be considered, including the palate, the lip, and the buccal mucosa.

Pleomorphic Adenoma

The terms "pleomorphic adenoma" and "mixed tumor" are equally satisfactory and interchangeable when describing this common minor salivary gland tumor. The designation "mixed" is based on the tumor's mixtures of neoplastic elements such that each mixed tumor has unique features (Melrose 1994). It has also been pointed out that the designation refers to the tumor showing combined features of epithelioid and connective tissue-like growth (Waldron 1991). There is universal agreement that the pleomorphic adenoma is the most common salivary gland tumor. The Armed Forces Institute of Pathology data of 13,749 salivary gland tumors showed 6,880 cases of pleomorphic adenoma, of which 4,359 were located in the parotid gland and 1,277 were located in minor salivary gland tissue (Auclair, Ellis, and Gnepp et al. 1991). The palate accounted for 711 of these 6,880 cases of pleomorphic adenoma (10.3%) and was the second most common site for this tumor in the AFIP data. The 711 cases in the palate represent 56% of cases located in the minor salivary glands. Interestingly, the AFIP data subclassified palatal pleomorphic adenomas into those occurring on the hard palate (118 cases) and those occurring in the soft palate (110 cases). There were 483 cases that were not specified as to location in the palate. The subclassification of specific anatomic location in the palate is of significance when working up these cases and planning surgical treatment for these patients. Those pleomorphic adenomas located primarily in the soft palate require investigation as to involvement of the parapharyngeal space.

Treatment of the palatal pleomorphic adenoma is based on the realization that this tumor does not possess a capsule. This notwithstanding, the tumor does exhibit a "pseudocapsule" represented by a loose fibrillar network surrounding the tumor. In addition, the periosteum on the superior aspect of the tumor does serve as a very competent anatomic barrier such that palatal bone may be preserved in this tumor surgery, even when the bone has been "cupped out" clinically and radiographically. Under such circumstances, the pleomorphic adenoma does not invade bone histologically such that bone resection is not warranted. In fact, it is reasonable to proceed with surgery without obtaining CT scans preoperatively. A periosteally sacrificing wide local excision is performed, observing a 5–10 mm linear margin surrounding the clinically apparent tumor (Figure 10.1). While these tumors are submucosal in nature, the mucosa must be sacrificed with the tumor due to the close proximity of the tumor and the overlying mucosa (Yih, Kratochvil, and Stewart 2005). The most appropriate linear margin of uninvolved soft tissue included at the periphery of the tumor seems to be a source of controversy (Carlson 1998; Ord 1994; Pogrel 1994). The soft palate musculature is dissected in a split thickness fashion so as to prevent an oral-nasal communication. A preoperatively fabricated palatal stent protects the exposed bone in the postoperative period until granulation tissue appears on the bone surface of the palate. There is no need to provide reconstruction of this exposed bone surface, as mucosalization ultimately occurs predictably. Negative soft tissue margins in the specimen predict a curative surgery without recurrence

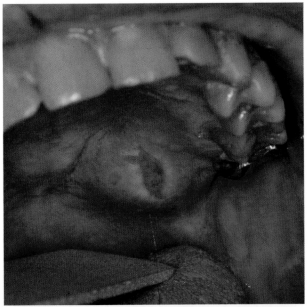

Figure 10.1a. The clinical appearance of a pleomorphic adenoma of the palate that has already undergone incisional biopsy.

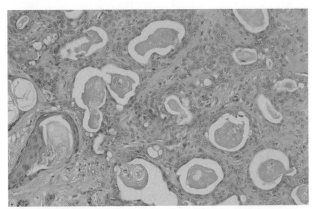

Figure 10.1b. An incisional biopsy was performed and showed an acanthomatous variant of the pleomorphic adenoma.

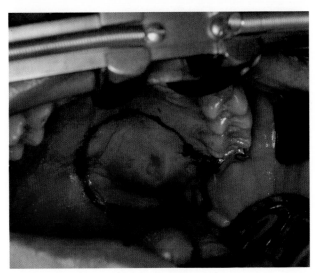

Figure 10.1c. A periosteal sacrificing, bone-sparing wide local excision with split thickness sacrifice of the soft palate was performed with a 5–10 mm linear mucosal margin.

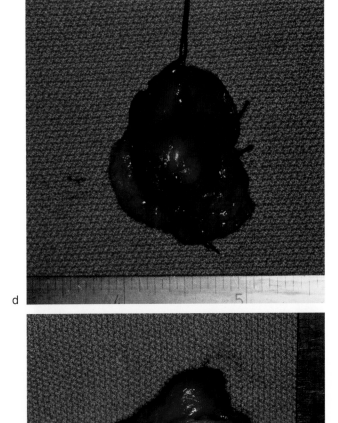

d

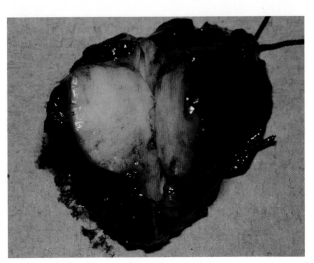

e

Figures 10.1d and 10.1e. In so doing, the periosteum serves as the superior anatomic barrier on the specimen.

Figure 10.1f. The cut specimen shows the characteristic appearance of a pleomorphic adenoma.

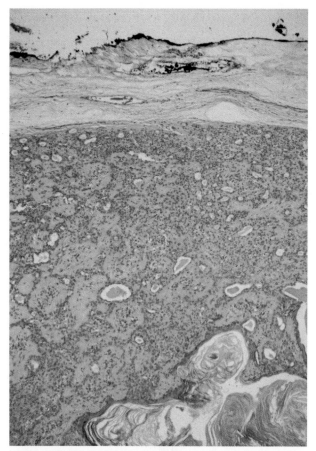

Figure 10.1g. The histopathology of the tumor specimen shows the tumor approaching but well contained within the pseudocapsule.

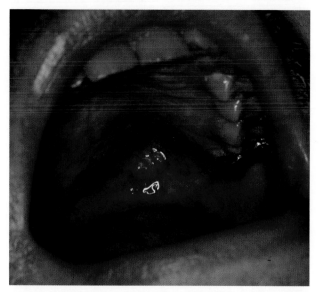

Figure 10.1i. The tissue bed is noted at 3 months postoperatively.

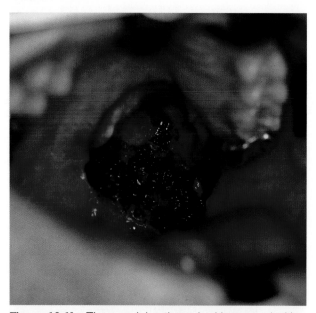

Figure 10.1h. The remaining tissue bed is covered with a surgical stent and allowed to heal with tertiary intention. No tissue coverage of the palate is required.

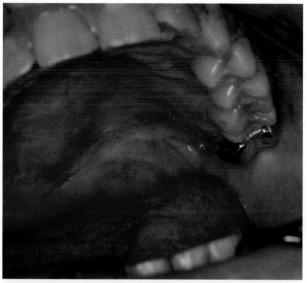

Figure 10.1j. The tissue bed is noted at 12 months postoperatively. Effective mucosalization of the exposed bone surface of the hard palate and exposed muscle surface of the soft palate has occurred.

of the tumor (Beckhardt, Weber, and Zane et al. 1995).

As previously mentioned, the pleomorphic adenoma that develops in the soft palate may be different from the pleomorphic adenoma of the hard palate, insofar as its anatomic progression is concerned. Tumors located on the hard palate will grow into the oral cavity (Figure 10.2), whereas tumors of the soft palate (Figure 10.3) may descend into the parapharyngeal space (Carlson 1998). As such, when considering the surgical treatment for a pleomorphic adenoma of the soft palate, the surgeon should obtain CT scans preoperatively so as to determine possible involvement of the parapharyngeal space. When dissection of the parapharyngeal space by the tumor is noted, a combined transoral/transcutaneous approach to tumor extirpation is indicated. A mandibular osteotomy for

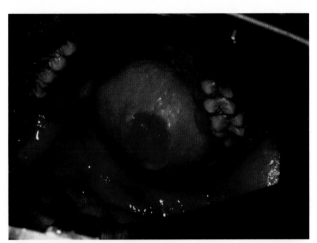

Figure 10.2. A large pleomorphic adenoma that is primarily located over the hard palate. As such, it is permitted to grow in an exophytic fashion, with cupping out of the palatal bone but no involvement of the parapharyngeal space. Reprinted with permission from Carlson ER. 1995. Salivary gland pathology—clinical perspectives and differential diagnosis. In: The Comprehensive Management of Salivary Gland Pathology, Oral and Maxillofacial Surgery Clinics of North America 7. Philadelphia: W.B. Saunders, pp. 361–386.

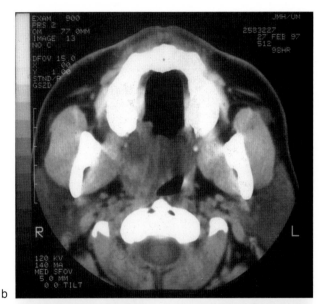

b

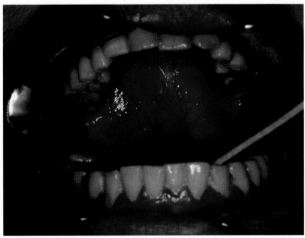

Figure 10.3a. The clinical appearance of a pleomorphic adenoma that is located primarily in the soft palate.

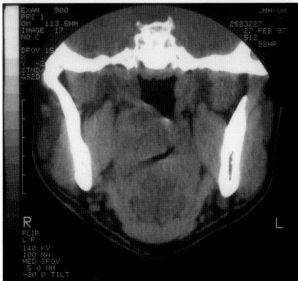

c

Figures 10.3b and 10.3c. Its chronic growth permitted entry into the parapharyngeal space, as noted on CT scans.

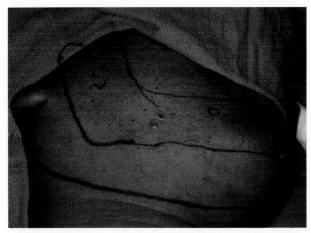

Figure 10.3d. Due to the relative inability to dissect this tumor bed entirely transorally, a decision was made to perform a combined transcutaneous and transoral approach to the tumor ablation with an Attia double osteotomy of the mandible. Wide transcutaneous access was accomplished for this tumor surgery.

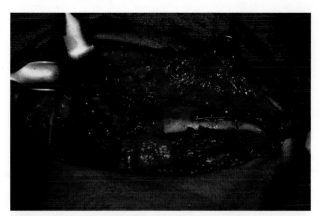

Figure 10.3f. Bone plates were placed on the mandible in preparation for the osteotomy. The plates were then removed and an Attia double osteotomy of the mandible was performed that involved a horizontal resection of the mandible superior to the mandibular foramen and a vertical resection of the mandible anterior to the mental foramen.

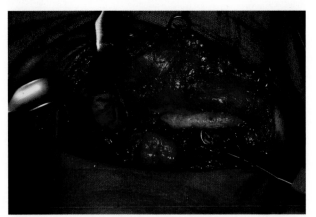

Figure 10.3e. Dissection of the mandible was performed in a subperiosteal fashion, while maintaining as much periosteum and muscle as possible on the lateral surface of the mandible.

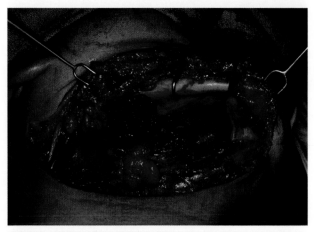

Figure 10.3g. Superior reflection of the mandibular segment was then able to be accomplished.

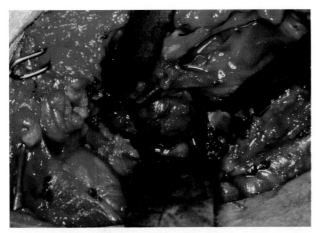

Figure 10.3h. Reflection of the medial surface of the medial pterygoid muscle permitted entry into the parapharyngeal space with identification of the tumor.

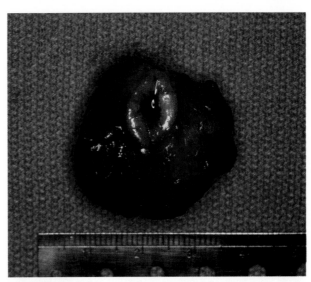

Figure 10.3j. The combination of transcutaneous access and transoral access permitted safe delivery of the specimen.

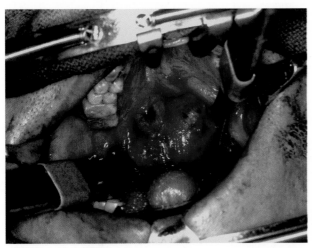

Figure 10.3i. With the great vessels of the neck protected, the tumor ablation continued intraorally with development of the tumor dissection surrounding the pseudocapsule.

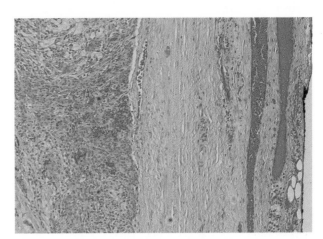

Figure 10.3k. Histopathology identified a pleomorphic adenoma with tumor present in the pseudocapsule, but with negative margins.

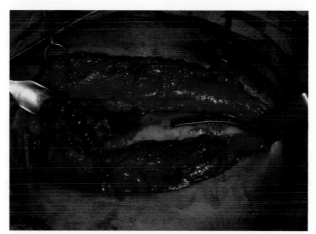

Figure 10.3l. Following delivery of the specimen, the plates are replaced on the mandible and closure occurred.

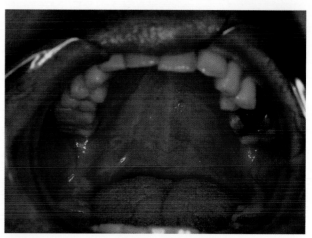

Figure 10.3m. The 6-month postoperative view of the palate is noted. This surgery was curative for this patient's tumor. Reprinted with permission from Carlson ER, Schimmele SR. 1998. The management of minor salivary gland tumors of the oral cavity. In: Surgical Management of Salivary Gland Disease, The Atlas of the Oral and Maxillofacial Surgery Clinics of North America 6. Philadelphia: W.B. Saunders, pp. 75–98.

effective dissection of the tumor bed and protection of the great vessels in the neck may be indicated.

Pleomorphic adenomas are known to occur in other minor salivary gland sites, including the lip, buccal mucosa, and tongue. Lip tumors accounted for 297 cases in the AFIP files, of which a majority occurred in the upper lip. Lower lip pleomorphic adenomas are very rare. The buccal mucosa accounted for 126 cases in the AFIP series. The surgery required for removal of pleomorphic adenomas in the lip and buccal mucosa involves an excision of the tumor and associated minor salivary gland tissue. The plane of dissection is "peri-pseudocapsular" in nature. This ensures an anatomic barrier of fascia surrounding the tumor. These tumor surgeries are curative as long as tumor spillage does not occur intraoperatively. Subtherapeutic ablation of these tumors in the form of an enucleation will certainly predispose the patient to persistent disease. Such recurrences are noted to be multifocal in nature as originally described in the major salivary glands (Foote and Frazell 1953).

Malignant pleomorphic adenomas of salivary gland origin are uncommon neoplasms. The broad heading, malignant mixed tumor, includes three different clinical and pathologic entities: *carcinoma ex-pleomorphic adenoma, carcinosarcoma,* and *metastasizing pleomorphic adenoma.* Carcinoma ex-pleomorphic adenoma, perhaps the most commonly referenced malignant pleomorphic adenoma, is a pleomorphic adenoma in which a second neo-

plasm develops from the epithelial component that fulfills the criteria for malignancy. These features include invasiveness, destruction of normal tissues, cellular anaplasia, cellular pleomorphism, atypical mitoses, and abnormal architectural patterns (Wenig and Gnepp 1991). The AFIP data showed 326 cases of carcinoma ex-pleomorphic adenoma, which accounted for 2.4% of their 13,749 cases. A significant majority of these were located in the parotid gland (64.4%); however, these malignancies occurred in the minor salivary glands, as well. The palate accounted for 36 of 57 cases in the minor glands, with the upper lip (6 cases), tongue (4 cases), and cheek (4 cases) also represented. A review of this tumor shows that preoperative duration of a benign pleomorphic adenoma is the main determining factor regarding malignant transformation. Specifically, the incidence of malignancy progressively increases from 1.6% for tumors present for less than 5 years to 9.4% for tumors present for periods longer than 15 years (Wenig and Gnepp 1991). The other predisposing condition for the development of this malignancy is recurrence of a benign pleomorphic adenoma. This fact supports a curative approach to the pleomorphic adenoma from the outset, with abandonment of the subtherapeutic enucleation of these tumors in the parotid gland or minor salivary gland tissues.

The prognosis for this malignancy is generally considered dismal, with 71% of patients exhibiting metastatic disease during the course of their disease.

Carcinosarcoma, also known as true malignant pleomorphic adenoma, is a tumor defined by histologic evidence of malignancy in both the epithelial and stromal elements of the tumor. These tumors are more rare than the carcinoma ex-pleomorphic adenoma, accounting for only 8 cases in the AFIP registry, and none occurred in the minor salivary glands. Other cases presented in the literature do identify the existence of this diagnosis in the minor salivary glands.

Metastasizing mixed tumor is a histologically benign pleomorphic adenoma, but located in distant sites. The pleomorphic adenomas are known to arise in major as well as minor salivary glands, and the metastatic foci have been identified in the cervical lymph nodes, spine, and liver (Wenig and Gnepp 1991). Data on the interval from removal of the primary tumor to the identification of the first metastasis is 1.5–51 years, with an average of 16.6 years.

Canalicular Adenoma

The canalicular adenoma is a benign tumor that has a significant predilection for the upper lip (Figure 10.4). In the past, this tumor was more commonly referred to as a "monomorphic adenoma." Gardner recommended that the term monomorphic adenoma be used as a nosologic group of epithelial salivary gland tumors that are not pleomorphic adenomas (Gardner and Daley 1983). The canalicular adenoma and basal cell adenoma identify specific forms of monomorphic

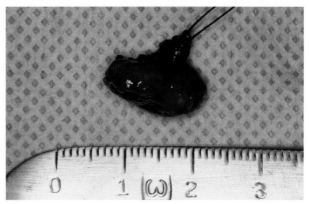

Figure 10.4b. Based on this assumption, an incisional biopsy is not required. A pericapsular dissection and excision of this mass was performed in association with surrounding minor salivary gland tissue, thereby allowing for delivery of the specimen.

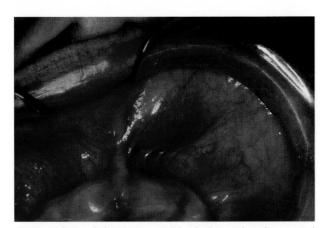

Figure 10.4a. A freely moveable, indurated, submucosal mass of the upper lip in an elderly woman, highly suggestive of a canalicular adenoma.

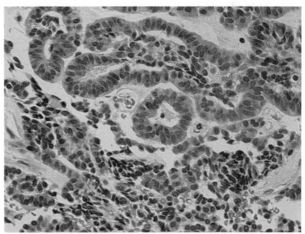

Figure 10.4c. The histopathology of the specimen confirms the clinical impression of canalicular adenoma. Reprinted with permission from Carlson ER, Schimmele SR. 1998. The management of minor salivary gland tumors of the oral cavity. In: Surgical Management of Salivary Gland Disease, The Atlas of the Oral and Maxillofacial Surgery Clinics of North America 6. Philadelphia: W.B. Saunders, pp. 75–98.

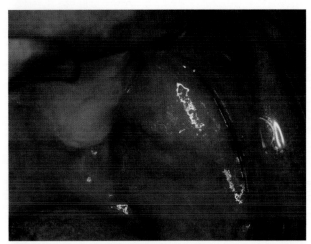

Figure 10.5a. A freely moveable, indurated, submucosal mass of the buccal mucosa is noted in this patient.

adenomas (Daley, Gardner, and Smout 1984). The canalicular adenoma classically occurs in the upper lip in elderly women (Kratochvil 1991). In fact, canalicular adenomas typically affect an older population compared to pleomorphic adenomas (Ord 1994). The canalicular adenoma is typically an asymptomatic, slow-growing, and freely moveable mass that uncommonly exceeds 2 cm in widest diameter. It may resemble mucoceles, which are uncommonly located in the upper lip. Of the 121 canalicular adenomas in the AFIP files, 89 of them occurred in the upper lip. The second most common site was the buccal mucosa (Auclair, Ellis, and Gnepp et al. 1991). The tumor is encapsulated such that an excision of the tumor in any anatomic site in a pericapsular fashion represents a curative surgery provided that tumor spillage does not occur (Figure 10.5). The canalicular adenoma is multifocal in 20% of cases (Ord 1994). If recurrence is believed to have occurred, it might actually represent a new primary tumor (Melrose 1994).

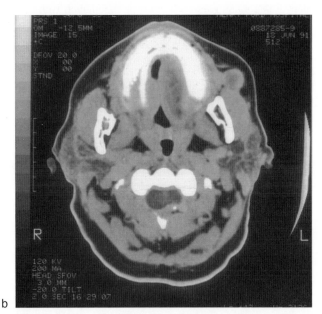

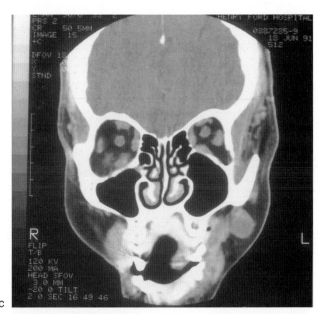

b   c

Figures 10.5b and 10.5c. The CT scans show a well-circumscribed mass of this region.

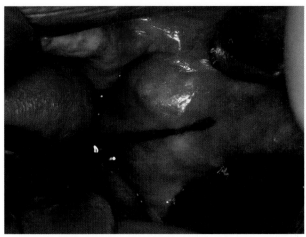

Figure 10.5d. A benign neoplastic process occupies a high position on the differential diagnosis such that a mucosal-sparing excision of the mass with transoral access is able to be performed without first obtaining an incisional biopsy.

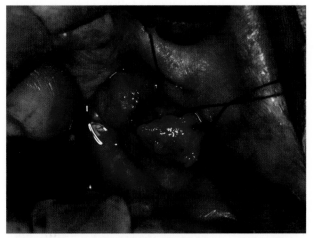

Figure 10.5e. A pericapsular dissection is performed.

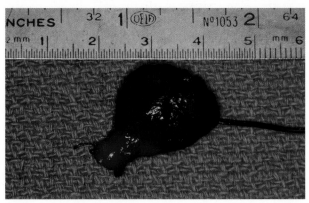

Figure 10.5f. This dissection permits delivery of the specimen. Stenson's duct was intimately attached to the tumor and therefore sacrificed with the tumor.

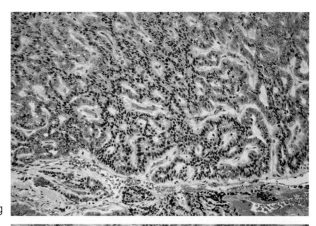

g

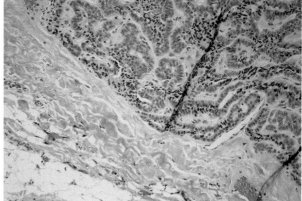

h

Figures 10.5g and 10.5h. Histopathology identified canalicular adenoma (g) with an uninvolved capsule (h).

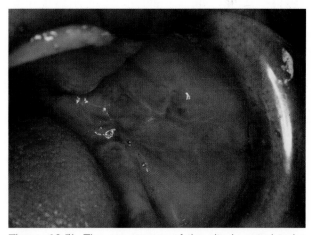

Figure 10.5i. The appearance of the site is noted to be well healed at 9 months postoperatively. Reprinted with permission from Carlson ER. 1995. Salivary gland pathology—clinical perspectives and differential diagnosis. In: The Comprehensive Management of Salivary Gland Pathology, Oral and Maxillofacial Surgery Clinics of North America 7. Philadelphia: W.B. Saunders, pp. 361–386.

SURGICAL TREATMENT OF MALIGNANT MINOR SALIVARY GLAND TUMORS

The malignant diagnoses in the minor salivary glands are more diverse than their benign counterparts. These malignant diagnoses may be low grade or high grade, and most represent histopathologic diagnostic challenges. As with the benign minor salivary gland tumors, surgery represents the hallmark of therapy for malignant minor salivary gland tumors, and the principles of surgery have not changed significantly over the past several decades (Bell et al. 2005). In addition to eradication of the primary malignancy, consideration should be given for neck dissection in very specific circumstances, as well as postoperative radiation therapy in this cohort of patients.

Mucoepidermoid Carcinoma

The mucoepidermoid carcinoma is the second most common tumor of the salivary glands overall, the most common salivary gland malignancy overall, and the most common minor salivary gland malignancy (Auclair and Ellis 1991). During the greater than 60 years since its first description, this neoplasm has generated significant debate regarding the possible existence of a benign variant, the optimal number of grades, and the proper treatment for certain minor salivary gland lesions. The term "mucoepidermoid tumor" was first introduced by Stewart, Foote, and Becker in 1945 in their publication of 45 cases (Stewart, Foote, and Becker 1945). In this report, only two grades were utilized, including relatively favorable (benign) and highly unfavorable (malignant) tumors. The authors indicated that the adjective "benign" was rarely ever applicable in an absolute sense and as used in their report did not imply innocent behavior. It did indicate, however, that the authors had not observed metastasis from these tumors. The designation "malignant" indicated a histologic structure that was associated with the ability to produce regional lymph node and distant metastases. This notwithstanding, the authors explicitly referred to and separated the benign and malignant tumors in their series of 45 cases in this report, of which there were 26 "benign" tumors and 19 "malignant" tumors. In 1953 this grading scheme was modified to include three grades due to the development of metastases related to tumors previously referred to as benign (Foote and Frazell 1953). These investigators accepted all of these tumors as malignant, and clinical and pathologic correlation suggested that separation into low-, intermediate-, and high-grade malignant subgroups might be useful, mainly due to histologically overlapping qualities. The designation of intermediate grade was recognized as behaving more like the low-grade tumors than the high-grade tumors. Interestingly, despite the authors' recognition that all of these tumors were malignant, the designation "mucoepidermoid tumor" persisted throughout their paper. Subsequent studies were undertaken to more objectively determine if a benign variant existed. One such study investigated 23 mucoepidermoid carcinomas with a malignant course, such as evidence of local extension of tumor outside the capsule, local recurrences, histologically verified metastases, or death due to the tumor (Eneroth et al. 1972). Fifteen patients showed local recurrences, 13 showed histologically verified metastases, and 22 patients died of their disease. In 7 of the 23 cases the histology revealed highly or moderately differentiated structures, and in 3 of these cases the primary tumor as well as the lymph node metastases were highly differentiated. Six of the 23 patients had tumors in the palate, with 2 of these patients developing recurrences, 1 with lymph node metastases, and 5 of the patients died due to their disease. The authors concluded by stating that well-differentiated metastases in cases with a malignant course contradicted the existence of a benign variety of mucoepidermoid carcinoma, such that all of these neoplasms should be considered cancers (Eneroth et al. 1972).

Of the 712 mucoepidermoid carcinomas occurring in the minor salivary glands in the AFIP registry, 305 (43%) of them were noted in the palate, 93 (13%) in the buccal mucosa, and 58 (8%) in the lip, with 37 specifically designated as the upper lip and 12 specifically designated as the lower lip (Auclair, Ellis, and Gnepp et al. 1991). While the AFIP data is generally recognized as being representative of the incidence of most salivary gland tumors, some authors have identified the mucoepidermoid carcinoma to be more common in minor salivary gland sites than in major salivary gland sites (Plambeck, Friedrich, and Schmelzle 1996).

Histologic grading of mucoepidermoid carcinomas is an important exercise. Histologic grade connotes biologic aggressiveness and prognosis and also provides the surgeon with important information with which to plan surgical treatment (Brandwein, Ivanov, and Wallace et al. 2001; Evans 1984). Mucoepidermoid carcinomas are composed of three cell types: mucous secreting, epidermoid, and intermediate. The intermediate cell is appropriately named because it is likely the progenitor of the two other cells (Batsakis and Luna 1990). Three grading schemes have found general acceptance among pathologists, and differences in biologic behavior could be demonstrated as a function of grade, even though clinical stage has also been considered an important prognosticator. Indeed, Brandwein, Ivanov, and Wallace et al. (2001) found that only 5% of low-grade mucoepidermoid carcinomas of the major glands, and only 2.5% of low-grade mucoepidermoid carcinomas of the minor glands, metastasized to regional lymph nodes or resulted in death. Spiro indicated that survival of patients with minor salivary gland carcinoma is significantly influenced by the clinical stage and the histologic grade, but the applicability of grading to survival was limited to patients with mucoepidermoid carcinoma or adenocarcinoma in their study (Spiro, Thaler, and Hicks et al. 1991). They determined that staging was important in all patients regardless of the histologic diagnosis.

The mucoepidermoid carcinoma is the most common salivary gland malignancy in children (Auclair, Ellis, and Gnepp et al. 1991; Luna, Batsakis, and El-Naggar 1991; Ord 1994; Rogerson 1995). Although most of these tumors are noted in the parotid gland, the palate is the second most common site of involvement. Most appear to occur in teenagers, and the majority are low-grade or intermediate-grade histology. Mucoepidermoid carcinoma in children appears to follow a more favorable course with cure rates of 98–100% (Ord 1994).

Surgical treatment of the mucoepidermoid carcinoma of minor salivary gland origin is primarily a function of the anatomic site of the tumor and its histologic grade. Those arising in the palate are not only the most common but also the most variable insofar as surgical treatment is concerned. It is the histologic grade that is of utmost importance when determining treatment in the palate. Large series show that low-grade cancer is most common in this anatomic site (Pires et al. 2007). Incisional biopsy is clearly essential to establish the histopathologic diagnosis, as previously described. Computerized tomograms are essential in planning surgical treatment of palatal mucoepi-

dermoid carcinomas, as they assess the involvement of the underlying palatal bone. When the palatal bone does not appear to be involved by the cancer, a bone-sparing, periosteal sacrificing wide local excision with split thickness sacrifice of the soft palate musculature is the surgical treatment of choice (Figure 10.6). Similar to the surgery for the palatal pleomorphic adenoma, the periosteum serves as the anatomic barrier on the superior aspect of the tumor specimen, and tumor-free peri-

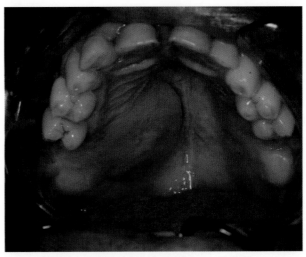

Figure 10.6a. A mass of the palate in a 45-year-old man.

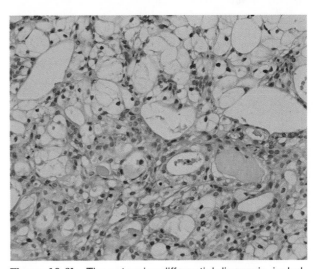

Figure 10.6b. The extensive differential diagnosis, including benign and malignant entities, requires an incisional biopsy for diagnosis prior to performing definitive tumor surgery. The biopsy identifies low-grade mucoepidermoid carcinoma.

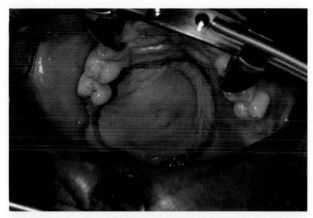

Figure 10.6c. A periosteal sacrificing, bone-sparing wide local excision with split thickness sacrifice of the soft palate is planned with 1 cm mucosal linear margins.

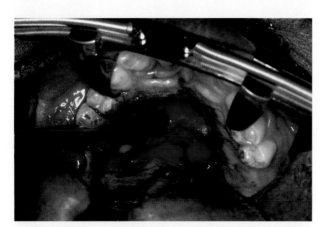

Figure 10.6d. A sharp dissection is performed with a periosteal elevator between the periosteum on the superior aspect of the tumor specimen and the overlying palatal bone.

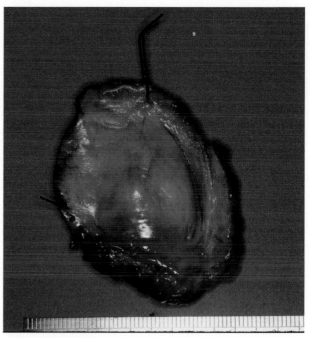

Figure 10.6e. The specimen is delivered and oriented for the pathologist with sutures. Histopathology shows low-grade mucoepidermoid carcinoma with negative margins.

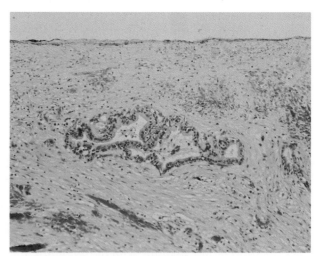

Figure 10.6f. The association of the superior aspect of the tumor and the periosteum is noted histologically.

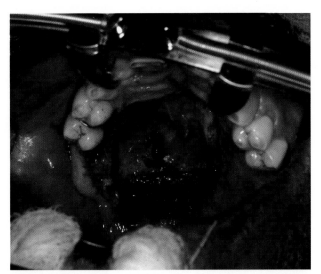

Figure 10.6g. The remaining tissue bed is temporarily covered with a palatal stent.

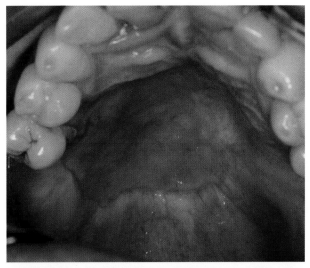

Figure 10.6h. Mucosalization of the exposed bone and soft palate musculature is noted at 9 months postoperatively. This surgery provided curative care for this patient's tumor. Reprinted with permission from Carlson ER, Schimmele SR. 1998. The management of minor salivary gland tumors of the oral cavity. In: Surgical Management of Salivary Gland Disease, The Atlas of the Oral and Maxillofacial Surgery Clinics of North America 6. Philadelphia: W.B. Saunders, pp. 75–98.

osteal frozen and permanent sections should be obtained so as to confirm this concept. When the periosteum has not been invaded by the cancer and all radial soft tissue margins are free of tumor, this surgery has a high frequency of cure.

The designation of an intermediate mucoepidermoid carcinoma of the palate may change the recommended surgical treatment of the tumor in this and other anatomic sites, with a more aggressive surgical procedure required for curative intent (Figure 10.7). This is particularly true if the designation of intermediate grade is made by the pathologist based on the worst microscopic pattern observed in the tumor. For example, a mucoepidermoid carcinoma that is predominantly low grade, but that shows a component of intermediate-grade cancer, will likely be designated intermediate grade. The behavior of such a tumor is likely to be low grade in nature. This scenario is different from a cancer that is designated intermediate grade that shows a predominantly intermediate-grade pattern with intermixed low-grade cancer. The surgeon may wish to offer more aggressive surgical therapy in the form of a partial maxillectomy for the mucoepidermoid carcinoma of the palate that is predominantly intermediate grade on microscopic sections. While rare, a high-grade mucoepidermoid carcinoma of the palate would require a partial maxillectomy, and prophylactic surgical treatment of the neck in the case of an N0 neck, or a therapeutic neck dissection in the case of an N+ neck. Postoperative radiation

therapy would also be administered in such circumstances.

Mucoepidermoid carcinoma of the buccal mucosa is the second most common minor salivary gland site affected. In contrast to benign neoplasms of this anatomic site, a mucosal-sacrificing tumor surgery is required, with attention to the sacrifice of surrounding submucosal anatomic barriers. The same is true of the lip (Figure 10.8).

Survival of patients with mucoepidermoid carcinomas of the minor salivary glands is clearly related to grade. Five-year survival rates have been estimated at 90% and 15-year survival rates have been estimated at 82% for low-grade mucoepidermoid carcinomas (Ord 1994).

Adenoid Cystic Carcinoma

Like the mucoepidermoid carcinoma, the adenoid cystic carcinoma is a very diverse tumor with three histologic variants. These have been described morphologically rather than by grade as is the case with the mucoepidermoid carcinoma, and include the tubular, cribriform, and solid variants. The adenoid cystic carcinoma is characteristically slow growing, with a high propensity for recurrent disease. It is highly infiltrative, exhibits profound neurotropism, and is associated with a dismal long-term survival rate. This malignancy was first described by Theodor Billroth in 1859 and referred to as "cylindroma" (Tomich 1991). In 1953 Foote and Frazell proposed the currently accepted nomenclature, adenoid cystic carcinoma. Of the 600 cases of adenoid cystic carcinoma in the AFIP files, 312 were noted in the major salivary glands, and 288 were noted in the minor salivary glands. The palate was the most common site affected in the minor salivary glands, followed by the tongue. Adenoid cystic carcinoma accounts for 8.3% of all palatal salivary gland tumors and 17.7% of all malignant palatal salivary gland tumors in the AFIP series (Tomich 1991).

From a surgical standpoint, adenoid cystic carcinoma is probably the most challenging salivary gland tumor for the surgeon (Ord 1994). While straightforward to perform in most cases,

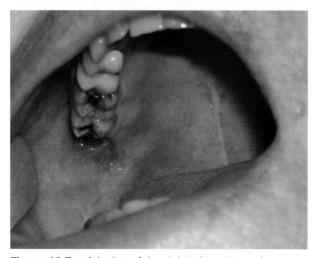

Figure 10.7a. A lesion of the right tuberosity region.

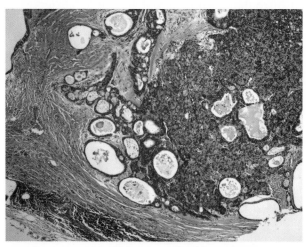

Figure 10.7b. The biopsy of the lesion from Figure 10.7a showed intermediate-grade mucoepidermoid carcinoma.

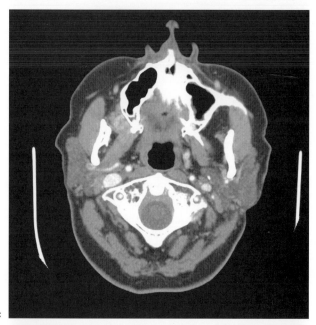

c

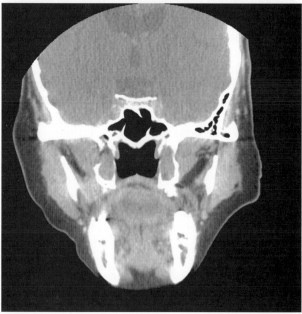

d

Figures 10.7c and 10.7d. Computerized tomograms identified an enhancing mass located lateral to the right tuberosity.

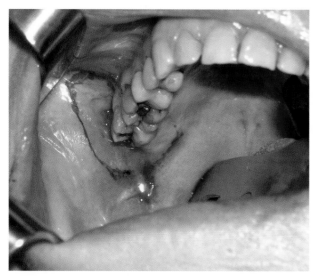

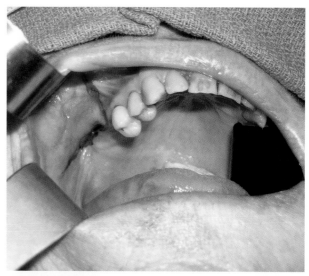

Figure 10.7e. Definitive tumor surgery involved a transoral partial maxillectomy and coronoidectomy en bloc.

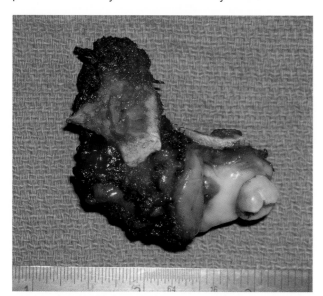

Figure 10.7f. The cancer from Figure 10.7e.

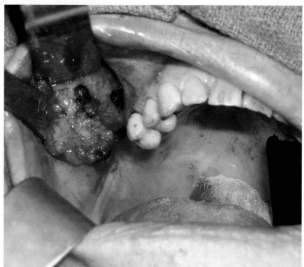

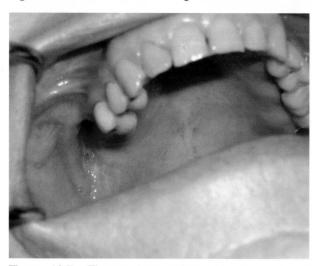

Figure 10.7g. The resultant defect was obturated and allowed to contract significantly over time.

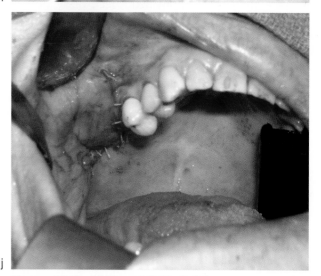

Figures 10.7h, 10.7i, and 10.7j. Soft tissue reconstruction was accomplished with a buccal fat flap and advancement of the mucosa.

237

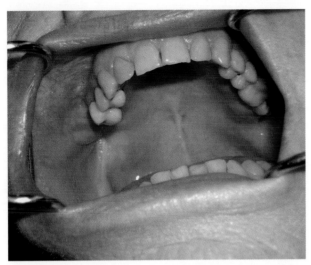

Figure 10.7k. The reconstruction healed well as noted at 1 year postoperatively.

radical resection is fraught with recurrences and ultimate distant metastases. This notwithstanding, palatal tumors should be managed with radical maxillectomy, observing 1–2 cm linear margins, and with resection of the greater palatine neurovascular bundle to foramen rotundum with frozen section guidance (Figure 10.9). The presence or absence of tumor in association with this nerve should be documented as far superior as possible. Cervical lymph node metastases are considered to be rare such that prophylactic neck dissection is not required in the patient with an N0 neck. Postoperative radiation therapy is generally considered advisable for all patients with adenoid cystic carcinoma of the minor salivary glands, regardless of the adequacy of the resection (Dragovic 1995; Ord 1994; Triantafillidou et al. 2006). The prognosis associated with adenoid cystic carcinoma of the minor salivary glands is inferior to that of the major salivary glands (Ampil and Misra 1987; Nascimento, Amaral, and Prado et al. 1986). In addition, it has been found that the best prognosis for the adenoid cystic carcinoma is associated with the tubular variant, while the solid variant is associated with the worst prognosis (Perzin, Gullane, and Clairmont 1978). It has also been pointed out that perineural invasion of major nerves and positive margins at surgery, in addition to the solid variant of adenoid cystic carcinoma, are associated with increased treatment failures (Fordice et al. 1999). Typical survival statistics for adenoid cystic carcinoma in general include 60% for 5-year sur-

vival, 30% for 10-year survival, and 7% for survival at 20 years (Ord 1994). It has been pointed out that adenoid cystic carcinoma of minor salivary gland sites has a worse prognosis, with a 0% survival at 20 years (Ord 1994). The presence of perineural spread has a significant impact on survival. Five-year survival rates of patients with perineural spread have been found to be 36.9%, while 5-year survival rates have been found to be 93.8% in patients without perineural spread (Ord 1994).

Polymorphous Low-Grade Adenocarcinoma

In 1983 two separate investigations reported on low-grade adenocarcinomas of minor salivary glands referred to as "terminal duct carcinoma" (Batsakis, Pinkston, and Luna et al. 1983) and "lobular carcinoma" (Freedman and Lumerman 1983). Terminal duct carcinoma was suggested to specify the histogenesis of the tumor, which was thought to be the progenitor cell of the terminal duct. Lobular carcinoma was suggested due to the morphology of the tumor resembling lobular carcinoma of the breast. A review of these reports indicates that the authors were independently describing the same neoplasm (Wenig and Gnepp 1991). It is thought that, prior to this time, these neoplasms were classified as either adenoid cystic carcinoma or adenocarcinoma (Regezi et al. 1991). High-power evaluation of polymorphous low-grade adenocarcinoma and adenoid cystic carcinoma may permit the distinction between the two malignancies, as adenoid cystic carcinoma shows ductal-type structures lined by multiple cells in thickness, while polymorphous low-grade carcinoma shows ductal-type structures more commonly lined by single cell layers (Figure 10.10). An Indian filing pattern is also seen in polymorphous low-grade adenocarcinoma. The common morphologic features of polymorphous low-grade adenocarcinoma and adenoid cystic carcinoma have led researchers to investigate methods of distinguishing these diagnoses (Beltran et al. 2006). In 1984 Evans and Batsakis described 14 cases of a distinctive minor salivary gland neoplasm that they named "polymorphous low-grade adenocarcinoma." This term emphasized the features of this neoplasm, including its cytologic uniformity and histologic diversity, variable growth patterns from solid to papillary to cribriform to fascicular, and relative lack of nuclear atypia (Evans and Batsakis 1984). Mitotic

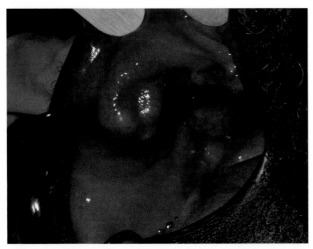

Figure 10.8a. An indurated upper lip mass that was fixed to the surrounding mucosa.

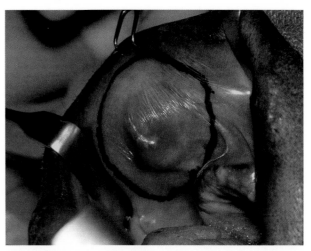

Figure 10.8c. A wide local excision of the mass with oral mucosal sacrifice observing 1 cm linear margins was planned.

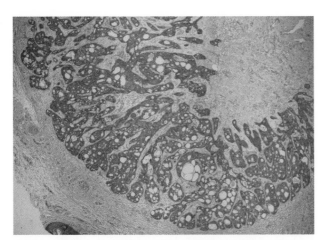

Figure 10.8b. Due to the likely but equivocal malignant nature of the mass, incisional biopsy is essential for the establishment of the diagnosis prior to definitive surgical therapy. The histopathology of the incisional biopsy identified intermediate-grade mucoepidermoid carcinoma.

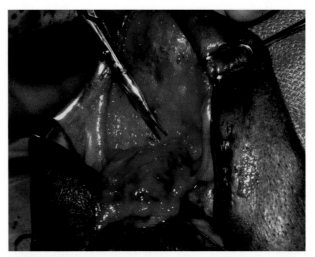

Figure 10.8d. A surgical plane was developed between the dermis of the upper lip and the musculature on the deep aspect of the tumor specimen.

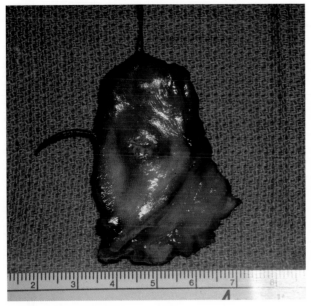

Figure 10.8e. The specimen was delivered and oriented for the pathologist with sutures.

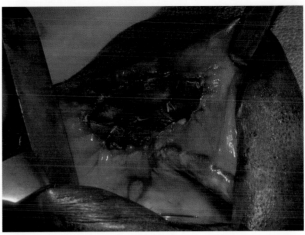

Figure 10.8g. The defect was reconstructed immediately with a full thickness skin graft.

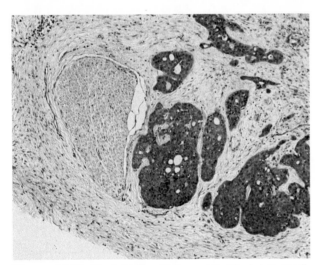

Figure 10.8f. Final histopathology identified intermediate-grade mucoepidermoid carcinoma with perineural invasion.

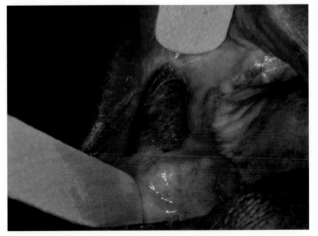

Figure 10.8h. A prophylactic neck dissection was not performed as part of this cancer surgery due to the low concern for occult neck disease associated with this diagnosis. The patient underwent postoperative radiation therapy and the surgical site was noted to be well healed at 1 year postoperatively without signs of recurrent disease. Reprinted with permission from Carlson ER. 1995. Salivary gland pathology—clinical perspectives and differential diagnosis. In: The Comprehensive Management of Salivary Gland Pathology, Oral and Maxillofacial Surgery Clinics of North America 7. Philadelphia: W.B. Saunders, pp. 361–386.

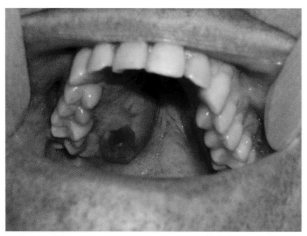

Figure 10.9a. A 52-year-old man with a 6-month history of a palatal mass.

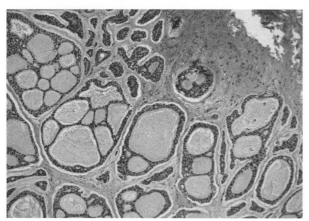

Figure 10.9b. Incisional biopsy showed adenoid cystic carcinoma.

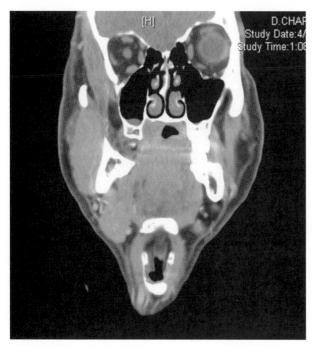

Figure 10.9c. Computerized tomograms identified a soft tissue mass and minimal invasion of the palatal bone.

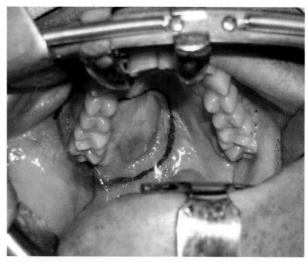

Figure 10.9d. A maxillectomy was planned for this patient observing 1 cm linear margins in bone and soft tissue.

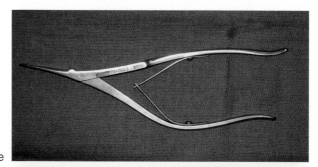

e

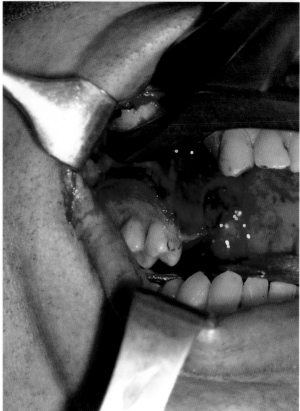

f

Figures 10.9e and 10.9f. The bony cuts were created throughout the maxilla and the Smith Ramus Separator (Walter Lorenz Surgical, a Biomet Company, Jacksonville, Florida) (e) was utilized to separate the specimen from the remaining facial skeleton (f).

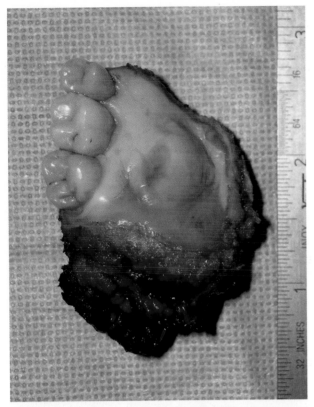

Figure 10.9g. The specimen was delivered and inspected from the palatal side so as to clinically confirm the efficacy of the resection.

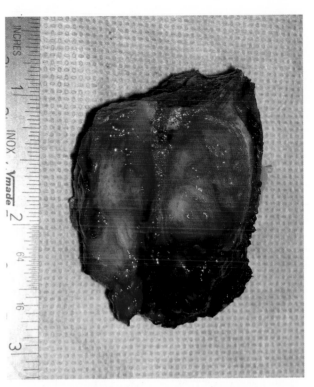

Figure 10.9h. The specimen was also inspected from the nasal/sinus side so as to confirm the adequacy of the resection.

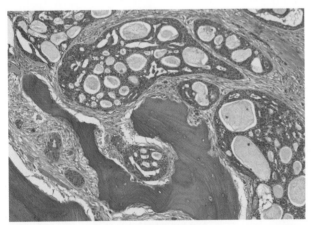

Figure 10.9i. Frozen sections were obtained to microscopically examine the soft tissue margins as well as a segment of the greater palatine nerve in the superior aspect of the defect near foramen rotundum. All frozen sections were negative, thereby not requiring additional sampling of the nerve or mucosa. The final decalcified histopathology showed the tumor invading the maxillary bone.

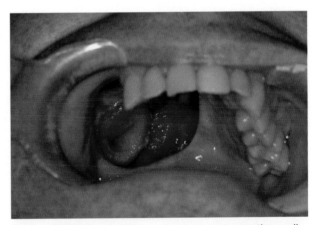

Figure 10.9j. The patient underwent postoperative radiation therapy and showed no evidence of cancer at 1 year postoperatively. This view provides anatomic delineation of the eustachian tube in the defect.

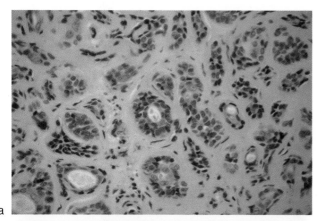

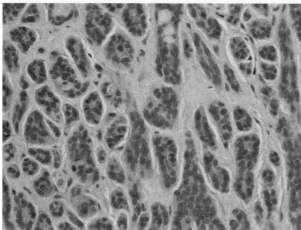

Figures 10.10a and 10.10b. Subtle differences between the adenoid cystic carcinoma (a) and the polymorphous low-grade adenocarcinoma (b). The adenoid cystic carcinoma characteristically shows multiple cell layered ductal structures, while the polymorphous low-grade adenocarcinoma shows single cell layered ductal structures. Reprinted with permission from Carlson ER. 1995. Salivary gland pathology—clinical perspectives and differential diagnosis. In: The Comprehensive Management of Salivary Gland Pathology, Oral and Maxillofacial Surgery Clinics of North America 7. Philadelphia: W.B. Saunders, pp. 361–386.

figures were infrequent and tumor necrosis was only seen in 1 case. Perineural invasion was and continues to be commonly noted in this malignancy. The tumors were distinctly unencapsulated and deeply infiltrative of bone and surrounding soft tissues. Radical surgical procedures were required for tumor control, but no distant metastases were noted. The authors judged from their survey of adenocarcinomas of the major salivary glands that the polymorphous low-grade adenocar-

cinoma was at least primarily an oral neoplasm. Since this report, Batsakis and El-Naggar (1991) have subclassified polymorphous low-grade adenocarcinomas (terminal duct adenocarcinomas) into papillary and nonpapillary forms. The papillary form was found to exhibit a more aggressive course with a higher rate of recurrence at the primary site, metastasis to cervical lymph nodes, and distant metastasis. The AFIP registry identified 75 cases of this neoplasm, and all were located in the minor salivary glands (Wenig and Gnepp 1991). Forty-four of these cases were located in the palate (58.6%), with the upper lip and buccal mucosa showing 12 cases each. Involvement of other oral minor salivary gland sites has been reported; however, this is quite rare (de Diego et al. 1996; Kennedy et al. 1987).

Since its original description in minor salivary gland sites, cases of polymorphous low-grade adenocarcinoma have been reported in the parotid gland, such that this tumor cannot be stated to be exclusive to minor salivary gland tissue (Barak, Grobbel, and Rabaja 1998; Merchant, Cook, and Eveson 1996).

Treatment of polymorphous low-grade adenocarcinoma requires surgery with curative intent. The surgical procedure is based on the anatomic site. Surgical removal of these tumors in the palate requires a thorough assessment of the palatal bone with computerized tomograms. Bone involvement by this tumor is not an inherent property of this neoplasm but rather a function of chronicity of the tumor. Since these malignancies are not fast growing, many patients have long histories of their presence, such that palatal bone infiltration by the tumor may occur over time. In addition, the characteristically deeply infiltrative nature of these tumors into surrounding soft tissues, regardless of the chronicity of the tumor, is such that the soft palate typically requires full thickness sacrifice in most cases. These features are clearly a departure from the treatment of mucoepidermoid carcinoma of the palate, where grade is the main determining factor in planning surgical treatment. Once a biopsy diagnosis of polymorphous low-grade adenocarcinoma of the palate has been established, therefore, CT scans should be obtained to examine the quality of the palatal bone. If the bone is unaltered by the tumor, a bone-sparing, periosteal sacrificing wide local excision with full thickness sacrifice of the soft palate may be performed (Figure 10.11). Due to the tumor's neurotropism, the greater palatine

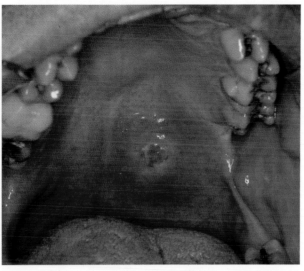

Figure 10.11a. A 51-year-old man with a mass of the soft palate that had reportedly been present for only 2 months.

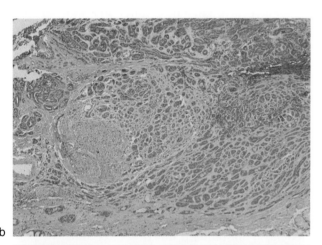

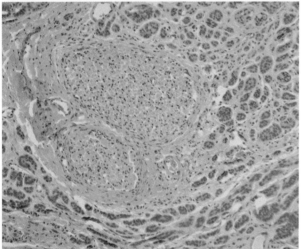

b

c

Figures 10.11b and 10.11c. Incisional biopsy showed a microscopically cribriform tumor with obvious perineural invasion. A diagnosis of polymorphous low-grade adenocarcinoma was made. Computerized tomograms did not reveal involvement of the palatal bone such that a periosteal sacrificing, bone-sparing wide local excision with full thickness sacrifice of the soft palate was performed.

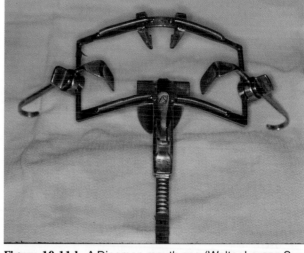

Figure 10.11d. A Dingman mouth gag (Walter Lorenz Surgical, a Biomet Company, Jacksonville, Florida) was utilized so as to provide acceptable retraction to perform this surgery.

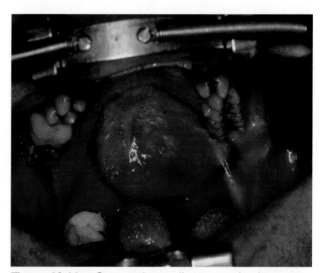

Figure 10.11e. One-centimeter linear margins in mucosa were planned.

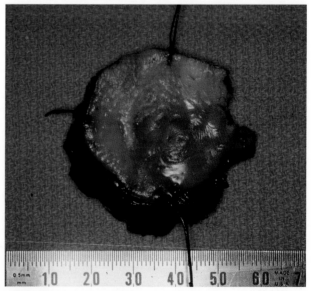

Figure 10.11f. The specimen is delivered.

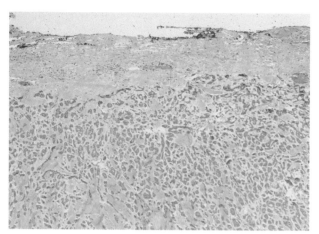

Figure 10.11g. Final histopathology identified a negative periosteal surface, thereby justifying the preservation of palatal bone.

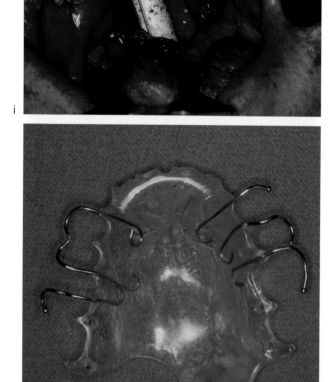

i

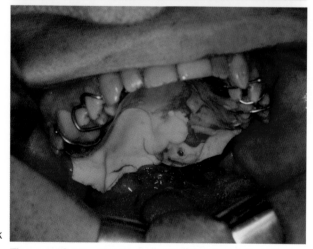

j

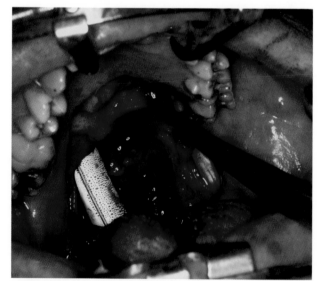

Figure 10.11h. The greater palatine neurovascular bundle was clamped prior to delivery of the specimen so as to procure a 1 cm segment of nerve for frozen section analysis. The hemostat remained on the nerve stump while the frozen section was being evaluated, which was negative for cancer. If the nerve had been positive for cancer, the nerve would have been pulled down to procure additional frozen sections so as to clear the cancer.

k

Figures 10.11i, 10.11j, and 10.11k. The defect (i) was addressed with an immediate obturator that had been fabricated preoperatively (j) and was placed intraoperatively (k).

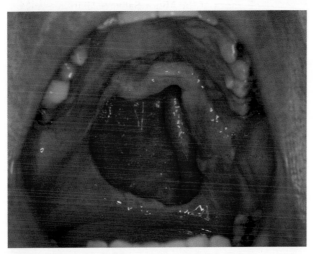

Figure 10.11l. The exposed palatal bone is covered with immature granulation tissue at 1 month postoperatively.

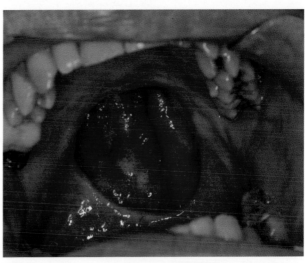

Figure 10.11n. At 1 year postoperatively, the patient's defect has demarcated well.

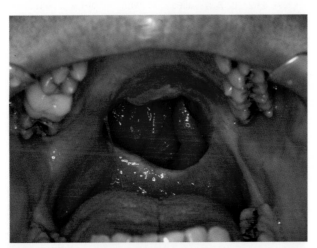

Figure 10.11m. Immature granulation tissue underwent maturation by 3 months postoperatively as seen in this image.

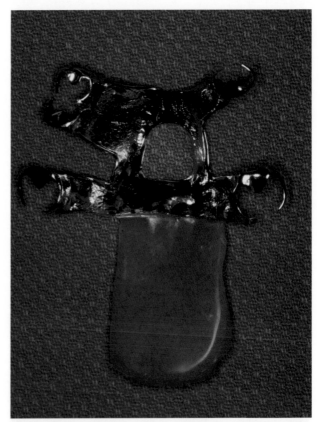

Figure 10.11o. A definitive obturator has been fabricated. Reprinted with permission from Carlson ER. 1995. Salivary gland pathology—clinical perspectives and differential diagnosis. In: The Comprehensive Management of Salivary Gland Pathology, Oral and Maxillofacial Surgery Clinics of North America 7. Philadelphia: W.B. Saunders, pp. 361–386.

246

neurovascular bundle should be sampled for frozen sections superiorly. Since perineural spread is not characteristic of this tumor, it is unlikely to find tumor tracking along the nerve, in contradistinction to adenoid cystic carcinoma, where tumor may be found surrounding this nerve at foramen rotundum. An immediate surgical obturator is fabricated preoperatively for insertion at the time of ablative surgery so as to permit the patient to begin taking a diet on the day of surgery. If the bone is eroded by the tumor, a traditional maxillectomy is necessary, also resulting in a full thickness sacrifice of the soft palate (Figure 10.12). An immediate surgical obturator must also be fabricated preoperatively for insertion at the time of surgery when a maxillectomy is planned for this diagnosis.

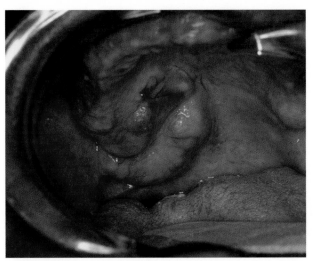

Figure 10.12a. A biopsy-proven polymorphous low-grade adenocarcinoma of the palate in a 53-year-old woman that had been present for several years, according to the patient.

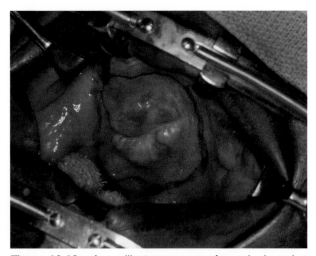

Figure 10.12c. A maxillectomy was performed, observing 1 cm linear margins in bone and soft tissue.

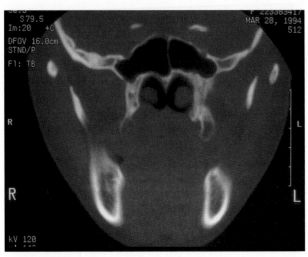

Figure 10.12b. Computerized tomograms were obtained that identified destruction of bone by the cancer.

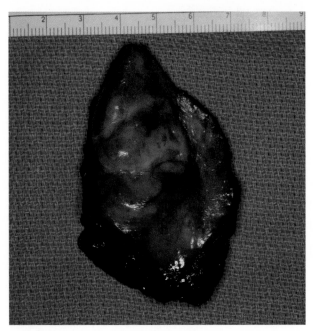

Figure 10.12d. The maxillectomy specimen delivered.

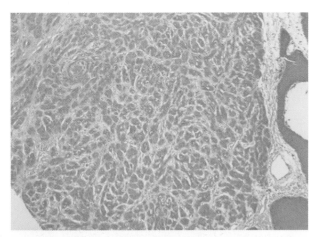

Figure 10.12e. The histopathology confirmed the involvement of the maxillary bone by the tumor.

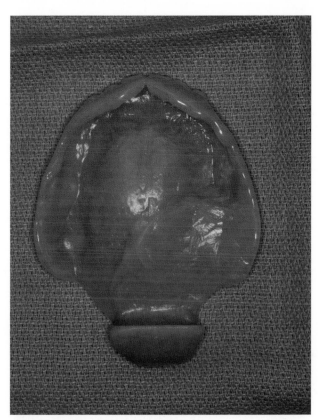

Figure 10.12g. The large ablative defect was addressed with an immediate obturator.

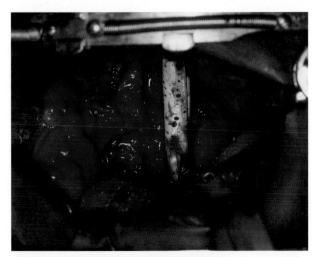

Figure 10.12f. The large ablative defect.

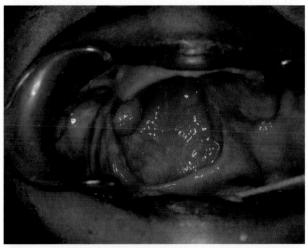

Figure 10.12h. At 1 year postoperatively, the patient showed no signs of recurrent disease.

The surgical treatment of polymorphous low-grade adenocarcinoma of the upper lip or buccal mucosa is similar to that of a mucoepidermoid carcinoma of these regions. The basic approach involves a mucosal-sacrificing wide local excision with attention to submucosal anatomic barriers being included on the specimen so as to ensure tumor-free margins (Figure 10.13).

The use of radiation therapy has been assessed in the management of polymorphous low-grade adenocarcinoma. In a clinicopathologic study of 164 cases of this malignancy, 17 patients underwent incisional, excisional, or wide local excision followed by radiation therapy (Castle, Thompson, and Frommelt et al. 1999). Adjuvant radiation therapy did not affect survival. Their study showed that patients who were treated with radiation therapy were more likely to have evidence of disease at last follow-up when compared with patients who did not have radiation therapy. Furthermore, there was no statistically significant difference in the overall patient outcome based on the type of initial treatment given or for any additional treatment rendered, whether it was additional surgery, radiation therapy, or chemotherapy. Based on this report and others (Crean et al. 1996), the treatment for polymorphous low-grade adenocarcinoma of minor salivary glands remains surgi-

cal. It has been estimated that approximately 80% of patients survive their disease without evidence of tumor at periods from between several months to 25 years after removal (Wenig and Gnepp 1991). One case has been reported where death occurred as a result of this neoplasm with direct extension to vital structures of the head (Aberle, Abrams, and Bowe et al. 1985). In addition, while rare, metastasis to cervical lymph nodes (Kumar, Stivaros, and Barrett et al. 2004) and to distant organs (Hannen, Bulten, and Festen et al. 2000) has been reported from polymorphous low-grade adenocarcinomas originating in the palate. These reports indicate that cervical lymph node involvement should be suspected in patients with papillary cystic change in the tumor, and that periodic chest X-ray examination should be performed postoperatively when this variant of tumor is diagnosed.

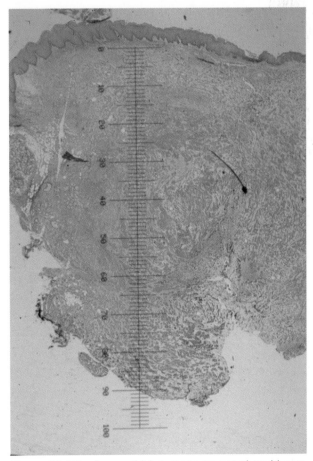

Figure 10.13b. A very thick tumor was noted on biopsy. The superimposed optical micrometer shows the tumor to be about 9 mm in thickness.

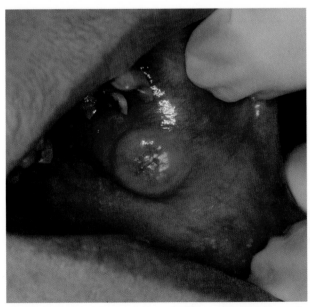

Figure 10.13a. A biopsy proved polymorphous low-grade adenocarcinoma of the buccal mucosa in a 45-year-old woman.

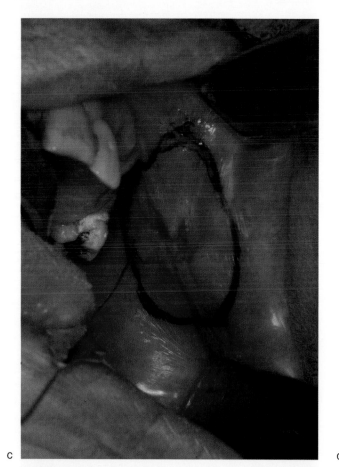

c

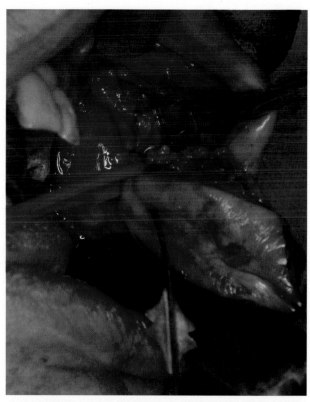

d

Figures 10.13c and 10.13d. A mucosal-sacrificing wide local excision with 1 cm linear margins and isolation of Stenson's duct was performed.

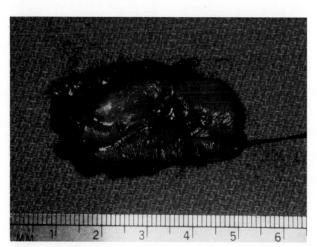

Figure 10.13e. The specimen was able to be delivered without tumor spillage.

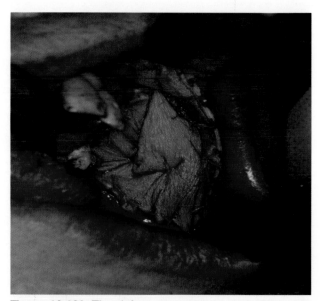

Figure 10.13f. The defect was reconstructed with a split thickness skin graft and a sialodochoplasty of Stenson's duct.

250

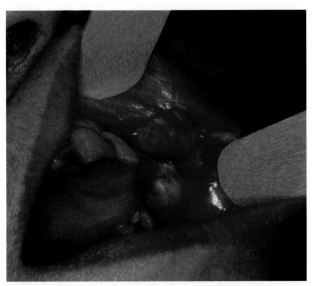

Figure 10.13g. Acceptable healing is noted without tumor recurrence at 6 months postoperatively. Reprinted with permission from Carlson ER. 1995. Salivary gland pathology—clinical perspectives and differential diagnosis. In: The Comprehensive Management of Salivary Gland Pathology, Oral and Maxillofacial Surgery Clinics of North America 7. Philadelphia: W.B. Saunders, pp. 361–386.

Acinic Cell Adenocarcinoma

Acinic cell adenocarcinoma is a very rare malignancy of the minor salivary glands. It has been estimated to represent approximately 2.5–3% of salivary gland tumors in general (Guimaraes et al. 1989; Spiro 1986) and about 4% of minor salivary gland tumors (Castellanos and Lally 1982). Indeed, acinic cell adenocarcinoma is not represented in many studies of minor salivary gland tumors (Chau and Radden 1986; Isacsson and Shear 1983; Jaber 2006), and other studies show only a very limited number of these cases (Lopes et al. 1999; Toida, Shimokawa, and Makita et al. 2005). The acinic cell adenocarcinoma behaves most similarly to the low-grade mucoepidermoid carcinoma (Ord 1994). In fact, like the low-grade mucoepidermoid carcinoma, the acinic cell adenocarcinoma was originally purported to be a benign neoplasm (Ellis and Auclair 1991a). For the first half of the twentieth century, these tumors were thought to be benign. In 1953, Buxton and his group were the first to ascribe a malignant character to many of these tumors (Buxton, Maxwell, and French 1953). These were identified as serous cell adenocarcinomas, after which time Foote and Frazell classified these

tumors as acinic cell adenocarcinomas (Foote and Frazell 1953).

The AFIP registry shows 886 acinic cell adenocarcinomas, of which 753 were located in the major salivary glands (85%), and 133 (15%) in the minor salivary glands. The most common site of minor salivary gland involvement was the buccal mucosa, accounting for 43 cases (32%), followed by the lip (38 cases, 29%). Tumors in the upper lip were three times more common than tumors in the lower lip. The palate was the only other significant anatomic site to be affected by this tumor, and accounted for 22 cases (17%). A female preponderance was noted, with a mean age of 44 years.

Surgery for acinic cell adenocarcinoma is performed in a similar fashion as that of low-grade mucoepidermoid carcinoma. Tumors of the buccal mucosa and upper lip are treated with mucosal-sacrificing wide local excisions, including 1 cm linear margins, with attention to the necessary sacrifice of surrounding anatomic barriers (Figure 10.14). Tumors of the palate can be treated with bone-sparing, periosteally sacrificing wide local excisions with split thickness sacrifice of the soft palate. Computerized tomograms may be obtained preoperatively to confirm the lack of bone erosion. Recurrences and regional and distant metastases are rare when these malignancies are treated according to these recommendations. Five and 10-year survival rates are generally quite favorable and reported as 82% and 68%, respectively (Hickman, Cawson, and Duffy 1984).

Epithelial-Myoepithelial Carcinoma

The epithelial-myoepithelial carcinoma of minor salivary gland origin has been categorized as an intermediate-grade malignancy according to the AFIP classification (Ellis and Auclair 1991b). Only 57 cases were identified in their series, with 50 cases diagnosed in the major salivary glands (88%), and 7 cases (12%) in the minor salivary glands (Corio 1991). Of the 7 cases in the minor salivary glands, 4 were located in the palate, 1 in the tongue, and 2 cases were not specified as to anatomic location. A mean age of 59 years was noted in these 57 cases. This tumor is known to be highly differentiated, yet it is malignant due to infiltrative and destructive growth patterns, the presence of necrosis, perineural involvement, and metastases (Corio et al. 1982). Corio et al. pre-

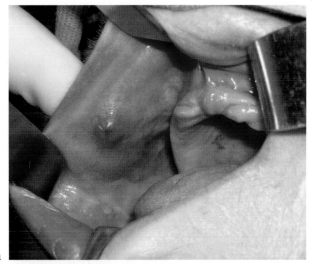

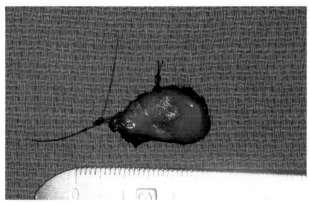

Figure 10.14d. Excision of the specimen occurred without tumor spillage.

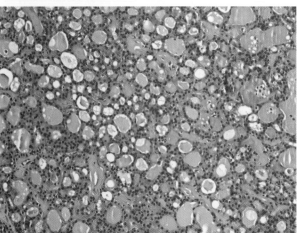

Figures 10.14a and 10.14b. An acinic cell adenocarcinoma of the right buccal mucosa in a 52-year-old patient. The histopathology of the biopsy shows a typical blue dot tumor (b).

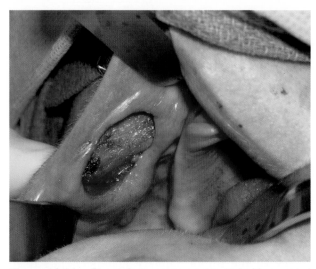

Figure 10.14e. The defect was reconstructed with mucosal flaps so as to not distort the appearance of the upper lip.

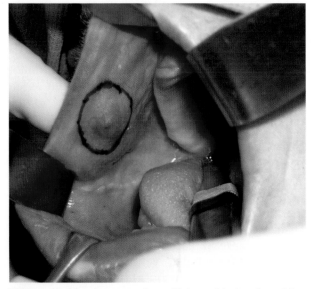

Figure 10.14c. A mucosal-sacrificing wide local excision observing 1 cm linear margins is performed.

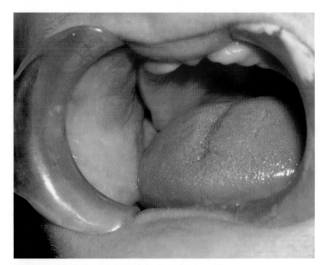

Figure 10.14f. Acceptable healing without tumor recurrence is noted at 1 year postoperatively.

sented 16 cases of this neoplasm and found 12 cases to involve the parotid gland, 3 cases in the submandibular gland, and 1 case in the buccal mucosa (Corio et al. 1982).

Standardized recommendations for surgery for the epithelial-myoepithelial carcinoma are difficult to make due to the rare nature of this malignancy. Nonetheless, evaluation of involved anatomic barriers with physical examination and

CT scans generally permits an effective approach to eradication of these malignancies in various minor salivary gland sites (Figure 10.15). In such circumstances, the surgeon respects well-established principles of linear and anatomic barrier margins when operating on salivary gland tumors, while also relying on past experience with other low- and intermediate-grade minor salivary gland malignancies. In so doing, tumor-free margins can

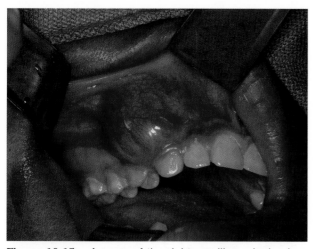

Figure 10.15a. A mass of the right maxillary gingiva in a 12-year-old girl.

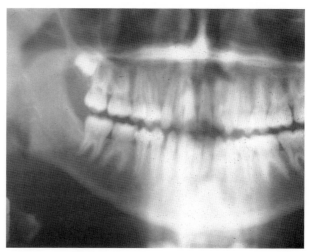

Figure 10.15b. Panoramic radiograph demonstrates tumor involvement of the bone between the first premolar and canine teeth with divergence of the roots of these teeth.

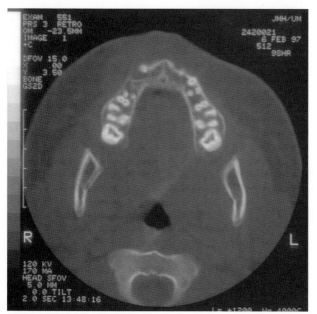

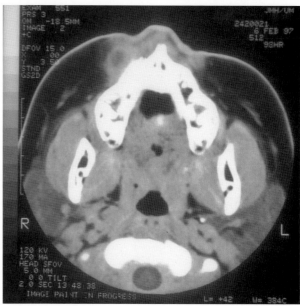

Figures 10.15c and 10.15d. Computerized tomograms demonstrate a soft tissue mass with involvement of the maxillary bone.

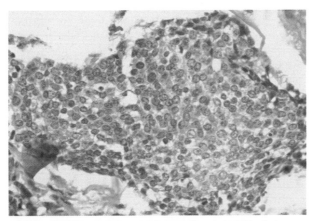

Figure 10.15e. Incisional biopsy showed epithelial-myo-epithelial carcinoma.

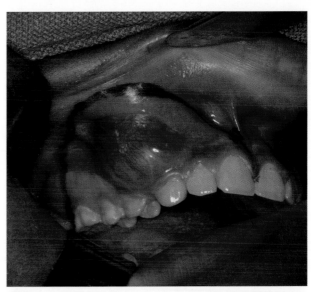

Figure 10.15f. A partial maxillectomy observing 1 cm linear margins in bone and soft tissue was performed.

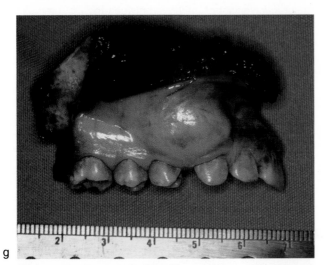

g

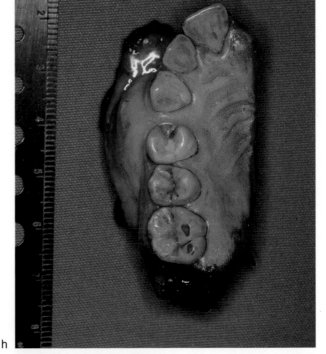

h

Figures 10.15g and 10.15h. The specimen was able to be removed without tumor spillage.

254

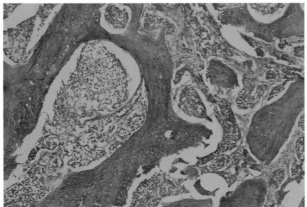

Figure 10.15i. Final histopathology showed destruction of bone by the cancer.

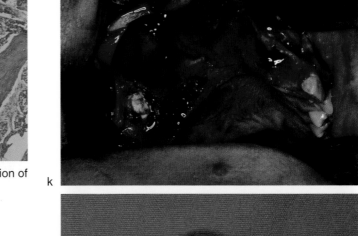

k

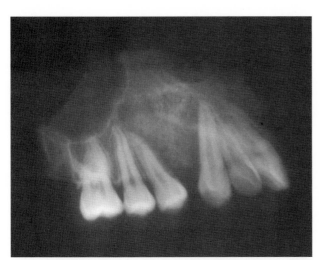

Figure 10.15j. The specimen radiograph demonstrated acceptable bone margins.

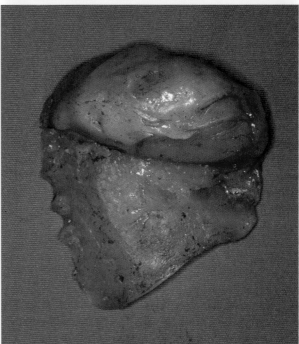

l

Figures 10.15k and 10.15l. The resultant ablative defect of the maxilla (k) was reconstructed with an immediate obturator device (l).

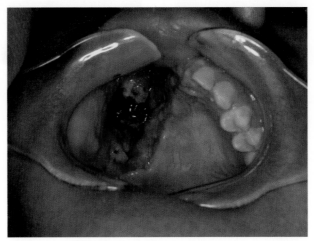

Figure 10.15m. The use of the obturator permitted contracture of the defect as noted at 1 month postoperatively.

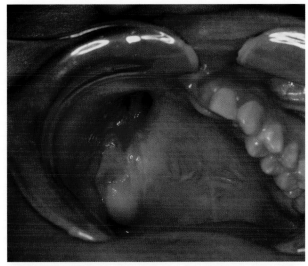

Figure 10.15n. By 3 months postoperatively, the defect had demarcated significantly.

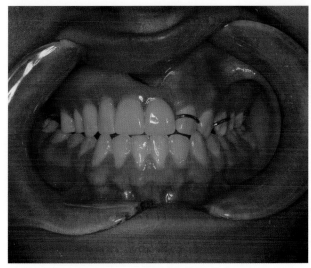

Figures 10.15p. This interim obturator allowed for seal of the defect and function with teeth.

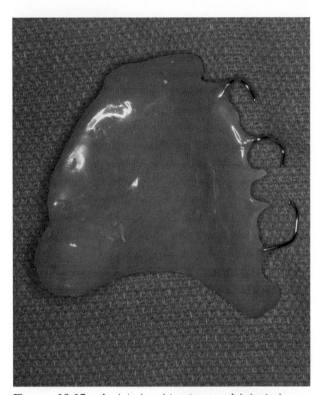

Figures 10.15o. An interim obturator was fabricated.

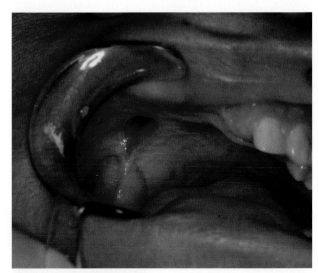

Figure 10.15q. The patient functioned well with the definitive obturator, which permitted additional contracture of the maxillary defect.

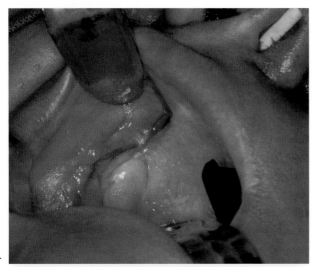

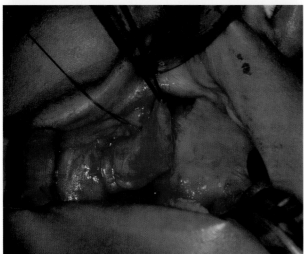

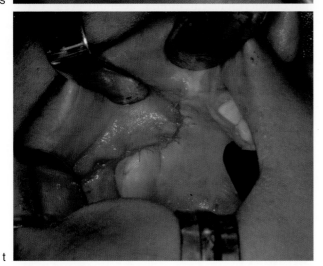

Figures 10.15r, 10.15s, and 10.15t. Soft tissue reconstruction was accomplished with a buccal fat flap and advancement of the buccal mucosa.

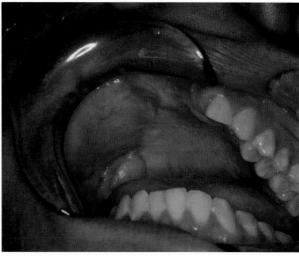

Figure 10.15u. The appearance of the healed flap is noted at 1 year postoperatively.

be obtained while performing surgery similar to that for a diagnosis of low- or intermediate-grade mucoepidermoid carcinoma. Recurrences have been reported (Corio 1991), but appropriate surgical management of epithelial-myoepithelial carcinomas of the minor salivary glands should be performed with curative intent. Quantitative survival statistics are not published in the literature.

SURGICAL MANAGEMENT OF THE NECK FOR MINOR SALIVARY GLAND MALIGNANCIES

Surgical management of the neck is a controversial and intriguing concept for surgeons managing oral/ head and neck malignant disease. At the core of this discipline is an assessment of occult disease in patients with clinically negative necks. To this end, there seems to be a consensus in the literature that occult neck disease is relatively uncommon related to minor salivary gland malignancies compared to squamous cell carcinoma of the oral/head and neck region. Moreover, it is also uncommon for patients with minor salivary gland malignancies to present with clinically palpable neck disease related to these tumors. Spiro found 53 patients presenting with cervical metastases among 378 patients (14%) with minor salivary gland malignancies (Spiro, Thaler, and Hicks et al. 1991). Another 26 patients (7%) developed subsequent cervical metastases for an overall rate of nodal involvement of 21%. Interestingly, 9 patients underwent an elective neck dissection, all of whom showed histologically confirmed metastatic disease. The authors do not, however, discuss the incidence of occult and clinically apparent metastases as a function of anatomic site of the primary minor salivary gland malignancy. Sadeghi et al. identified 9 patients presenting with cervical metastases related to minor salivary gland malignancies, 5 of which were present in the tongue base (Sadeghi, Tran, and Mark et al. 1993). Beckhardt et al. found N+ necks in only 3% of their patients with malignant minor salivary gland tumors of the palate, while Chung identified only 2 of 20 patients with malignant salivary gland tumors of the palate presenting with cervical metastases (Beckhardt, Weber, and Zane et al. 1995; Chung, Rahman, and Constable 1978). The latter three studies only discussed clinical staging of the neck without comments regarding their histology such that limited information is available regarding the true rate of metastasis to the cervical lymph nodes. In the final analysis, it seems that the incidence of occult neck disease related to a minor salivary gland malignancy of the oral cavity is sufficiently low to negate the need for elective neck dissection. Indications for neck dissection in these patients, therefore, are limited to patients who present with cervical metastases, those patients whose preoperative imaging studies document changes in the cervical lymph nodes consistent with metastatic disease, and those patients with high-grade malignancies, regardless of the clinical and radiographic imaging results.

THE ROLE OF RADIATION THERAPY IN THE MANAGEMENT OF MINOR SALIVARY GLAND MALIGNANCIES

It was once thought that salivary gland malignancies were radioresistant (Dragovic 1995). This previously stated misconception can no longer be considered valid. As such, radiation therapy is indicated in the postoperative management of all high-grade malignant minor salivary gland tumors, as well as in patients with positive surgical margins, positive regional lymph nodes, and recurrent tumor (Dragovic 1995). This being the case, it is important to remember that surgery is the primary therapy for minor salivary gland malignancies. Shingaki et al.'s review of the role of radiation therapy in 44 patients with salivary gland cancers, 34 of whom were treated for minor salivary gland cancers, examined the results of surgery vs. surgery and postoperative radiation therapy in these patients (Shingaki et al. 1992). Interestingly, no patients experienced recurrent disease when negative surgical margins were found in the specimen, regardless of whether surgery or surgery and postoperative radiation therapy was performed. All patients with positive surgical margins developed recurrent disease when surgery was the modality of treatment, and 8 of 15 patients (53%) with positive surgical margins developed recurrent disease when their salivary gland cancer was treated with a combination of surgery and postoperative radiation therapy. While not broken down to major vs. minor salivary gland primary sites, these results do point to the significant benefit of obtaining negative margins in the resected specimen.

THE ROLE OF CHEMOTHERAPY IN THE MANAGEMENT OF MINOR SALIVARY GLAND MALIGNANCIES

There are few reports on the benefit of systemic chemotherapy in the management of salivary gland cancers. Chemotherapy is generally reserved for the palliative management of advanced, nonresectable disease where radiation therapy has already been administered. Most patients for whom chemotherapy is considered will have diagnoses of mucoepidermoid carcinoma, adenoid cystic carcinoma, or high-grade adenocarcinoma (Laurie and Licitra 2006). The expression of c-kit in adenoid cystic carcinoma, overexpression of her-2 in mucoepidermoid carcinoma, overexpression of epithelial growth factor receptor in adenocarcinoma, and androgen receptor positivity in salivary duct carcinoma makes the use of imatinib, trastuzumab, cetuximab, and antiandrogen therapy at least theoretically beneficial (Laurie and Licitra 2006). While these agents may be of value in treating difficult cases of minor salivary gland malignancies, there is a need to conduct high-quality clinical trials in patients with these cancers.

Summary

- Approximately 10% of all salivary gland tumors arise in the minor glands.

- Approximately 1% of head and neck tumors occur within the minor salivary glands, although some authors believe that this figure is somewhat higher.
- 70% of minor salivary gland tumors arise in the oral cavity.
- 50% of oral minor salivary gland tumors are found in the palate.
- 50% of oral minor salivary gland tumors are benign and 50% are malignant.
- Inconclusive evidence exists for cause and effect relationships with minor salivary gland tumors.
- An incisional biopsy is almost always indicated prior to definitive management of a palatal minor salivary gland tumor.
- An excisional biopsy of a buccal mucosal or upper lip minor salivary gland tumor may be acceptable without first obtaining the histopathologic diagnosis, provided signs of benign disease exist.
- Benign tumors of the palate, buccal mucosa, and upper lip may be excised without special imaging studies.
- When present, ulceration predicts a malignant diagnosis, although many minor salivary gland malignancies do not create ulceration of the oral mucosa.
- Pain is associated with perineural invasion, most commonly seen with adenoid cystic carcinoma.
- Malignant tumors of the palate should undergo special imaging studies so as to determine involvement of the palatal bone.
- Malignant tumors of the buccal mucosa and upper lip may not require imaging prior to ablative surgery.
- Surgery represents the primary treatment of minor salivary gland tumors.
- Surgical removal of minor salivary gland tumors requires a scientific approach to the surrounding anatomic barriers.
- High cure rates are anticipated following removal of pleomorphic adenomas and canalicular adenomas of minor salivary gland sites.
- High cure rates are anticipated following removal of low-grade mucoepidermoid carcinomas and polymorphous low-grade adenocarcinomas of minor salivary gland sites.
- Variable cure rates are associated with surgery for intermediate and high-grade mucoepidermoid carcinomas and adenoid cystic carcinomas of minor salivary glands.

References

Abbey LM, Schwab BH, Landau GC, Perkins ER. 1984. Incidence of second primary breast cancer among patients with a first primary salivary gland tumor. *Cancer* 54:1439–1442.

Aberle AM, Abrams AM, Bowe R et al. 1985. Lobular (polymorphous low-grade) carcinoma of minor salivary glands: A clinicopathologic study of 20 cases. *Oral Surg Oral Med Oral Pathol* 60:387–395.

Ampil FL, Misra RP. 1987. Factors influencing survival of patients with adenoid cystic carcinoma of the salivary glands. *J Oral Maxillofac Surg* 45:1005–1010.

Ansari MH. 2007. Salivary gland tumors in an Iranian population: A retrospective study of 130 cases. *J Oral Maxillofac Surg* 65:2187–2194.

Auclair PL, Ellis GL. 1991. Mucoepidermoid carcinoma. In: Ellis GL, Auclair PL, Gnepp DR (eds.), Surgical Pathology of the Salivary Glands. Philadelphia: W.B. Saunders, pp. 269–298.

Auclair PL, Ellis GL, Gnepp DR et al. 1991. Salivary gland neoplasms: General considerations. In: Ellis GL, Auclair PL, Gnepp DR (eds.), Surgical Pathology of the Salivary Glands. Philadelphia: W.B. Saunders, pp. 135–164.

Barak AP, Grobbel M, Rabaja DR. 1998. Polymorphous low-grade adenocarcinoma of the parotid gland. *Am J Otolaryngol* 19:322–324.

Batsakis JG, El-Naggar AK. 1991. Terminal duct adenocarcinomas of salivary tissues. *Ann Otol Rhinol Laryngol* 100:251–253.

Batsakis JG, Luna MA. 1990. Histopathologic grading of salivary gland neoplasms: I. Mucoepidermoid carcinomas. *Ann Otol Rhinol Laryngol* 99:835–838.

Batsakis JG, Pinkston GR, Luna MA, et al. 1983. Adenocarcinomas of the oral cavity: A clinicopathologic study of terminal duct carcinomas. *J Laryngol Otol* 97:825–835.

Beckhardt RN, Weber RS, Zane R et al. 1995. Minor salivary gland tumors of the palate: Clinical and pathologic correlates of outcome. *Laryngoscope* 105:1155–1160.

Bell RB, Dierks EJ, Homer L, Potter BE. 2005. Management and outcome of patients with malignant salivary gland tumors. *J Oral Maxillofac Surg* 63:917–928.

Beltran D, Faquin WC, Gallagher G, August M. 2006. Selective immunohistochemical comparison of polymorphous low-grade adenocarcinoma and adenoid cystic carcinoma. *J Oral Maxillofac Surg* 64:415–423.

Brandwein MS, Ivanov K, Wallace DI et al. 2001. Mucoepidermoid carcinoma: A clinicopathologic study of 80 patients with special reference to histological grading. *Am J Surg Pathol* 25:835–845.

Buxton RW, Maxwell JH, French AJ. 1953. Surgical treatment of epithelial tumors of the parotid gland. *Surg Gynecol Obstet* 97:401–416.

Carlson ER. 1998. The management of minor salivary gland tumors of the oral cavity. *Atlas Oral Maxillofac Surg Clin North Amer* 6:75–98.

Castellanos JL, Lally ET. 1982. Acinic cell tumor of the minor salivary glands. *J Oral Maxillofac Surg* 40:428–431.

Castle JT, Thompson LDR, Frommelt RA et al. 1999. Polymorphous low grade adenocarcinoma: A clinicopathologic study of 164 cases. *Cancer* 86:207–219.

Chau MNY, Radden BG. 1986. Intra-oral salivary gland neoplasms: A retrospective study of 98 cases. *J Oral Pathol* 15:339–342.

Chidzonga MM, Lopez-Perez VM, Portilla-Alvarez AL. 1995. Salivary gland tumours in Zimbabwe: Report of 282 cases. *Int J Oral Maxillofac Surg* 24:292–297.

Chung CK, Rahman SM, Constable WC. 1978. Malignant salivary gland tumors of the palate. *Arch Otolaryngol* 104:501–504.

Corio RL. 1991. Epithelial-myoepithelial carcinoma. In: Ellis GL, Auclair PL, Gnepp DR (eds.), Surgical Pathology of the Salivary Glands. Philadelphia: W.B. Saunders, pp. 412–421.

Corio RL, Sciubba JJ, Brannon RB, Batsakis JG. 1982. Epithelial-myoepithelial carcinoma of intercalated duct origin: A clinicopathologic and ultrastructural assessment of sixteen cases. *Oral Surg Oral Med Oral Pathol* 53:280–287.

Crean SJ, Bryant C, Bennett J, Harris M. 1996. Four cases of polymorphous low-grade adenocarcinoma. *Int J Oral Maxillofac Surg* 25:40–44.

Daley TD, Gardner GD, Smout MS. 1984. Canalicular adenoma: Not a basal cell adenoma. *Oral Surg Oral Med Oral Pathol* 57:181–188.

de Diego JI, Bernaldez R, Prim MP, Hardison D. 1996. Polymorphous low-grade adenocarcinoma of the tongue. *J Laryngol Otol* 10:700–703.

Dragovic J. 1995. The role of radiation therapy in the management of salivary gland neoplasms. *Oral Maxillofac Surg Clin North Amer* 7:627–632.

Ellis GL, Auclair PL. 1991a. Acinic cell carcinoma. In: Ellis GL, Auclair PL, Gnepp DR (eds.), Surgical Pathology of the Salivary Glands. Philadelphia: W.B. Saunders, pp. 299–317.

Ellis GL, Auclair PL. 1991b. Classification of salivary gland neoplasms. In: Ellis GL, Auclair PL, Gnepp DR (eds.), Surgical Pathology of the Salivary Glands. Philadelphia: W.B. Saunders, pp. 129–134.

Eneroth CM, Hjertman L, Moberger G, Soderberg G. 1972. Mucoepidermoid carcinomas of the salivary glands with special reference to the possible existence of a benign variety. *Acta Otolaryng* 73:68–74.

Epker BN, Henny FA. 1969. Clinical, histopathological and surgical aspects of intraoral minor salivary gland tumors: Review of 90 cases. *J Oral Surg* 27:792–804.

Evans HL. 1984. Mucoepidermoid carcinoma of salivary glands: A study of 69 cases with special attention to histologic grading. *Am J Clin Pathol* 81:696–701.

Evans HL, Batsakis JG. 1984. Polymorphous low-grade adenocarcinoma of minor salivary glands: A study of 14 cases of a distinctive neoplasm. *Cancer* 53:935–942.

Eveson JW, Cawson RA. 1985. Salivary gland tumors: A review of 2410 cases with particular reference to histological types, site, age and sex distribution. *J Pathol* 146:51–58.

Foote FW, Frazell EL. 1953. Tumors of the major salivary glands. *Cancer* 6:1065–1133.

Fordice J, Kershaw C, El-Naggar A, Goepfert H. 1999. Adenoid cystic carcinoma of the head and neck: Predictors of morbidity and mortality. *Arch Otolaryngol Head Neck Surg* 125:149–152.

Freedman PD, Jones AC. 1994. A pathologist's approach to tissue diagnosis. *Oral Maxillofac Surg Clin North Amer* 6:357–375.

Freedman PD, Lumerman H. 1983. Lobular carcinoma of intraoral minor salivary glands. *Oral Surg Oral Med Oral Pathol* 56:157–165.

Gardner DG, Daley TD. 1983. The use of the terms monomorphic adenoma, basal cell adenoma, and canalicular adenoma as applied to salivary gland tumors. *Oral Surg Oral Med Oral Pathol* 56:608–615.

Guimaraes DS, Amaral AP, Prado LF, Nascimento AG. 1989. Acinic cell carcinoma of salivary glands: 16 cases with clinicopathologic correlation. *J Oral Pathol Med* 18:396–399.

Hannen EJM, Bulten J, Festen J et al. 2000. Polymorphous low grade adenocarcinoma with distant metastases and deletions on chromosome 6q23-qter and 1q23-qter: A case report. *J Clin Pathol* 53:942–945.

Hickman RE, Cawson RA, Duffy SW. 1984. The prognosis of specific types of salivary gland tumors. *Cancer* 54:1620–1624.

Isacsson G, Shear M. 1983. Intraoral salivary gland tumors: A retrospective study of 201 cases. *J Oral Pathol* 12:57–62.

Ito RA, Ito K, Vargas PA et al. 2005. Salivary gland tumors in a Brazilian population: A retrospective study of 496 cases. *Int J Oral Maxillofac Surg* 34:533–536.

Jaber MA. 2006. Intraoral minor salivary gland tumors: A review of 75 cases in a Libyan population. *Int J Oral Maxillofac Surg* 35:150–154.

Katz AD, Preston-Martin S. 1984. Salivary gland tumors and previous radiotherapy to the head or neck: Report of a clinical series. *Am J Surg* 147:345–348.

Kennedy KS, Healy KM, Taylor RE, Strom CG. 1987. Polymorphous low-grade adenocarcinoma of the tongue. *Laryngoscope* 97:533–536.

Kratochvil FJ. 1991. Canalicular adenoma and basal cell adenoma. In: Ellis GL, Auclair PL, Gnepp DR (eds.), *Surgical Pathology of the Salivary Glands*. Philadelphia: W.B. Saunders, pp. 202–224.

Kumar M, Stivaros N, Barrett AW et al. 2004. Polymorphous low-grade adenocarcinoma—a rare and aggressive entity in adolescence. *Br J Oral Maxillofac Surg* 42:195–199.

Laurie SA, Licitra L. 2006. Systemic therapy in the palliative management of advanced salivary gland cancers. *J Clin Oncol* 24:2673–2678.

Lopes MA, Kowalski LP, Santos GC, Almeida OP. 1999. A clinicopathologic study of 196 intraoral minor salivary gland tumours. *J Oral Pathol Med* 28:264–267.

Luna MA, Batsakis JG, El-Naggar AD. 1991. Salivary gland tumors in children. *An Otol Rhinol Laryngol* 100:869–871.

MacIntosh RB. 1995. Minor salivary gland tumors: Types, incidence and management. *Oral Maxillofac Surg Clin North Amer* 7:573–589.

Melrose RJ. 1994. Clinicopathologic features of intraoral salivary gland tumors. *Oral Maxillofac Surg Clin North Amer* 6:479–497.

Merchant WJ, Cook MG, Eveson JW. 1996. Polymorphous low-grade adenocarcinoma of parotid gland. *Br J Oral Maxillofac Surg* 34:328–330.

Nascimento AG, Amaral ALP, Prado LAF et al. 1986. Adenoid cystic carcinoma of salivary glands: A study of 61 cases with clinicopathologic correlation. *Cancer* 57:312–319.

Ord RA. 1994. Management of intraoral salivary gland tumors. *Oral Maxillofac Surg Clin North Amer* 6:499–522.

Perzin KH, Gullane P, Clairmont AC. 1978. Adenoid cystic carcinomas arising in salivary glands: A correlation of histologic features and clinical course. *Cancer* 42:265–282.

Pires FR, Pringle GA, de Almeida OP, Chen SY. 2007. Intraoral minor salivary gland tumors: A clinicopathological study of 546 cases. *Oral Oncology* 43:463–470.

Plambeck K, Friedrich RE, Schmelzle R. 1996. Mucoepidermoid carcinoma of salivary gland origin: Classification, clinical-pathological correlation, treatment results and long-term follow-up in 55 patients. *J Craniomaxillofac Surg* 24:133–139.

Pogrel MA. 1994. The management of salivary gland tumors of the palate. *J Oral Maxillofac Surg* 52:454–459.

Potdar GG, Paymaster JC. 1969. Tumors of minor salivary glands. *Oral Surg Oral Med Oral Pathol* 28:310–319.

Regezi JA, Lloyd RV, Zarbo RJ, McClatchey KD. 1985. Minor salivary gland tumors: A histologic and immunohistochemical study. *Cancer* 55:108–115.

Regezi JA, Zarbo RJ, Stewart JCB, Courtney RM. 1991. Polymorphous low-grade adenocarcinoma of minor salivary gland: A comparative histologic and immunohistochemical study. *Oral Surg Oral Med Oral Pathol* 71:469–475.

Rivera-Bastidas H, Ocanto RA, Acevedo AM. 1996. Intraoral minor salivary gland tumors: A retrospective study of 62 cases in a Venezuelan population. *J Oral Pathol Med* 25:1–4.

Rogerson KC. 1995. Salivary gland pathology in children. *Oral Maxillofac Surg Clin North Am* 7:591–598.

Sadeghi A, Tran LM, Mark R et al. 1993. Minor salivary gland tumors of the head and neck: Treatment strategies and prognosis. *Am J Clin Oncol* 16:3–8.

Saku T, Hayashi Y, Takahara O et al. 1997. Salivary gland tumors among atomic bomb survivors, 1950–1987. *Cancer* 79:1465–1475.

Satko I, Stanko P, Longauerova I. 2000. Salivary gland tumours treated in the stomatological clinics in Bratislava. *J Craniomaxillofac Surg* 28:56–61.

Shingaki S, Ohtake K, Nomura T, Nakajima T. 1992. The role of radiotherapy in the management of salivary gland carcinomas. *J Craniomaxillofac Surg* 20:220–224.

Spiro RH. 1986. Salivary neoplasms: Overview of a 35-year experience with 2,807 patients. *Head & Neck Surg* 8:177–184.

Spiro RH, Thaler HT, Hicks WF et al. 1991. The importance of clinical staging of minor salivary gland carcinoma. *Am J Surg* 162:330–336.

Spitz MR, Tilley BC, Batsakis JG et al. 1984. Risk factors for major salivary gland carcinoma: A case-comparison study. *Cancer* 54:1854–1859.

Stewart FW, Foote FW, Becker WF. 1945. Mucoepidermoid tumors of salivary glands. *Ann Surg* 122:820–844.

Stuteville OH, Corley RD. 1967. Surgical management of tumors of intraoral minor salivary glands: Report of eighty cases. *Cancer* 20:1578–1586.

Toida M, Shimokawa K, Makita H et al. 2005. Intraoral minor salivary gland tumors: A clinicopathological study of 82 cases. *Int J Oral Maxillofac Surg* 34:528–532.

Tomich CE. 1991. Adenoid cystic carcinoma. In: Ellis GL, Auclair PL, Gnepp DR (eds.), Surgical Pathology of the Salivary Glands. Philadelphia: W.B. Saunders, pp. 333–349.

Triantafillidou K, Dimitrakopoulos J, Iordanidis F, Koufogiannis D. 2006. Management of adenoid cystic carcinoma of minor salivary glands. *J Oral Maxillofac Surg* 64:1114–1120.

Waldron CA. 1991. Mixed tumor (pleomorphic adenoma) and myoepithelioma. In: Ellis GL, Auclair PL, Gnepp DR (eds.), Surgical Pathology of the Salivary Glands. Philadelphia: W.B. Saunders, pp. 165–186.

Waldron CA, El-Mofty SK, Gnepp DR. 1988. Tumors of the intraoral minor salivary glands: A demographic and histologic study of 426 cases. *Oral Surg Oral Med Oral Pathol* 66:323–333.

Wenig BM, Gnepp DR. 1991. Polymorphous low-grade adenocarcinoma of minor salivary glands. In: Ellis GL, Auclair PL, Gnepp DR (eds.), Surgical Pathology of the Salivary Glands. Philadelphia: W.B. Saunders, pp. 390–411.

Yih WY, Kratochvil FJ, Stewart JCB. 2005. Intraoral minor salivary gland neoplasms: Review of 213 cases. *J Oral Maxillofac Surg* 63:805–810.

Chapter 11
Non-salivary Tumors of the Salivary Glands

Outline

Introduction

This chapter will review the non-salivary tumors that occur in the major salivary glands, having discussed the primary epithelial salivary gland tumors in chapters 8, 9, and 10. Essentially the chapter will be divided into primary benign and malignant mesenchymal tumors and metastatic lesions, primarily epithelial, in the lymph nodes or substance of the major glands. As the epidemiology and etiology of these tumors is extremely variable, they will be discussed in relation to individual tumors and groups of tumors.

Mesenchymal Tumors

BENIGN MESENCHYMAL TUMORS

Hemangiomas

Hemangiomas and hemangioendotheliomas are most commonly seen in the parotid gland and in children, where they account for up to 35% of salivary tumors (Ord 2004). These tumors are most commonly seen under the age of 1 year and may be present at birth, where they may exhibit aggressive growth. Hemangioendotheliomas are more aggressive and rapidly growing and occur in the <6 month infant, while the older children tend to present with the slower-growing cavernous lesions (Figure 11.1). In the past surgical removal was advocated, but as the majority of tumors involute over time, and because of the morbidity of surgery in infants, this has largely been abandoned in favor of medical therapy. Previous papers have indicated that vascular malformations of the parotid respond poorly to medical therapy; however, this has been disproved by Greene, Rogers, and Mulliken (2004). These authors reviewed 100 consecutive children with a 4.5 : 1 female to male ratio with 59% ulcerating during the proliferating phase and 89% involving nearby structures. Seventy of the patients were treated medically, 67 primarily with corticosteroids and 3 with interferon. Initially 56/67 of the patients treated with steroids showed regression or stabilization, but 18 required further treatment with interferon. The overall response to steroids/alfa-2a or -2b interferon was 98%, and the authors concluded that parotid gland vascular tumors respond in the same way as hemangiomas elsewhere. Interestingly, 66% of the children required some form of reconstructive surgery during the involuted phase. In adults vascular lesions of the parotid are less common, but intramuscular hemangiomas of the masseter muscle can be a diagnostic challenge (Figure 11.2).

Vascular lesions of the submandibular gland are seen rarely and like vascular lesions elsewhere will be treated depending on their flow characteristics and the vessel(s) affected (Figure 11.3).

Lymphangiomas

Lymphangiomas may be capillary or cavernous (and associated with vascular malformations) or

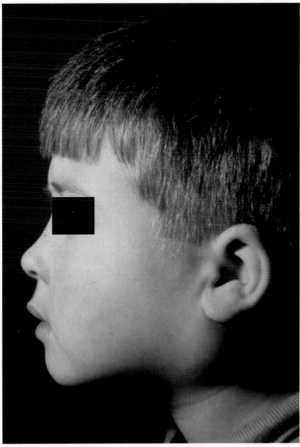

Figure 11.1a. A 3-year-old boy with prominent cavernous vascular neoplasm of the parotid gland.

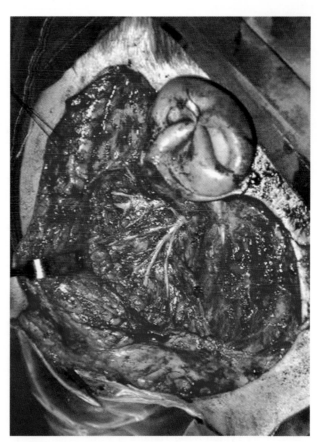

Figure 11.1c. The vascular neoplasm is removed in total with the superficial lobe of the parotid gland after complete facial nerve dissection.

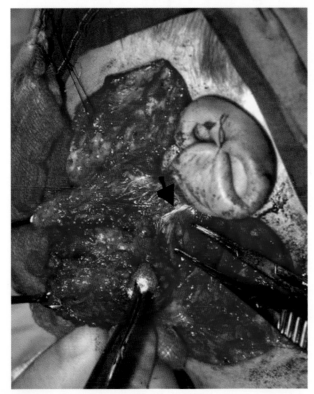

Figure 11.1b. Operative sequence shows the neoplasm is mobilized forward after ligating feeding vessels and is being peeled off the main trunk of the facial nerve (arrow).

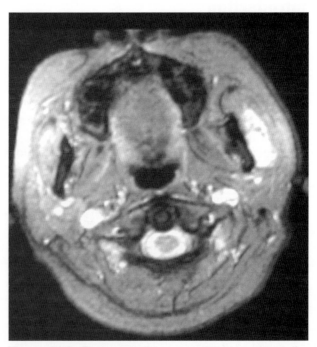

Figure 11.2. The magnetic resonance scan shows the vascular malformation to be located intramuscularly in the left masseter muscle deep to the parotid.

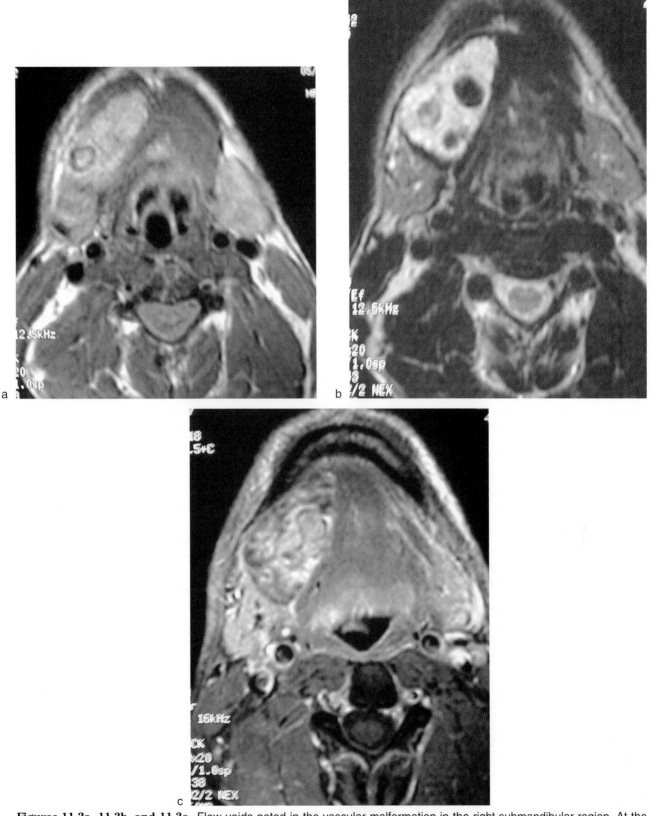

Figures 11.3a, 11.3b, and 11.3c. Flow voids noted in the vascular malformation in the right submandibular region. At the time of surgery this was found to be cavernous and primarily venous.

be cystic in nature. They are common in the neck and seen more in the submandibular (37%) than parotid glands (31%) (Orvidas and Kasperbauer 2000). They may be prominent at birth as cystic hygromas and may pose a threat to the airway (Figure 11.4). In children they can increase considerably in size during upper respiratory tract infections. Some authors have documented the posterior triangle to be a more common site in the neck than the submandibular space, 54% versus 17%, respectively (Fageeh, Manoukian, and Tewfik et al. 1997). In a series of 324 pediatric patients with salivary gland masses, 89 (27.5%) were lymphangiomas compared to 192 (59.2%) being hemangiomas (Bentz et al. 2000). Many of these lesions are treated surgically, but persistence and recurrence are problematic (Orvidas and Kasperbauer 2000). Especially in the infiltrating lesions, complete excision may be impossible and debulking is performed. Surgery can be combined with sclerosing injections or these can be used as a single modality. Sclerosing agents are most effective in macrocystic lymphangiomas, and in 54 of these cases 49% had excellent results, 35% good, and 16% poor using sclerosant injection (Emran, Dubois, and Laberge et al. 2006).

Neural Tumors

In Siefert and Oehne's (1986) review of 150 benign mesenchymal tumors of the salivary glands, 16% were neurogenic in origin distributed over the fourth to seventh decade. These were divided into neurilemmomas (neurinomas) in 12 of 27 cases, neurofibromas in 12 of 27 cases, and neurofibromatosis in 3 of 27 cases. There was a predominance of males, 75% for neurofibromas but 65% females for neurilemmomas. Both MR and CT scan may be useful in imaging. In the parotid gland extension of the tumor in the gland and in the petrous bone is well defined by MR imaging, while CT scan shows bone erosion and relationship to the inner ear. A combination of CT and MR is recommended when surgical resection is planned (Martin et al. 1992).

Complete removal of these lesions, especially the plexiform neurofibroma, can be extremely difficult due to their infiltrating nature and often increased vascularity (Figure 11.5). Although approximately one-third of neurilemmomas occur in the head and neck (Almeyda et al. 2004), they are comparatively rare in the salivary glands published as isolated case reports. However, as they may be mistaken for a malignant parotid tumor due to facial nerve dysfunction—for example, progressive weakness, sudden facial paralysis, hemifacial spasm and pain (Balle and Greisen 1984)—it is important to make the diagnosis to avoid inappropriate radical surgery. Regarding intra-parotid neurofibromas, a "conservative course of treatment with limited tumor excision and emphasis on retaining facial nerve function" is advocated (McGuirt, Johnson, and McGuirt 2003). Indeed, once the histologic diagnosis is made, because of the slow growth of the tumor and the unlikelihood of malignant change, conservative treatment of leaving the tumor in situ to preserve the nerve has been recommended (Fierke, Laskawi, and Kunze 2006).

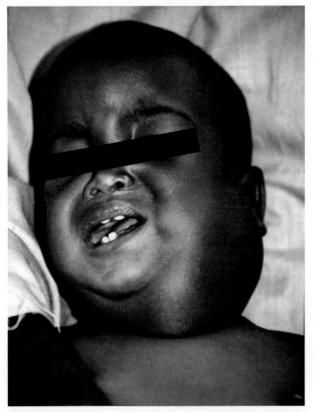

Figure 11.4. Lymphangioma involving both the parotid and submandibular glands in an 8-month-old infant.

Lipomas

Approximately 15–20% of lipomas occur in the head and neck region (Weiss and Goldblum 2001),

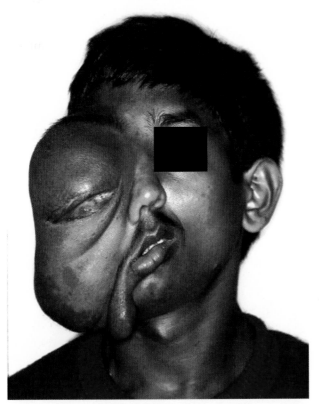

Figure 11.5a. Massive plexiform neurofibroma involving the parotid gland and orbit.

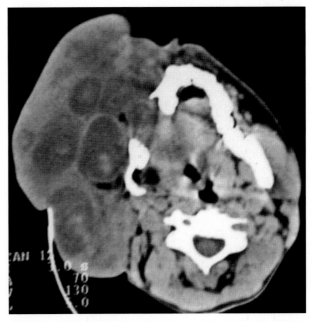

Figure 11.5b. CT scan shows extensive soft tissue involvement.

and in reviewing 125 lipomas in the oral and max-illofacial region, 30 (24%) were parotid and 17 (13.6%) were submandibular in orgin (Furlong, Fanburg-Smith, and Childers 2004). In this series there was a 3:1 male to female gender ratio and a mean age of 51.9 years. Histologically almost half (62/125) were classic lipomas, while 59 were spindle cell/pleomorphic, 2 were fibrolipomas, and 2 chondroid lipomas. Spindle cell lipomas comprised the majority of parotid lipomas. In a review of 167 mesenchymal salivary gland tumors, Seifert and Oehne (1986) found lipomas comprised 22.5% of 150 benign tumors and 95% were in the parotid. Again 85% occurred in males. A report of 660 parotid neoplasms found only 8 patients had lipomatous tumors (1.3%), 5 with focal lipoma and 3 with diffuse lipomatosis (Ethunandan, Vura, and Umar et al. 2006). Only one tumor of 8 was in the deep lobe, but small series of parotid lipomas in the deep lobe have been reported (Gooskens and Mann 2006).

Lipomas are comparatively rare in the oral cavity, but in one paper with 46 cases, 2 patients were classified as having minor salivary gland lipomas (Fregnani, Pires, and Falzoni et al. 2003).

Salivary lipomas usually present as slow-growing painless masses, and their appearance on CT or MR is diagnostic (Figure 11.6). Surgical excision is the treatment of choice, and although easy in classic lipoma, it can be challenging in the infiltrating variety (Figure 11.7).

Recently a designation of sialolipoma has been proposed for lipomas containing glandular elements, for example, ductal or acinar tissue (Nagao, Sugano, and Ishida et al. 2001). In their series of 2,051 salivary tumors, 7 sialolipomas, 5 in the parotid, and 2 palatal, were reported. Excision as for classic lipoma is curative. Since the initial report other cases both in major and minor glands have been published (Lin, Lin, and Chen et al. 2004; Michaelidis, Stefanopoulos, and Sambaziotis et al. 2006).

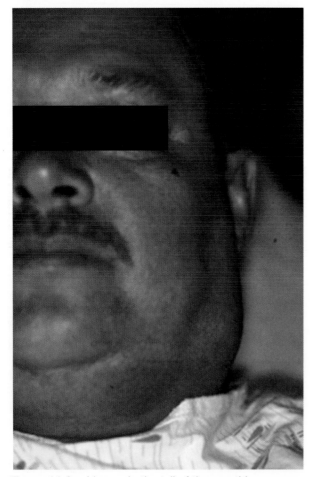

Figure 11.6a. Lipoma in the tail of the parotid.

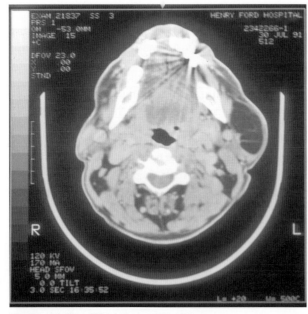

Figure 11.6b. CT is diagnostic of lipoma.

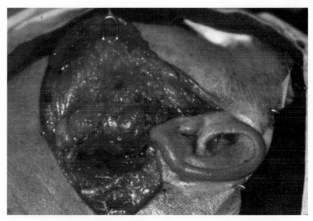

Figure 11.6c. Intraoperative view of parotidectomy with parotid tail lipoma.

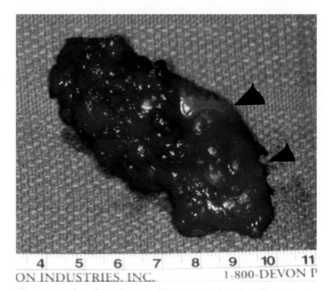

Figure 11.6d. Specimen with arrows showing lipoma.

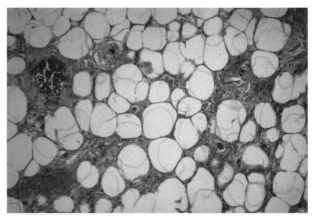

Figure 11.6e. Histopathology confirms the presence of lipoma.

268

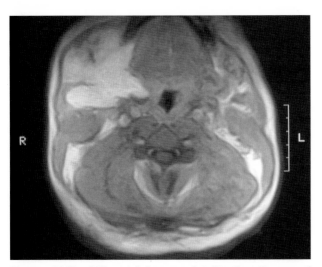

Figure 11.7a. MR axial image of infiltrating lipoma of right submandibular region extending between the cervical muscles.

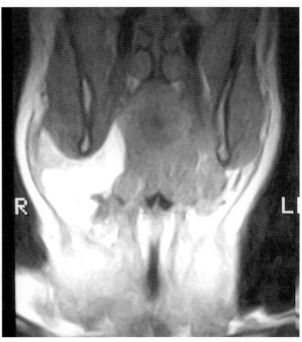

Figure 11.7b. Coronal MR image shows the lipoma extending medial to the right medial pterygoid muscle into the lateral pharyngeal space.

MALIGNANT MESENCHYMAL TUMORS

Sarcomas

Sarcomas of the salivary glands are very rare and case reports of virtually all histologic types have been reported. In Siefert and Oehne's 1986 review of 167 mesenchymal tumors of the salivary glands, only 17 were sarcomas (10%). In this series, 5 cases were malignant fibrous histiocytomas, 5 cases were malignant schwannomas, 4 cases were embryonal rhabdomyosarcoma, and single cases of myxoid liposarcoma, leiomyosarcoma, and malignant hemangioendothelioma were reviewed. In reviewing salivary masses in children, rhabdomyosarcomas were the most common malignant mesenchymal tumor (7%) (Bentz et al. 2000), and in 137 children with rhabdomyosarcomas of the head and neck the parotid was the site for 6% of these tumors (Hicks and Flaitz 2002). Obviously treatment plans will be dictated by the individual sarcoma type, with initial chemotherapy for rhabdomyosarcoma in children followed by radiation therapy or surgery for residual disease. Rhabdomyosarcoma of the salivary glands appears locally aggressive with a poor prognosis (BenJelloun,

Jouhadi, and Maazouzi et al. 2005). In malignant fibrous histiocytoma, clear surgical margins appear to be the most important prognostic factor (Sachse, August, and Alberty 2006). Angiosarcoma may affect the parotid as a primary or metastatic tumor, and in a series of 29 angiosarcomas of the oral and salivary gland region there were 4 primary parotid and 3 primary submandibular gland angiosarcomas with a further 3 metastatic to the parotid (Fanburg-Smith, Furlong, and Childers 2003).

All of the metastatic patients died, but patients with primary salivary gland angiosarcoma appear to have a better prognosis than those with cutaneous or deep tissue angiosarcomas. Malignant neural sarcomas are treated with wide excision and facial nerve grafting or reanimation (McGuirt, Johnson, and McGuirt 2003). Other sarcomas of the salivary glands are rare; for example, Chadan et al. (2004) found only 11 reported cases of salivary gland liposarcoma in the literature.

Sarcomas can involve any of the major salivary glands although the parotid is most common, and due to its rarity, treatment is usually on an individual and empiric basis (Figure 11.8).

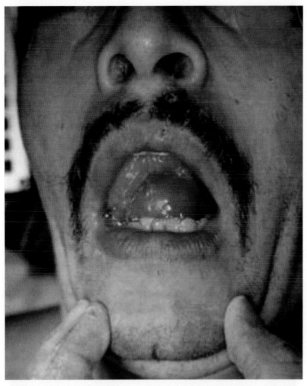

Figure 11.8a. Rapidly growing sublingual gland tumor diagnosed as synovial cell sarcoma on biopsy and immunohistochemistry.

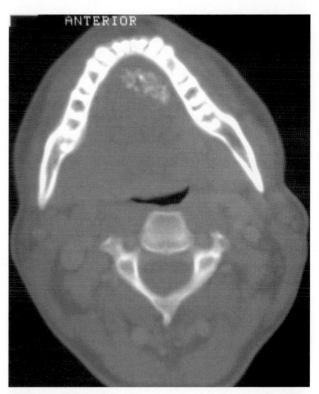

Figure 11.8c. CT bone window shows calcifications throughout the mass.

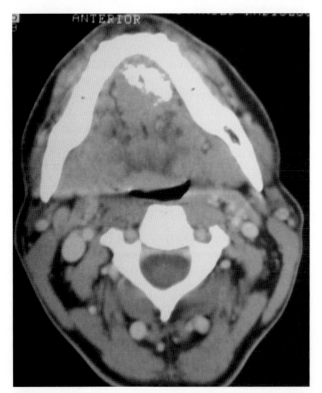

Figure 11.8b. CT image reveals calcification in the mass leading to an initial clinical diagnosis of a high-grade malignant carcinoma ex-pleomorphic adenoma.

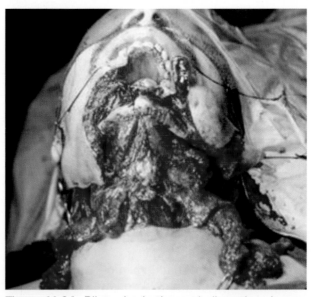

Figure 11.8d. Bilateral selective neck dissections in continuity with lip split to access the mandible.

270

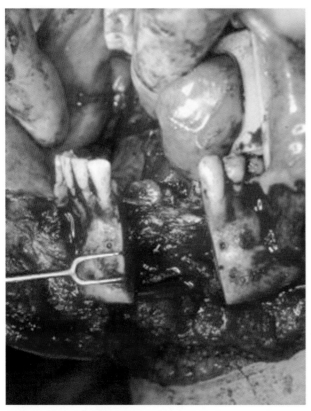

Figure 11.8e. Midline mandibulotomy prior to excision of the floor of mouth and ventral tongue.

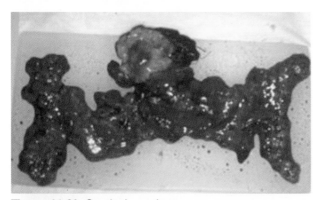

Figure 11.8f. Surgical specimen.

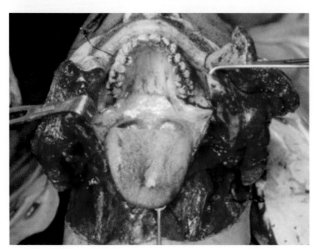

Figure 11.8g. Post-resection—the reconstruction will be a microvascular forearm flap.

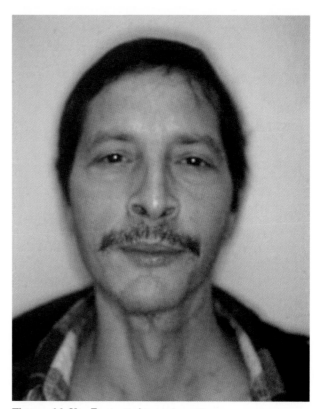

Figure 11.8h. Four weeks post-surgery.

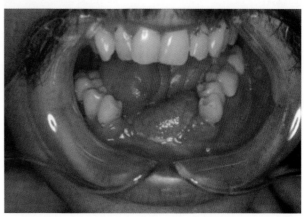

Figure 11.8i. Intraoral view showing the forearm flap reconstruction of the floor of the mouth.

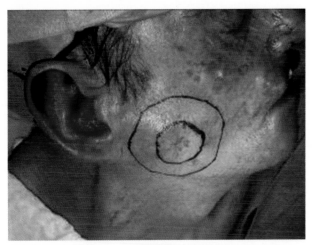

Figure 11.9a. Elderly man with primary desmoid melanoma of the parotid gland. A 2 cm margin is marked; the light blue staining of the skin around the lesion is from dye injection for sentinel node biopsy (patient had lymphoscintigraphy immediately preoperatively).

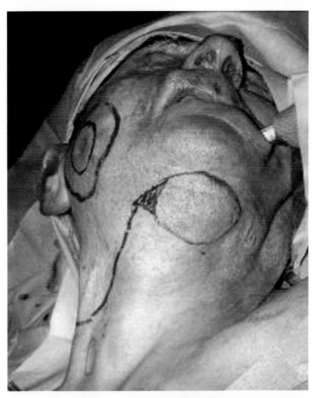

Figure 11.9b. Markings for the proposed surgery involving a total parotidectomy with left supraomohyoid neck dissection (unless sentinel nodes are found at levels IV or V). Reconstruction with a submental flap based on the submental vessels.

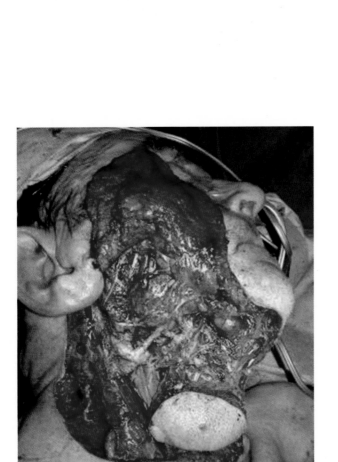

Figure 11.9c. The neck dissection and parotidectomy with preservation of the facial nerve is complete. The submental flap is pedicled on its vascular supply prior to being rotated into the defect.

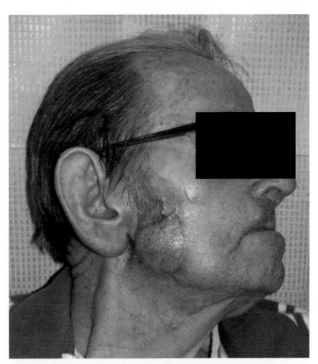

Figure 11.9d. Three months postoperatively.

EPITHELIAL NON-SALIVARY TUMORS

The major salivary glands may be infiltrated by squamous cell carcinoma from the overlying skin or be primarily involved by melanoma. Surgical resection with a margin of normal tissue preserving the facial nerve and utilizing neck dissection and adjuvant radiotherapy as indicated by the tumor stage is the appropriate treatment (Figure 11.9).

Tumors of Salivary Gland Lymph Nodes

PRIMARY LYMPH NODE TUMORS

Lymphomas

Primary lymphoma of the salivary glands is rare. Eighty percent of lymphomas of the salivary glands are found in the parotid gland and 20% in the submandibular gland, with only case reports of sublingual and minor gland involvement (Eraso, Lorusso, and Palacios 2005) (Figure 11.10).

Other authors have found a higher incidence of submandibular involvement (39%) (Dunn, Kuo, and Shih et al. 2004). In 121 parotid tumors 8.3% were lymphomas (Shine, O'Leary, and Blake 2006), and in 51 submandibular tumors 14% were lymphomas (Preuss, Klussman, and Wittekindt et al. 2007).

Patients with Sjogren's syndrome, AIDS, and hepatitis C have an increased risk of developing salivary lymphomas. In a review of 463 cases of Sjogren's syndrome, 27 patients had a diagnosis of lymphoma (5.8%) (Tonami, Matoba, and Kuginuki et al. 2003). In this series 26 of the 27 patients had non-Hodgkin's lymphoma [including 6 mucosa-associated lymphoid tissue (MALT) lymphomas] and only 1 patient had Hodgkin's lymphoma. At the initial presentation 14 (52%) of patients had extranodal disease, with 9 of 27 (33%) in the salivary glands. However, 21 patients (78%) had nodal involvement, mostly in the cervical nodes. Masaki and Sugai (2004) also reported a figure of 5% of Stage III Sjogren's patients developing lymphomas that are thought to arise from lymphoepithelial lesions. The B cells in these lesions become activated by interactions between CD40L and CD40 with progression from polyclonal lymphoproliferation, to monoclonal lymphoproliferation, to MALT lymphoma, and finally to high-grade lymphoma as a multistep process. Other authors have highlighted

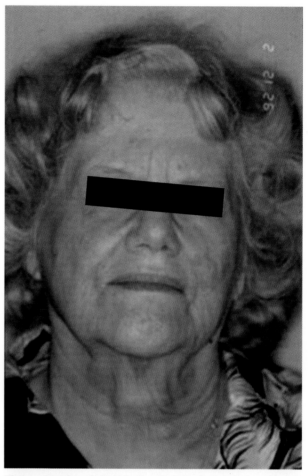

Figure 11.10a. Elderly lady with itchy facial and neck rash who complains of an intraoral swelling.

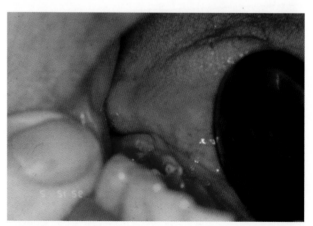

Figure 11.10b. A red fleshy swelling of the sublingual gland is appreciated with retraction of the commissure by the patient's finger and retraction of the tongue by the mirror. Biopsy showed a non-Hodgkin's lymphoma of the sublingual gland.

the difficulty in diagnosing true lymphoma from the other lymphoproliferative disorders occurring in Sjogren's syndrome, although there is a forty-fold increased risk in developing B-cell lymphomas (Prochorec-Sobieszek and Wagner 2005). Clinical features associated with lymphoma include persistent major salivary enlargement (>2 months), persistent lymphadenopathy or splenomegaly, monoclonal gammopathy, and type II mixed cryoglobulinemia.

Hepatitis C is also associated with MALT lymphomas of the salivary glands. In a series of 33 cases of primary salivary MALT lymphomas, 15 patients had a history of Sjogren's syndrome (45.5%), 2 (6%) other autoimmune disease, and 7 (21%) hepatitis C infection (Ambrossetti, Zanotti, and Passaro et al. 2004). There is an increase in lymphoma in AIDS, however, although in 51% of patients in a study of 100 patients who died with AIDS without salivary gland symptoms who showed histologic signs of parotid disease, only 1 case of lymphoma was found (Vargas, Mauad, and Bohm et al. 2003) (Figure 11.11).

Not all primary salivary lymphomas fall into the MALT group, and follicular lymphomas comprise 30% and 22% of two recently published series (Kojima, Nakamura, and Ichimura et al. 2001; Nakamura, Ichimura, and Sato et al. 2006) (Figure 11.12). These lymphomas have a younger age of onset than MALT lymphomas, do not occur in patients with autoimmune disease, and appear relatively more common in the submandibular gland.

Most salivary lymphomas present as unilateral, painless masses, usually with a history of <4 months, and although CT scans show poorly

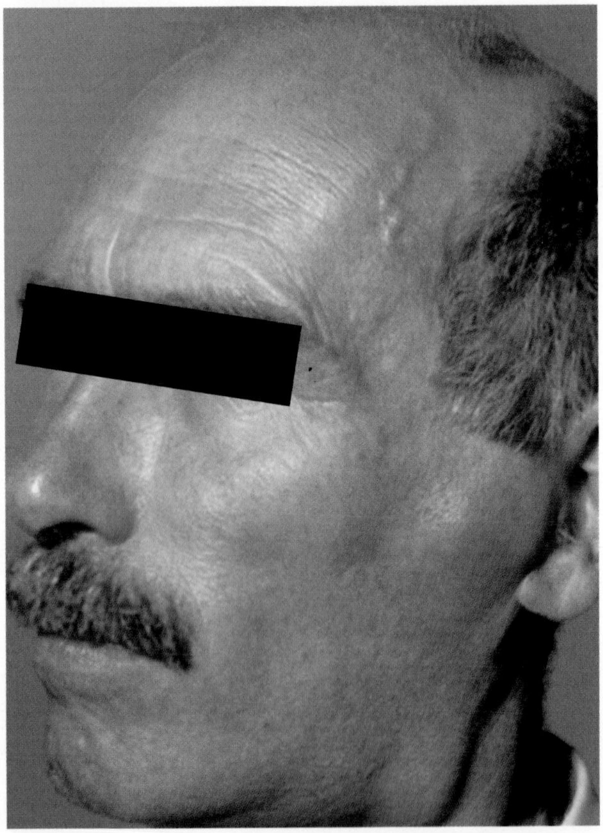

Figure 11.11. A 52-year-old man with a left parotid mass and a firm level II node who has a salivary lymphoma as a presenting sign of previously undiagnosed AIDS.

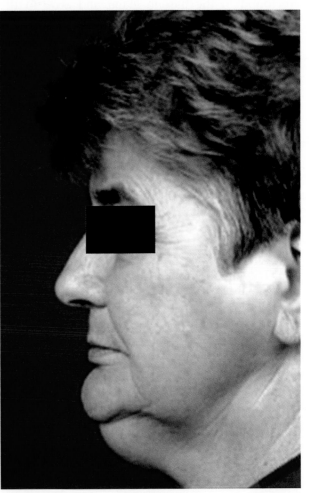

Figure 11.12. Non-Hodgkin's lymphoma of the left parotid gland and submental nodes.

defined indistinct margins, there is no pathognomic sign for salivary lymphoma (Shine, O'Leary, and Blake 2006). The lesions may be multiple in the ipsilateral gland and associated lymphadenopathy can be noted. The use of FNAB in diagnosing salivary lymphoma has been questioned as inaccurate with high rates of false negative results.

Zurrida, Alasio, and Tradati et al. (1993) were only able to identify 2 of 7 lymphomas (28.6%), and Hughes, Volk, and Wilbur (2005) found a 57% false negative rate in salivary lymphomas in reviewing the data from the College of American Pathologists Interlaboratory Comparison Program in Nongynecologic Cytology. In the absence of Sjogren's syndrome or clinical suspicion of lymphoma, these lesions are frequently diagnosed following surgical removal.

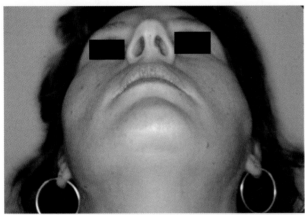

Figure 11.13a. A 35-year-old lady with MALT lymphoma of Waldeyer's ring controlled by chemotherapy. Now has bilateral parotid involvement that is not responding to medical therapy and she is concerned regarding her appearance.

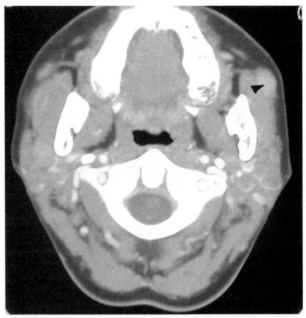

Figure 11.13c. CT scan shows smaller mass of MALT lymphoma in the anterior left parotid gland.

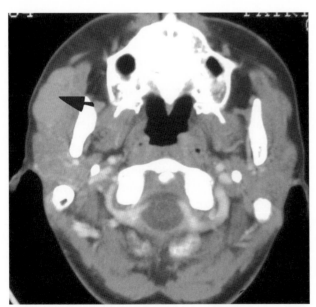

Figure 11.13b. CT scan shows homogenous mass of MALT lymphoma in the anterior portion of the right parotid (arrow), which has slowly increased in size over a 3-year period.

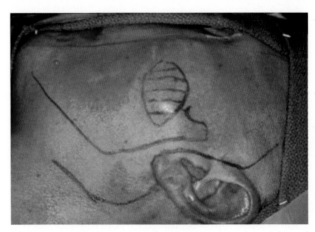

Figure 11.13d. Proposed parotidectomy and excision of MALT lymphoma.

Treatment is by chemotherapy, medical therapy, and radiation therapy depending on the histologic diagnosis and the clinical staging. MALT lymphomas of salivary glands appear to have a low-grade indolent course with 5-year overall survival, case-specific survival, and progression-free survival of 85% (±8%), 94% (±6%), and 65% (±10%), respectively (Ambrossetti, Zanotti, and Passaro et al. 2004). These results were noted despite 42% of their patients being Stage IV, and local therapy was often adequate (Figure 11.13). Dunn, Kuo, and Shih et al. (2004) in 23 primary salivary lymphomas, 19 MALT, 3 diffuse large cell, and 1 follicular found overall 5-year survival of 94.7% and relapse-free survival of 51.4%. Only 2 patients died; MALT lymphoma in 1 patient transformed into diffuse large cell lymphoma and the patient died. Kojima, Nakamura, and Ichimura et al. (2001) noted that follicular lymphomas arising from salivary glands appeared to share some of the characteristics of MALT lymphoma with an indolent prognosis.

SECONDARY LYMPH NODE TUMORS

Regional Metastases

The lymph nodes associated with the major glands may all become involved by regional metastases. In the parotid gland, skin cancer, particularly squamous cell carcinoma (SCC) and malignant melanoma (MM) of the scalp, forehead, temple, upper lip, cheek, and ear is most common, although Merkel cell tumors, malignant syringomas, and other more unusual skin cancers can be seen (Figure 11.14).

The largest experience with these tumors is in Australia, where squamous cell carcinoma and melanoma of the facial skin is epidemic and metastatic cutaneous cancer is the commonest parotid malignancy (O'Brien, McNeil, and McMahon et al. 2002). Although less than 5% of patients with cutaneous SCC do metastasize to lymph nodes, certain features may give these tumors an increased risk of metastasizing. In a review of 266 patients, 61% having parotid lymph node involvement ± cervical involvement, tumor thickness >4–5 mm, and proximity to the parotid (temple/forehead, cheek, or ear) were high risks, and increasing tumor size and recurrence contributed to an increased risk (Veness, Palme, and Morgan 2006) (Figure 11.15). In 2002 O'Brien, McNeil, and

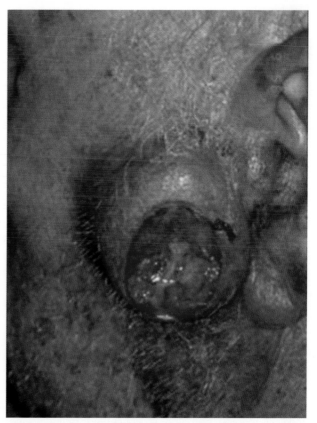

Figure 11.14. Malignant syringoma of forehead metastatic to the left parotid gland and fungating through preauricular skin.

McMahon et al. suggested that the TNM system of designating all nodal metastases from cutaneous cancer N1 was limited and did not accurately delineate the extent of disease. They suggested separating disease in the parotid P1 <3 cm, P2 >3 cm and <6 cm, P3 >6 cm from neck disease: N0 no nodal disease, N1 a single node <3 cm, N2 multiple nodes or any node >3 cm for staging. In a multivariate analysis of 87 patients they found that increasing P stage, positive margins, and lack of adjuvant RT independently predicted for decreased local control in the parotid. Clinical and pathologic N stage both significantly impacted survival. They concluded that patients with positive nodes in both parotid and neck had the worst prognosis, and that prognosis was worse for nodal disease > N1 (Figure 11.16). A much smaller study from Israel showed a zero overall survival for patients with both parotid and cervical nodes positive for metastatic cutaneous SCC (Barzilai et al. 2005). Using the separate staging system for parotid disease (P) and neck disease (N) proposed by

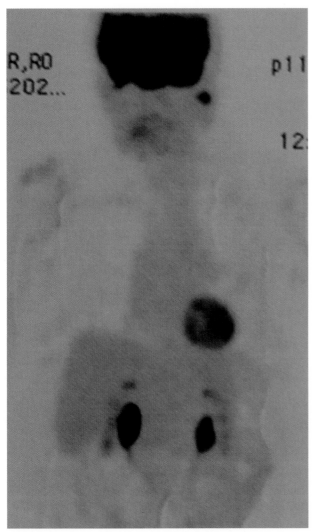

Figure 11.15a. PET scan of elderly woman with left pre-auricular mass post-resection of squamous cell carcinoma of the cheek. Scan shows a hot spot (SUV 6.7).

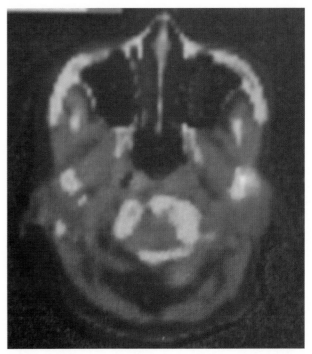

Figure 11.15b. Fused PET/CT confirms positive node in the parotid gland.

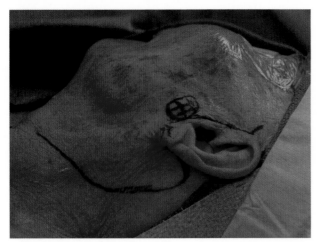

Figure 11.15c. Proposed surgery of superficial parotidectomy with extended Blair incision to allow for supraomohyoid neck dissection.

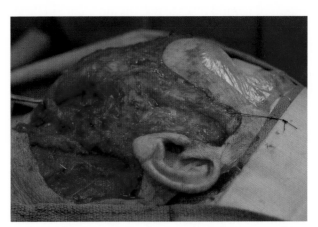

Figure 11.15d. Incision allows wide access down to level III of the neck.

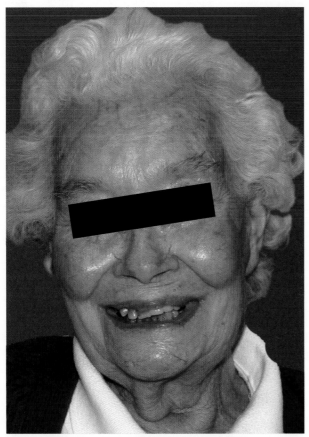

Figure 11.15e. Postoperatively the patient has no nerve weakness.

O'Brien, McNeil, and McMahon et al. (2002), two recent studies have been published. One series of 67 patients from New Zealand found again that the extent of parotid disease was an independent prognostic factor and that patients with both parotid and neck disease did worst, although interestingly adjuvant RT did not influence survival in their data (Ch'ng, Maitra, and Lea et al. 2006). The second paper was a retrospective multi-center trial from three Australian and three U.S. centers with 322 patients with metastatic cutaneous SCC to the parotid and/or neck. Results from this study show a significantly worse 5-year survival for patients with advanced P stage, 69%, vs. 82% for early P stage; and 61% with parotid + neck disease vs. 79% for parotid alone. This study supported the adoption of the new staging system separating parotid and neck disease (Andruchow, Veness, and Morgan et al. 2006).

In terms of behavior of metastatic cancer to the parotid, Bron et al. (2003) reviewed 232 cases of which 54 were primary parotid cancers, 101 were metastatic cutaneous SCC, 69 MM, and 8 other metastatic cancers. Patients were treated with primary surgery sparing the facial nerve where indicated, with 54 therapeutic and 110 elective neck dissections, and 78% of the patients had adjuvant RT. Five-year survival rates were 77% for primary cancers, 65% for metastatic SCC, 46% for MM, and 56% for other metastatic cancers. As expected, local failure was highest in metastatic SCC and distant failure in MM.

In treating patients with nodal involvement of the parotid, superficial parotidectomy with wide excision to obtain negative margins is indicated with facial nerve sacrifice if it is infiltrated. When the neck is also involved level II is the commonest site, and in these cases a comprehensive neck dissection is recommended (Figure 11.17). If the neck is clinically uninvolved (N0), and the primary cancer anterolateral to the parotid, then a supraomohyoid neck dissection including the external jugular nodes is indicated, and with a posterior primary level V should be dissected as well (Vauterin, Veness, and Morgan et al. 2006). Adjuvant RT is given in node positive necks for close margins or perineural invasion. In the case of MM where sentinel lymph nodes are identified in the parotid by scintigraphy, intraparotid sentinel lymph node biopsy is a reliable, accurate, and safe procedure (Loree, Tomljanovich, and Cheney et al. 2006).

In addition to regional metastasis from cutaneous primary cancers, metastasis can occur from noncutaneous head and neck carcinomas. Metastasis to the parotid from other head and neck sites—for example, the oral cavity—is more common if the usual lymphatic drainage pattern has been disrupted by previous neck dissection or radiation therapy (Ord, Ward-Booth, and Avery 1989). It is also possible for mucosal melanoma to metastasize to the parotid region (Figure 11.18).

There are fewer reports of involvement of the submandibular gland being directly involved by lymph node metastases, although it is routinely removed during neck dissection. The lymph nodes are not usually found within its capsule; however, Preuss, Klussman, and Wittekindt et al. (2007) found that in 24 malignant submandibular gland

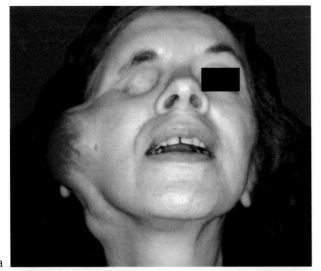

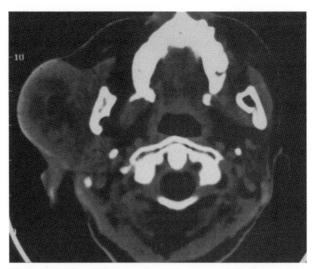

Figure 11.16c. CT scan shows huge parotid mass.

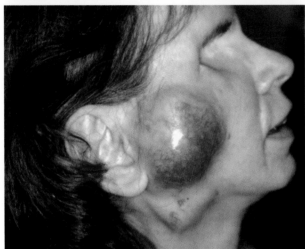

Figures 11.16a and 11.16b. An elderly lady who had excision of eyelids and orbital exenteration for advanced squamous cell carcinoma of the eyelids. She was lost to follow-up and now presents with massive disease in the parotid nodes (P3) and level II neck nodes (N2).

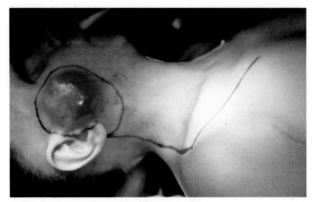

Figure 11.16d. Proposed surgery with radical parotidectomy and radical neck dissection.

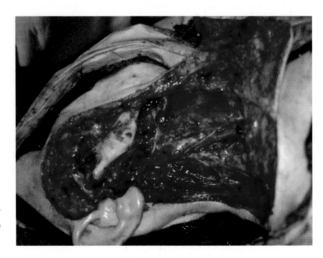

Figure 11.16e. Post-resection the masseter muscle is sacrificed along with the facial nerve and a total parotidectomy. The mandible was uninvolved by tumor and was preserved.

279

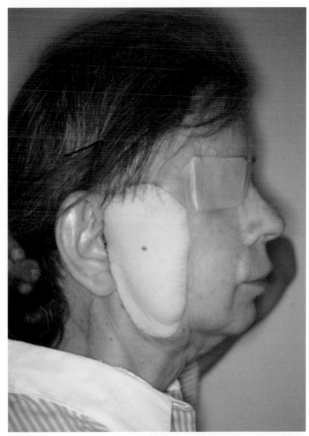

Figure 11.16f. Reconstruction is with a latissimus dorsi flap. The patient developed chest metastases 18 months post-surgery. Figures 11.16a, 11.16b, and 11.16f reprinted with permission from Ord RA. Local and regional flap reconstruction. In: Ward-Booth P, Schendel SA, Hausamen JE (eds.), Maxillofacial Surgery (2nd ed.). New York: Elsevier, 2007, pp. 643–665.

tumors, 30% were metastatic, 3 from the oropharynx, 2 from the nasopharynx, and 2 with unknown primaries.

In the sublingual gland metastatic spread from tongue cancer to sublingual nodes is not common and was first reported in 3 cases in 1985 (Ozeki et al. 1985). In one study of 253 patients with 326 neck dissections, 5 cases of lingual lymph node metastases were found and in all of these cases bilateral cervical nodes were found (Woolgar 1999). Whether these may explain some cases of "local" recurrence with previous negative margins is unclear. Certainly these lingual nodes would be removed in composite or "commando" resections where the tongue primary is removed in continuity

with the neck dissection, but they may be left in cases where the primary cancer is resected from an intraoral approach and the neck dissection is performed separately. One study reports a 5-year actuarial survival of 80% for patients treated with incontinuity neck dissection compared to 63% for those with discontinuity dissection (Leemans et al. 1991). Whether some of this difference in survival is attributable to involvement of sublingual gland nodes is unknown.

Distant Metastases

The major salivary glands can also be a site for distant metastatic disease, especially the parotid gland, although these cases are rare. In a literature review of over 800 patients with metastatic disease in the parotid, 80% were from cutaneous SCC or melanoma (as described above), while 66 were noncutaneous head and neck tumors and 87 from a distant primary site (Pisani et al. 1993). In their personal series of 38 patients, 10 had noncutaneous head and neck cancers, while 4 were from distant sites (2 renal and 2 lung). Nuyens et al. (2006) found 34 of 520 parotid tumors to be metastatic, 31 from cutaneous primaries, 2 from ductal breast cancer, and 1 from an extremity rhabdomyosarcoma. Although rare, these distant metastases can provide a diagnostic challenge, as the two commonest primary sites appear to be lung and kidney. Small cell lung cancer is very difficult to differentiate from primary small cell carcinoma of the salivary glands, such that CT scan of the lungs is an essential part of the workup (Figure 11.19). Salivary glands are the second commonest head and neck site for primary small cell carcinomas (larynx being the most common), and these are aggressive tumors with an overall poor prognosis (Renner 2007). They are divided into neuroendocrine and ductal types, and according to cytokeratin 20 immunoreactivity the ductal sites can be subdivided into pulmonary and Merkel types (Nagao, Gaffey, and Olsen et al. 2004). This study indicated that negative immunostain for cytokeratin 20 could be a marker for poor prognosis and also that salivary gland small cell carcinoma may have a better prognosis than extrasalivary sites.

In a single case report, immunohistochemical study of estrogen receptors was used to identify a parotid tumor as a breast metastasis (Perez-Fidalgo, Chirivella, and Laforga et al. 2007). Regarding distant metastases from renal cell cancer the same

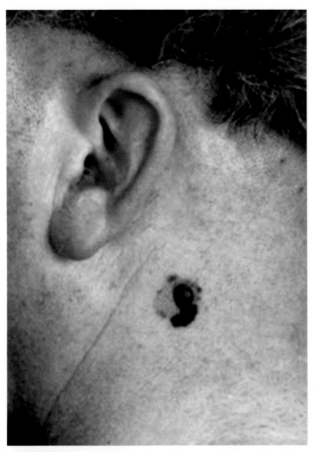

Figure 11.17a. Patient with nodular melanoma of posterior neck with palpable parotid lymph nodes.

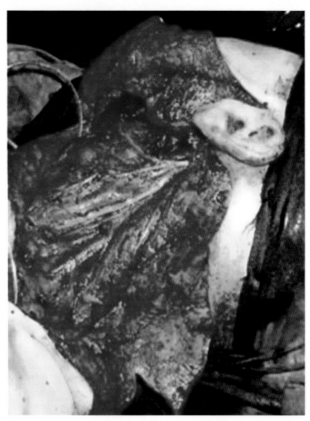

Figure 11.17b. Post–total parotidectomy and radical neck dissection.

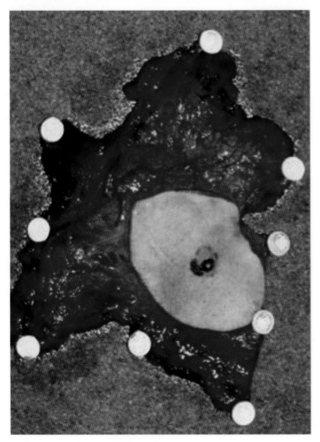

Figure 11.17c. Surgical specimen with 5 cm skin margins. Patient developed lung metastases within 6 months and died of disease. Figures 11.17a, 11.17b, and 11.17c reprinted with permission from Ord RA. Metastatic melanoma of the parotid lymph nodes. *Int J Oral Maxillofac Surg* 18:3, 1989.

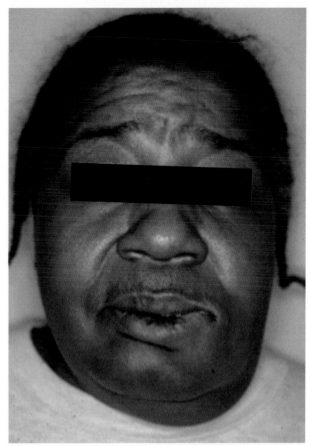

Figure 11.18a. Patient with large lymph node swelling at level I and pigmented melanoma of lower lip.

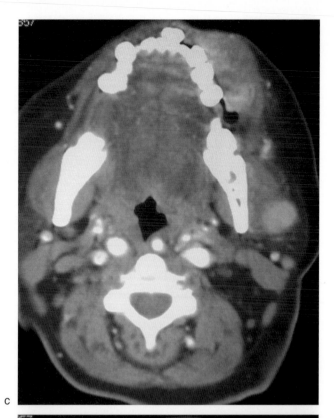

c

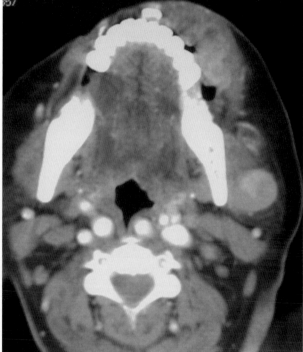

d

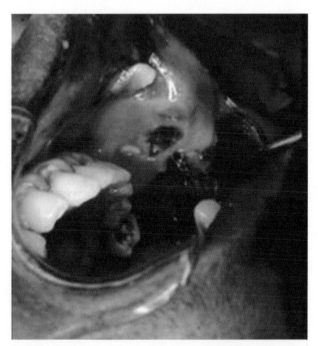

Figure 11.18b. Intraoral exam shows deeply pigmented melanoma involving the buccal mucosa and extending to the retromolar region.

Figures 11.18c and 11.18d. CT scans show primary melanoma as thickening of the left cheek and lip with nodal involvement of the left parotid gland.

282

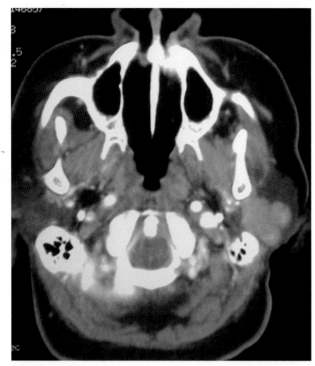

Figure 11.18e. CT scan at a more cephalad level now shows multiple positive nodes in the parotid gland.

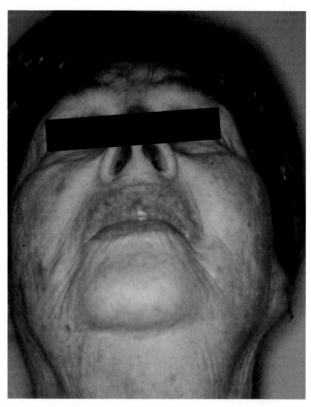

Figure 11.19a. An 80-year-old woman with known small cell carcinoma of the lung presenting with metastatic mass in the left parotid gland.

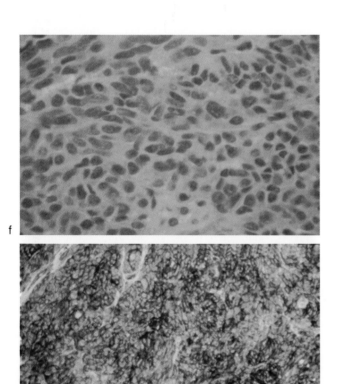

Figures 11.18f and 11.18g. Hematoxylin and eosin stain of the tumor (f) and HMB-45 stain (g) confirming the diagnosis of melanoma.

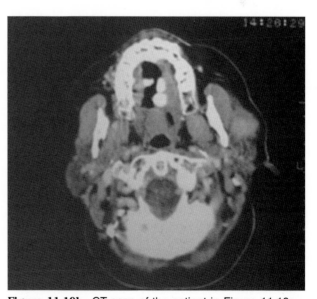

Figure 11.19b. CT scan of the patient in Figure 11.19a.

283

problem is found. Most of these will be from clear cell renal carcinoma and mimic the salivary clear cell adenocarcinoma or clear cell variant of MEC, which are both primary salivary gland cancers. In a case report and review of the literature, Park and Hlivko (2002) were able to find 25 cases of metastatic renal cell carcinoma to the parotid gland. In 14 of these cases (56%) the metastasis was the initial presenting sign of a previously undiagnosed renal carcinoma. None of the cases presented with facial paralysis and the authors were able to make the diagnosis in 3 of 6 cases with FNAB. In a small series of our own patients we were able to differentiate renal cell carcinoma from monomorphic clear cell salivary adenocarcinoma by immunohistochemistry and electron microscopic ultrastructural differences (Rezende, Drachenberg, and Kumar et al. 1997).

Distant metastasis to salivary glands other than the parotid appears to be extremely unusual, although a unique case of bilateral submandibular gland metastases from breast carcinoma was published in 2001 (Cain, Goodland, and Denholm 2001).

Summary

- The commonest parotid tumors in children are hemangiomas and hemangioendotheliomas.
- Medical therapy with steriods or alpha/beta interferon is preferred in the treatment of vascular parotid lesions in children.
- A combination of debulking and sclerosing injections to macrocystic areas is used for management of salivary lymphangiomas.
- Parotid lymphomas are usually associated with Sjogren's syndrome, hepatitis C, or AIDS.
- Most salivary lymphomas are MALT lymphomas, which follow a fairly indolent course.
- The parotid lymph node bed may be the first-echelon nodes for cutaneous cancers of the cheek, ear, scalp, forehead, and temple.
- Metastatic parotid nodes (P) and neck nodes (N) should be staged separately when involved by primary cutaneous cancers.
- Patients with both neck nodes and parotid nodes have the worst prognosis.
- Radiation therapy is given for close margins, perineural spread, and more than one positive node.

- When small cell carcinomas of the salivary glands are diagnosed, a full workup must be done to determine whether the tumor is a primary salivary gland cancer or a metastatic tumor from a distant site.

References

Almeyda R, Kothari P, Chau H, Cumberworth V. 2004. Submandibular neurilemmoma; a diagnostic dilemma. *J Laryngol Otol* 118(2):156–158.

Ambrossetti A, Zanotti R, Passaro C et al. 2004. Most cases of primary salivary mucosa-associated lymphoid tissue lymphoma are associated either with Sjogren's syndrome or hepatitis C virus infection. *Br J Haematol* 126(1): 43–49.

Andruchow JL, Veness MJ, Morgan GJ et al. 2006. Implications for clinical staging of metastatic cutaneous carcinoma of the head and neck based on a multicenter study of treatment outcomes. *Cancer* 106(5):1078–1083.

Balle VH, Greisen O. 1984. Neurilemmomas of the facial nerve presenting as parotid tumors. *Ann Otol Rhinol Laryngol* 93:70–72.

Barzilai G, Greenberg E, Cohen-Kermen R, Doweck I. 2005. Pattern of regional metastases from cutaneous squamous cell carcinoma of the head and neck. *Otolaryngol Head Neck Surg* 132(6):852–856.

BenJelloun H, Jouhadi H, Maazouzi A et al. 2005. Rhabdomyosarcoma of the salivary glands. Report of 3 cases. (Article in French.) *Cancer Radiother* 9(5):316–321.

Bentz BG, Hughes CA, Ludemann JP, Maddalozzo J. 2000. Masses of the salivary gland region in children. *Arch Otolaryngol Head Neck Surg* 126(12):1435–1439.

Bron LP, Traynor SJ, McNeil EB, O'Brien CJ. 2003. Primary and metastatic cancer of the parotid; comparison of clinical behavior in 232 cases. *Laryngoscope* 113(6):1070–1075.

Cain AJ, Goodland J, Denholm SW. 2001. Metachronous bilateral submandibular gland metastases from carcinoma of the breast. *J Laryngol Otol* 115(8):683–684.

Ch'ng S, Maitra A, Lea R et al. 2006. Parotid metastasis—an independent prognostic factor for head and neck cutaneous squamous cell carcinoma. *J Plast Reconstr Aesthet Surg* 59(12):1288–1293.

Chadan VS, Fung EK, Woods CI, de la Roza G. 2004. Primary pleomorphic liposarcoma of the parotid gland: A case report and review of the literature. *Am J Otolaryngol* 25:432–437.

Dunn P, Kuo TT, Shih LY et al. 2004. Primary salivary gland lymphoma: A clinicopathologic study of 23 cases in Taiwan. *Acta Hematol* 112(4):203–208.

Emran MA, Dubois J, Laberge L et al. 2006. Alcoholic solution of zein (Ethibloc) sclerotherapy for treatment of lymphangiomas in children. *J Pediatr Surg* 41(5): 975–979.

Eraso A, Lorusso G, Palacios E. 2005. Primary lymphoma of the parotid gland. *ENT-Ear Nose Throat J* 84(4):198–199.

Ethunandan M, Vura G, Umar T et al. 2006. Lipomatous lesions of the parotid gland. *J Oral Maxillofac Surg* 64(11):1583–1586.

Fageeh N, Manoukian J, Tewfik T et al. 1997. Management of head and neck lymphatic malformations in children. *J Otolaryngol* 26(4):253–258.

Fanburg-Smith JC, Furlong JC, Childers EL. 2003. Oral and salivary gland angiosarcoma: A clinicopathologic study of 29 cases. *Mod Pathol* 16(3):263–271.

Fierke O, Laskawi R, Kunze E. 2006. Solitary intraparotid neurofibroma of the facial nerve. Symptomatology, biology and management. (Article in German.) *HNO* 54(10):772–777.

Fregnani ER, Pires FR, Falzoni R et al. 2003. Lipomas of the oral cavity: Clinical findings, histological classification and proliferative activity of 46 cases. *Int J Oral Maxillofac Surg* 32(1):49–53.

Furlong MA, Fanburg-Smith JC, Childers EL. 2004. Lipomas of the oral and maxillofacial region: Site and subclassification of 125 cases. *Oral Surg Oral Med Oral Pathol Oral Radiol Endod* 98(4):441–450.

Gooskens I, Mann JJ. 2006. Lipoma of the deep lobe of the parotid gland: Report of 3 cases. *ORL J Otorhinolaryngol Relat Spec* 68(5):290–295, epub May 6, 2007.

Greene AK, Rogers GF, Mulliken JB. 2004. Management of parotid hemangiomas in 100 children. *Plast Reconstr Surg* 113(1):53–60.

Hicks J, Flaitz C. 2002. Rhabdomyosarcoma of the head and neck in children. *Oral Oncol* 38(5):450–459.

Hughes JH, Volk EE, Wilbur DC. 2005. Pitfalls in salivary gland fine-needle aspiration cytology: Lessons from the College of American Pathologists Interlaboratory Comparison Program in Nongynecologic Cytology. *Arch Pathol Lab Med* 129(1):26–31.

Kojima M, Nakamura S, Ichimura K et al. 2001. Follicular lymphoma of the salivary gland: A clinicopathologic and molecular study of six cases. *Int J Surg Pathol* 94(4):287–293.

Leemans CR, Tiwari R, Nauta JJ, Snow GB. 1991. Discontinuous vs. in-continuity neck dissection in carcinoma of the oral cavity. *Arch Otolaryngol Head Neck Surg* 117(9):1003–1006.

Lin YJ, Lin LM, Chen YK et al. 2004. Sialolipoma of the floor of the mouth: A case report. *Kaohsiung J Med Sci* 20(8):410–414.

Loree TR, Tomljanovich PI, Cheney RT et al. 2006. Intraparotid sentinel lymph node biopsy for head and neck melanoma. *Laryngoscope* 116(8):1461–1464.

Martin N, Sterkers O, Mompoint D, Nahum H. 1992. Facial nerve neuromas: MR imaging. Report of four cases. *Neuroradiology* 34(1):62–67.

Masaki Y, Sugai S. 2004. Lymphoproliferative disorders in Sjogren's syndrome. *Autoimmun Rev* 3(3):175–182.

McGuirt WF Sr, Johnson PE, McGuirt WT. 2003. Intraparotid facial nerve neurofibromas. *Laryngoscope* 113(10):82–84.

Michaelidis IG, Stefanopoulos PK, Sambaziotis D et al. 2006. Sialolipoma of the parotid gland. *J Craniomaxillofac Surg* 34(1):43–46, epub Dec. 15, 2005.

Nagao T, Gaffey TA, Olsen KD et al. 2004. Small cell carcinomas of the major salivary glands: Clinicopathologic study with emphasis on cytokeratin 20 immunoreactivity and clinical outcomes. *Am J Surg Pathol* 28(6):762–770.

Nagao T, Sugano I, Ishida Y et al. 2001. Sialolipoma: A report of seven cases of a new variant of salivary gland lipoma. *Histopathol* 38:33–36.

Nakamura S, Ichimura K, Sato Y et al. 2006. Follicular lymphoma frequently originates in the salivary gland. *Pathol Int* 56(10):576–583.

Nuyens M, Schupbach J, Stauffer E, Zbaren P. 2006. Metastatic disease to the parotid gland. *Otolaryngol Head Neck Surg* 135(6):844–848.

O'Brien CJ, McNeil EB, McMahon JD et al. 2002. Significance of clinical stage, extent of surgery, and pathologic findings in metastatic cutaneous squamous cell carcinoma of the parotid gland. *Head Neck* 24(5):417–422.

Ord RA. 2004. Salivary gland tumors in children. In: Kaban LB, Troulis MJ (eds.), Pediatric Oral and Maxillofacial Surgery. Philadelphia: W.B. Saunders, p. 202.

Ord RA, Ward-Booth RP, Avery BS. 1989. Parotid lymph node metastases from primary intraoral carcinomas. *Int J Oral Maxillofac Surg* 18:104–106.

Orvidas LJ, Kasperbauer JL. 2000. Pediatric lymphangiomas of the head and neck. *Ann Otol Rhinol Laryngol* 109(4):411–421.

Ozeki S, Tashiro H, Okamamoto M, Matsushima T. 1985. Metatasis to the lingual lymph nodes in carcinoma of the tongue. *J Maxillofac Surg* 13(6):277–281.

Park YW, Hlivko TJ. 2002. Parotid gland metastasis from renal cell carcinoma. *Laryngoscope* 112(3):453–456.

Perez-Fidalgo JA, Chirivella I, Laforga J et al. 2007. Parotid gland metastasis of a breast cancer. *Clin Transl Oncol* 9(4):264–265.

Pisani P, Krengeli M, Ramponi A, Pia F. 1993. Parotid metastases: A review of the literature and case reports. (Article in Italian) *Acta Otorhinolaryngol Ital* 12 Suppl 37:1–28.

Preuss SF, Klussman JP, Wittekindt C et al. 2007. Submandibular gland excision: 15 years of experience. *J Oral Maxillofac Surg* 65(5):953–957.

Prochorec-Sobieszek M, Wagner T. 2005. Lymphoproliferative disorders in Sjogren's syndrome. (Article in Polish.) *Otolaryngol Pol* 59(4):559–564.

Renner G. 2007. Small cell carcinomas of the head and neck: A review. *Semin Oncol* 34(1):3–14.

Rezende RB, Drachenberg CB, Kumar D et al. 1997. Differential diagnosis between monomorphic adenocarcinoma of the salivary glands and renal (clear) cell carcinoma. *Am J Surg Pathol* 23:1532–1538.

Sachse F, August C, Alberty J. 2006. Malignant fibrous histiocytoma in the parotid gland. Case series and literature review. (Article in German.) *HNO* 54(2):116–120.

Seifert G, Oehne H. 1986. Mesenchymal (non-epithelial) salivary gland tumors. Analysis of 167 tumor cases of the salivary gland register. *Laryngol Rhinol Otol* (Stuttg) 65(9):485–491.

Shine NP, O'Leary G, Blake SP. 2006. Parotid lymphomas—clinical and computed tomographic features. *S Afr J Surg* 44(2):62–64.

Tonami H, Matoba M, Kuginuki Y et al. 2003. Clinical and imaging findings of lymphoma in patients with Sjogren's syndrome. *J Comput Assist Tomogr* 27(4):517–524.

Vargas PA, Mauad T, Bohm GM et al. 2003. Parotid gland involvement in advanced AIDS. *Oral Dis* 9(2):55–61.

Vauterin TJ, Veness MJ, Morgan GJ et al. 2006. Patterns of lymph node spread of cutaneous squamous cell carcinoma of the head and neck. *Head Neck* 28:785–791.

Veness MJ, Palme CE, Morgan GJ. 2006. High-risk cutaneous squamous cell carcinoma of the head and neck: Results from 266 treated patients with metastatic lymph node disease. *Cancer* 106(11):2389–2396.

Weiss SW, Goldblum JR. 2001. In: Enzinger FM, Weiss SW (eds.), Soft Tissue Tumors (4th ed.). St. Louis: Mosby, p. 571.

Woolgar JA. 1999. Histological distribution of cervical lymph node metastases from intraoral/oropharyngeal squamous cell carcinomas. *Br J Oral Maxillofac Surg* 37(3):175–180.

Zbaren P, Schar C, Hotz MA et al. 2001. Value of fine-needle aspiration cytology of parotid gland masses. *Laryngoscope* 111(11 part 1):1989–2002.

Zurrida S, Alasio L, Tradati N et al. 1993. Fine needle aspiration of parotid masses. *Cancer* 72(8):2306–2311.

Chapter 12
Trauma and Injuries to the Salivary Glands

Outline

Introduction

The salivary glands may be subjected to a number of injuries and insults. Trauma to the parotid is relatively rare, noted to be present in only 0.21% of patients in a trauma unit (Lewis and Knottenbelt 1991). Penetrating trauma may be truly uncontrolled or accidental in nature; however, identical complications and injuries are seen after the intentional controlled trauma of surgery. This chapter will therefore deal with the complications of both salivary gland surgery and true traumatic injury. In addition, the injurious effects of radiation and barotrauma will be reviewed.

Penetrating Injuries

TRAUMA TO THE GLAND

Salivary Fistula
Penetrating injury to the substance of a major gland—for example, the parotid or submandibular gland—will cause direct damage to the gland and possible related structures and may lead to the formation of an external salivary fistula to the skin (Figure 12.1). When the substance of the gland is injured, suture of the parenchyma is recommended (Lewkowicz, Hasson, and Nablieli 2002). In addition to direct closure of the parotid capsule, a pressure dressing for 48 hours is applied to reduce the chances of sialocele formation. In 51 cases of parotid complications following trauma, 15 (29.4%) developed parotid fistula, treated by intravenous fluids and nil by mouth, with faster healing of parenchymal injuries alone than when the ductal system was involved (Parkeh, Glezerson, and Stewart et al. 1989). Similarly, Ananthakrishnan and Parkash (1982) reported that their 3 cases of fistula from the parotid gland parenchyma resolved without treatment, unlike the 14 fistulae related to parotid ductal injury. In a study of 13 patients with traumatic parotid fistulae, 54% resolved with conservative management within 3 weeks and the remainder were cured by internal drainage with a catheter (Cant and Campbell 1991). Landau and Stewart (1985) advocated conservative management of post-traumatic parotid fistulae and sialoceles and found that parenchymal injuries alone resolved in 5 days, whereas ductal injuries took 14 days. Morestin (1917), in a series of 62 war injuries with parotid fistula, 30 glandular and 32 ductal, reported good success with the creation of an intraoral fistula. In more extensive avulsive injuries with gross scarring, conservative treatment may be less successful (Figure 12.2), and established epithelialized fistulae require excision with repair of the parotid capsule and closure.

The submandibular gland is less liable to be involved in the development of traumatic fistulae, perhaps because it is protected by the mandible and its smaller size. Few cases of submandibular gland fistulae have been reported. A case report of submandibular gland fistula secondary to a gunshot wound was reported in 1995, where the authors also reviewed the literature and found only one

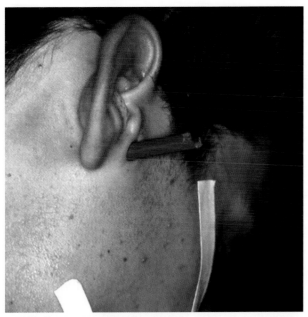

Figure 12.1a. Penetrating injury of the parotid after stabbing with a pencil.

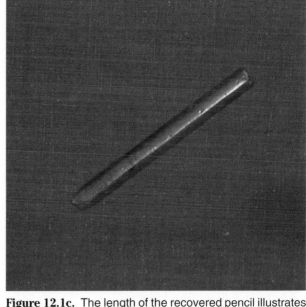

Figure 12.1c. The length of the recovered pencil illustrates the depth of the wound. Patient treated by Mr. B.S. Avery, Consultant OMS, Middlesborough, England.

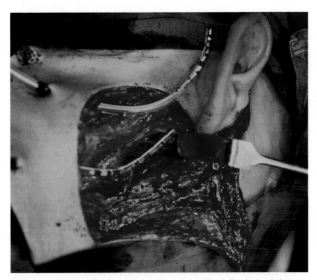

Figure 12.1b. Exploration via a modified Blair incision to check for damage to the external carotid artery and facial nerve and to suture the parotid capsule.

other case from 1976 (Singh and Shaha 1995). In their 1995 case the fistula resolved without active treatment in 10 days.

Rarely internal parotid fistulae can occur presenting as rhinorrhea or rhinorrhea related to food,

usually as a result of maxillary fracture with parotid fistula into the maxillary antrum (Faussat, Ghiassi, and Princ 1993; Scher and Poe 1988). In a recent report of parotid fistula into the maxillary antrum (and a very rare case of a sublingual gland fistula to the skin), excellent results were achieved with botulinum toxin injection (Breuer, Ferrazzini, and Grossenberger 2006). Although the authors state that primary surgical repair should be carefully considered, they found the injection of botulinum toxin to be effective, to shorten fistula closure time, and to be minimally invasive. The current management of fistulae from the parotid gland parenchyma is therefore conservative, as cases that do not involve the duct will resolve. In recalcitrant cases botulinum toxin appears a good option. True fistula post-surgery—for example, superficial parotidectomy—is not common but may occur through the surgical skin incision. Usually management with antisialogogues, nil by mouth, or botulinum toxin will lead to resolution. In a report of 3 cases post-parotidectomy treated with injection of botulinum toxin under electromyographic control, all resolved with no recurrence 14–21 months after therapy (Marchese-Ragona et al. 2006).

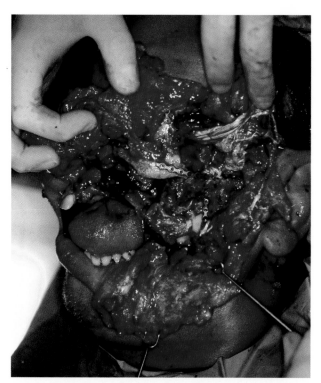

Figure 12.2a. Extensive avulsive injury from self-inflicted shotgun blast.

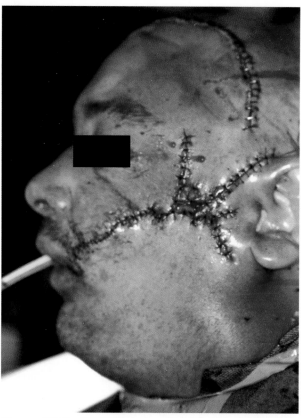

Figure 12.2b. Post-surgical reduction of facial fractures and wound closure.

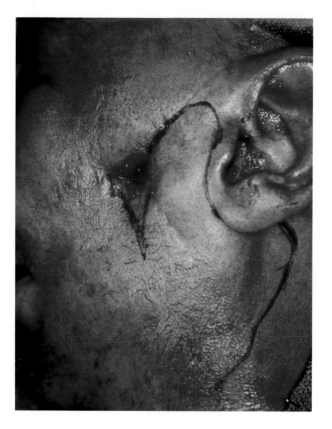

Figure 12.2c. A rotation advancement flap is marked out for skin coverage following excision of the parotid fistula.

Sialocele

A sialocele is formed by the extravasation of saliva into glandular or periglandular tissues due to disruption of the parenchymal or ductal structures of the salivary gland. This is most commonly seen following trauma, and the usual sites are the sublingual gland (ranula) or minor salivary glands (mucocele). Ranulae and mucoceles were discussed in chapter 4, and this section will concentrate largely on parotid sialoceles. Parotid sialoceles are usually seen after penetrating trauma to the parotid region and will present as painless, cystic swellings that are gradually increasing in size. Aspiration of the sialocele with fluid positive for amylase >10,000 units/liter will confirm the diagnosis. Computerized tomograms will show a cystic mass with smooth margins and a density lower than the surrounding tissues. After 2 weeks there will be enhancing borders due to the development of a capsule (Cholankeril and Scioscia 1993) (Figure 12.3).

Traditional management has been conservative, the same as for parotid parenchymal fistulae (Cant and Campbell 1991; Landau and Stewart 1985; Parkeh, Glezerson, and Stewart et al. 1989), with resolution reported in approximately the same time period as for fistulae. Most sialoceles develop 8–14 days post-injury, and the development of a late capsulated sialocele is more difficult to treat. Literature reviews show that treatments proposed include multiple aspirations, pressure dressings, secondary duct repair if this is the etiology, creation of an intraoral fistula, sectioning the auriculotemporal nerve, the use of antisialogogues (atropine, probanthine, glycopyrolate), duct ligation, and even radiation or parotidectomy (Canosa and Cohen 1999; Lewkowicz, Hasson, and Nablieli 2002) (Figures 12.4 and 12.5).

In recent years the use of botulinum toxin has caused a paradigm shift in the way these injuries can be managed. In 1999 Ragona, Blotta, and Pastore et al. reported a case of post-traumatic parotid sialocele resistant to conservative therapy that was successfully cured using botulinum injection. These authors used botulinum F due to its earlier and shorter efficacy compared to botulinum A, and injected the gland with electromyographic control. Botulinum toxin works by causing a chemical denervation of the gland by blocking the cholinergic neurotransmitter. Following this paper a

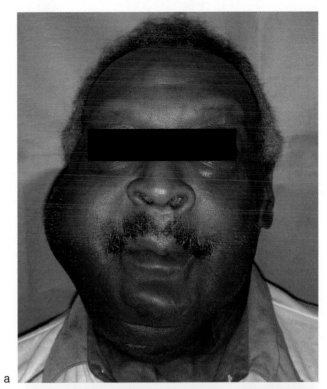

a

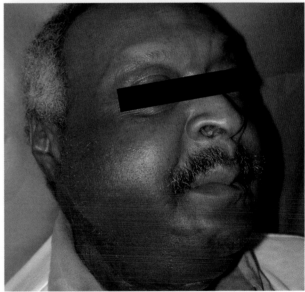

b

Figures 12.3a and 12.3b. Frontal and three-quarter views of patient with right parotid sialocele post-surgery.

report of 4 cases of recurrent post-parotidectomy sialoceles treated with botulinum A toxin injected subcutaneously with 100% success was published (Vargas, Galati, and Parnes 2000), as well as other

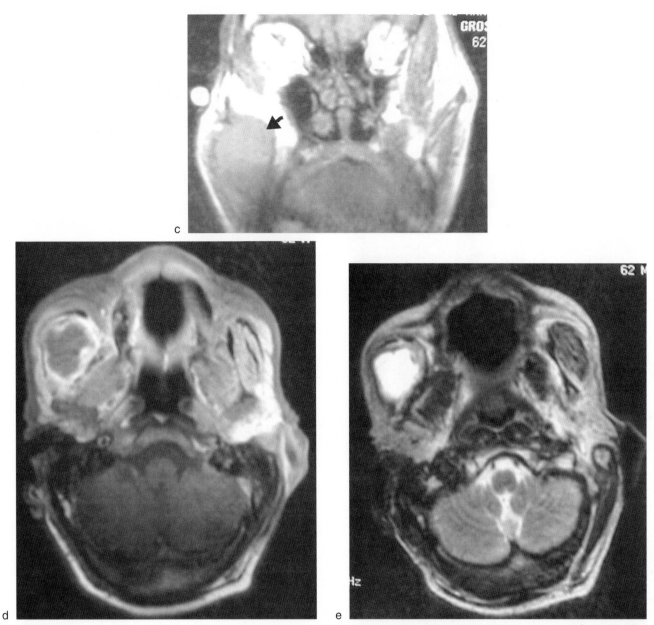

Figures 12.3c, 12.3d, and 12.3e. MR views of sialocele with enhancing capsule on Figure 12.3d.

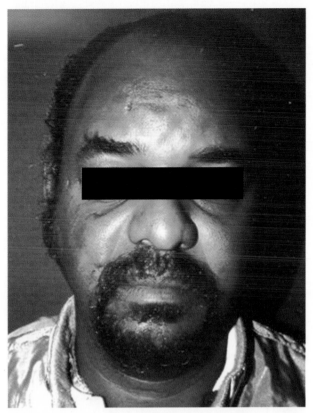

Figure 12.4a. A 41-year-old male post-gunshot wound that entered in the left parotid region and traversed to the right parotid region with fracture of both left and right condyles. He developed an increasing sialocele in the right parotid gland.

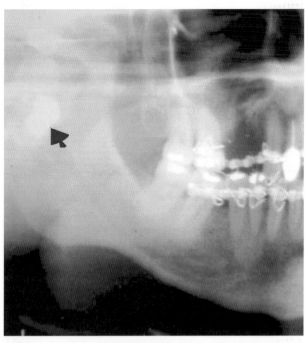

Figure 12.4b. Panoramic film shows the retained bullet in the right parotid gland (arrow).

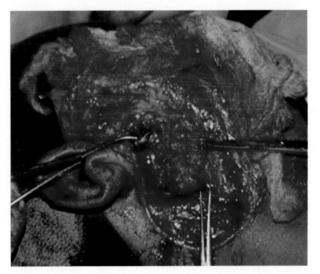

Figure 12.4c. Modified Blair incision and partial parotidectomy, with mosquito forceps indicating the bullet. The bullet was situated between the superior and inferior branches of the facial nerve, which was intact with no weakness. The capsule of the parotid gland was repaired and the sialocele resolved. Reprinted with permission from Blanchaert R, Ord RA. 1997. Management of late complications of penetrating injuries to the parotid gland. *Pan American Journal of Trauma* 6(1):52–57.

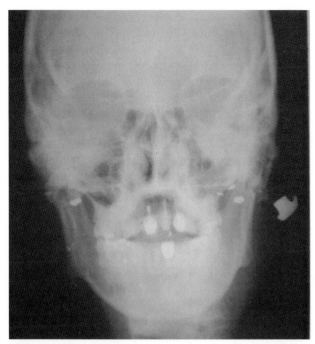

Figure 12.5a. Plain film of a 20-year-old man following a gunshot wound shows the bullet "floating" in parotid sialocele.

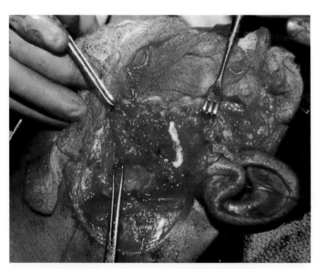

Figure 12.5b. Surgical exploration to remove the bullet revealed an abscess cavity where the bullet had lodged. Note draining pus. Reprinted with permission from Blanchaert R, Ord RA. 1997. Management of late complications of penetrating injuries to the parotid gland. *Pan American Journal of Trauma* 6(1):52–57.

case reports (Chow and Kwok 2003). There is a single case of a submandibular sialocele treated with resolution using botulinum toxin A (Capaccio, Cuccarini, and Benicchio et al. 2006).

Nerve Injury

The facial nerve is at risk from penetrating injury to the facial region both in the parotid and in the distribution of its peripheral branches to the facial musculature. It is stated that damage to branches distal to a line drawn from the lateral canthus to the commissure does not require repair and may be managed expectantly. All patients with facial wounds should have a careful clinical examination of facial nerve function. Where this is not possible—for example, in the unconscious patient or the uncooperative infant (Figure 12.6)—the wound should be carefully explored at the time of surgery to exclude transaction of the branches of

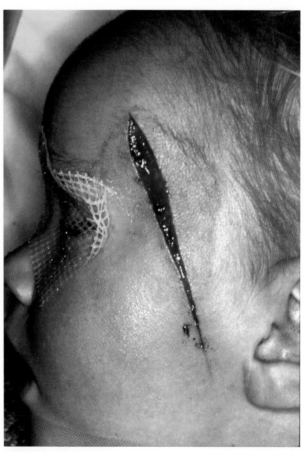

Figure 12.6. Infant with laceration from broken glass. No facial nerve damage was present.

the facial nerve. Primary repair soon after the injury with end to end anastomosis is the ideal scenario, as paralysis of the facial nerve is a devastating injury for the patient, and even when "successful" nerve repair has been carried out with satisfying results (based on House-Brackmann, Stennert, and May grading), patients experience a reduced quality of life (Guntinas-Lichius, Straesser, and Streppel 2007) (Figures 12.7 and 12.8). This section will discuss the management of the primary nerve injury and will not discuss the techniques for facial reanimation or static slings, which are beyond the scope of this text. The interested reader will find many recent review articles addressing these topics (Guntinas-Lichius, Streppel, and Stennert 2006; Malik, Kelly, and Ahmed et al. 2005).

Classically the nerve is sutured under the microscope using 9-0 or 10-0 nylon sutures attempting to coapt the nerve ends without tension (Figure

12.9). The suturing can be epineural or fasicular. In epineural suture less damage is caused to the neural bundles with less foreign body reaction in the fasicles due to the suture materials; however, fasicular suturing should allow better adaptation of the fasicles and trimming back the epineurium to prevent fibrous tissue in-growth. However, anatomic studies have shown the fasicular and connective tissue anatomy of the facial nerve to be complex, with the number of fasicles increasing in a proximo-distal way from the geniculate ganglion

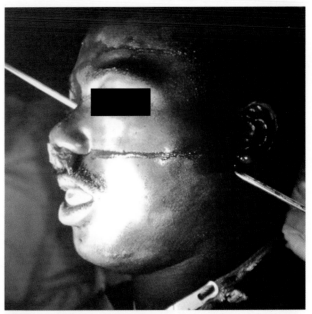

Figure 12.7b. Bougie placed through track of bullet to demonstrate entrance and exit.

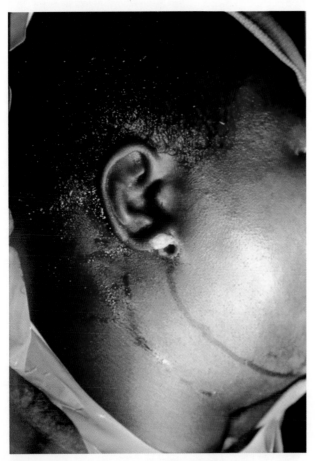

Figure 12.7a. Entrance wound for bullet below ear lobe.

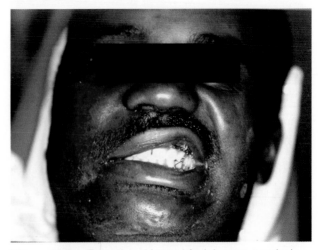

Figure 12.7c. Frontal and buccal facial nerve paralysis.

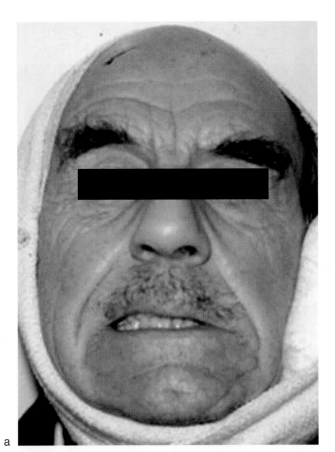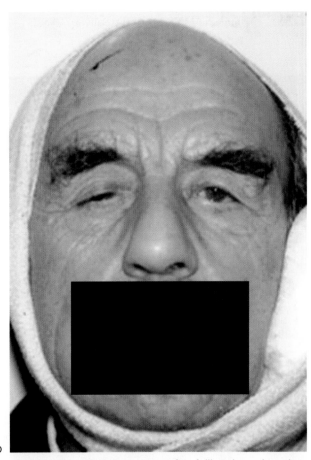

Figures 12.8a and 12.8b. A 72-year-old man diagnosed with a stroke in the emergency room after falling through a plate glass window. The diagnosis was made due to the dense facial nerve palsy.

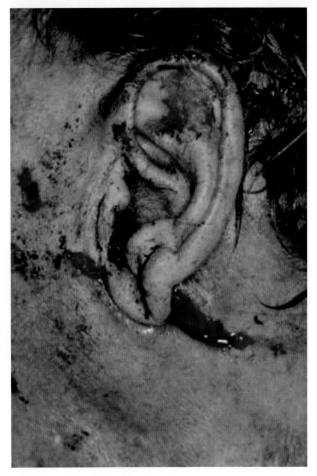

Figure 12.8c. After removing the dressings the deep penetrating wound in the region of the facial nerve trunk is appreciated.

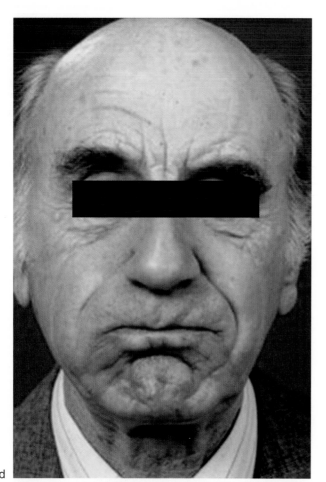

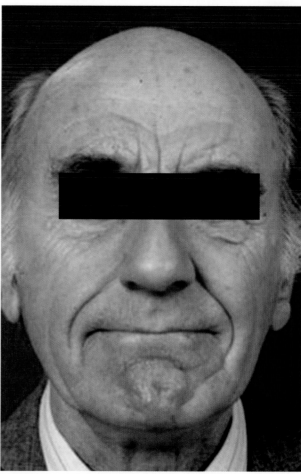

d

e

Figures 12.8d and 12.8e. One year post-repair of nerve trunk and microneural suture the patient still has some weakness of the upper lid and cannot "blow out" his cheek on the left side, but has good facial symmetry and function.

with diminishing diameter (Figure 12.10). This variability in number of fasicles and structure along the extratemporal facial nerve constitutes a difficulty in facial nerve repair (Captier, Canovas, Bonnel, Seignarbieux 2005). The use of tubes (e.g., collagen) to support the anastomosis and prevent connective tissue in-growth and also tissue glues (e.g., fibrin) to replace sutures and their foreign body reactions have been advocated. However, the tubes can themselves cause foreign body reactions and possible compression. Regarding the tissue glues, animal experiments appear to show sutures to be superior. In the rabbit model axonal growth was faster and greater with epineural suture than fibrin adhesive (Junior, Valmaseda-Castellon, and Gay-Escoda 2004). Although the rate and amount of reduction in conduction velocity was equivalent between the two methods, the authors concluded that epineural suture appears to

be the method of choice. In another study in the rat model looking at suture and the effects of platelet rich plasma (PRP) and fibrin sealant, the best return of function for the facial nerve was again with suture (Farrag, Lehar, and Verhaegen et al. 2007). The authors did note a favorable neurotrophic effect for the PRP but no benefit for the fibrin sealant. As it is vital that the anastomosis be tension free, difficulty is encountered when a gap between the nerve ends exists. In a cadaver study, Gardetto, Kovacs, and Piegger et al. (2002) showed that removal of the superficial part of the parotid gland could allow overlap of the cut branches of the facial nerve. They found it possible to bridge gaps of 15 mm in the temporo-zygomatic branches, 23 mm in the buccal-mandibular branches, and 17 mm in the nerve trunk. Following this experimental work the authors have reported successful clinical results on 3 patients, recommending the

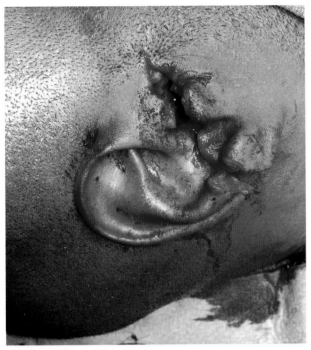

Figure 12.9a. Penetrating wound through ear and parotid gland.

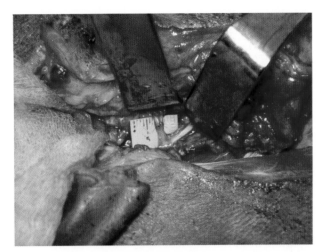

Figure 12.9c. Post-microsurgical repair.

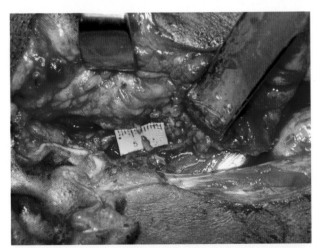

Figure 12.9b. Exploration of wound reveals transection of the superior branch of the facial nerve. (Ruler from surgical marker makes a good background for microsuture if custom microsurgical background material is unavailable.)

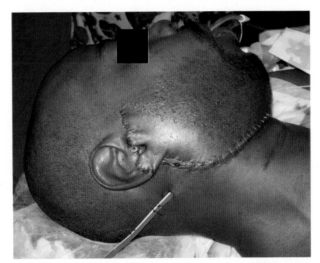

Figure 12.9d. Post-suturing of wounds. This case treated by Dr. J. Caccamese, Dept. OMS, University of Maryland.

technique for gaps up to 15 mm but cautioning against its use in the presence of infection or nerve defects (Piza-Katzer et al. 2004). In another approach the use of a rapid nerve expander (2 cm/30 minutes) was used to bridge gaps up to 3 cm (Ya, Gao, and Wang 2007). In 9 patients 5 achieved good results with EMG peak value of mimetic muscles 82–95%, of the normal side, 3 cases were fair with EMG 60–90%, and 1 case poor with EMG 55%. Other surgical options in this situation are the use of a tube as a conduit and grafting. In 7 patients with post-traumatic defects up to 3 cm the use of a bioabsorbable polyglycolic acid tube was reported as giving very good results in 1 case, good in 4, and fair in 2 (Navissano et al. 2005). The two commonest sites for donor nerves for the facial nerve are the greater auricular, which is adjacent to the surgical field, and the sural nerve. Surgical principles for repair follow those for direct anastomosis. As expected, facial nerve function from cable nerve graft interposition is not as good as end to end anastomosis (Malik, Kelly, and Ahmed et al. 2005). If there is widespread destruction of multiple branches from an injury such as a gunshot the entire superficial cervical plexus can be used to supply multiple grafts.

Frey's Syndrome

Although Frey's syndrome is now most commonly seen in relation to parotid surgery, it was originally described after a shotgun injury to the parotid gland (Frey 1923); however, despite Frey's landmark paper, gustatory sweating was probably first described by Baillarger in 1853 (Dulguerov, Marchal, and Gusin 1999). In the trauma situation obviously the problem is management and treatment of the condition, whereas in the post-parotidectomy cases much work has been done on prevention.

Previously reported treatments of Frey's syndrome have included topical and systemic anticholinergics, tympanic neurectomy, sectioning of the auriculotemporal or glossopharyngeal nerves, or interposition of fascia lata between the parotid bed and overlying skin. Currently the use of botulinum toxin is the most frequently reported therapeutic modality for Frey's syndrome. A report of 33 patients with Frey's syndrome treated by intracutaneous injection of 16–80 IU of botulinum toxin A showed all symptoms to resolve within a week (Eckardt and Kuettner 2003). In a prospective

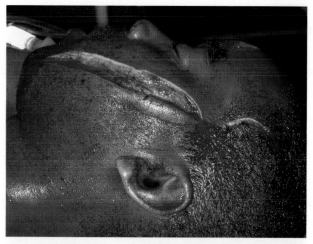

Figure 12.10a. Extensive penetrating wound anterior to the parotid gland, which involves the peripheral branches of the facial nerve.

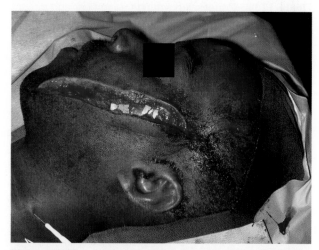

Figure 12.10b. Nerve branches identified for microneural repair.

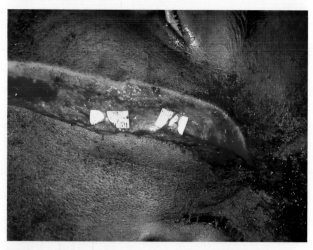

Figure 12.10c. High-power view of completed repair.

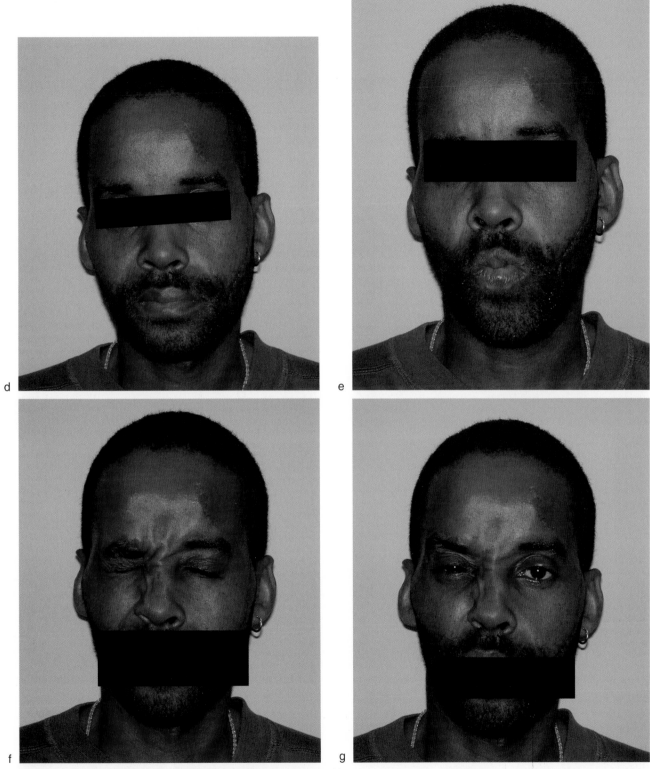

Figures 12.10d, 12.10e, 12.10f, and 12.10g. Post-repair. Note upper branch weakness persists. This case treated by Dr. J. Caccamese, Dept. OMS, University of Maryland.

nonrandomized, nonblinded study of 11 patients treated with botulinum toxin A with follow-up 6–23 months, only 1 patient recurred and was successfully retreated (Kyrmizakis, Pangalos, and Papadakis et al. 2004). A prospective randomized trial to establish the ideal dosage and length of effect of botulinum toxin A was carried out on 20 patients divided into two groups receiving either $2\ MU/cm^2$ or $3\ MU/cm^2$. In the $3\ MU/cm^2$ group a single injection resulted in nearly complete absence of gustatory sweating during the 12 month follow-up period. In the $2\ MU/cm^2$ group 44% of the total skin areas were still sweating and required a second injection, and the authors concluded that $3\ MU/cm^2$ is the recommended dose (Nolte, Gollmitzer, and Loeffelbein et al. 2004). Some authors have cautioned that the effect of botulinum toxin

in Frey's syndrome is often temporary and further injections may be necessary depending upon the initial dose and the length of time followed (Ferraro et al. 2005).

In regards to parotidectomy patients, probably 100% will have gustatory sweating if tested with starch and iodine (Laage-Hellman 1957) (Figure 12.11). However, few patients clinically notice this problem and most do not wish for treatment, so that this condition will be underestimated in clinical reports. Frey's syndrome is rarely reported after submandibular gland removal. Berini-Aytes and Gay-Escoda (1992) reviewed 206 submandibular gland excisions and found only 1 case of Frey's syndrome, while Teague, Akhtar, and Phillips (1998) reviewed the literature and could find 7 reported cases since 1934.

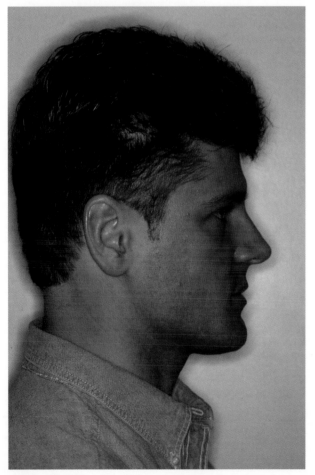

Figure 12.11a. Lateral facial view of patient complaining of gustatory sweating (Frey's syndrome).

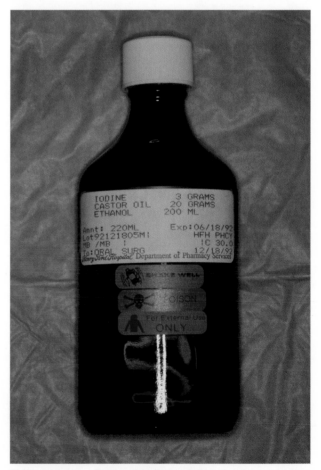

Figure 12.11b. Bottle of iodine solution that is painted on the patient's face and then covered in corn starch.

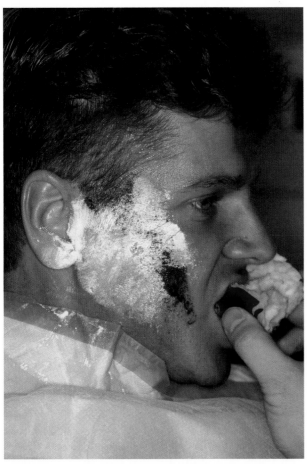

Figure 12.11c. While the patient eats an apple the cornstarch is discolored blue-black, indicative of gustatory sweating.

The techniques described for prevention of Frey's syndrome depend upon placing a barrier between the parotid bed and skin to prevent the growth of the secretory parasympathetic nerves from the parotid into the sweat glands, causing a paradoxical innervation. Acellular dermis has been used with success but with a higher complication rate (Govindaraj, Cohen, and Genden et al. 2001). Temporoparietal flaps and the superficial musculo-aponeurotic system (SMAS) have been used with good outcomes in 146 parotidectomy patients (Cesteleyn et al. 2002). In reviewing 160 patients followed from 5 to 22 years treated with an inter-positional SMAS layer at the time of parotidectomy and tested with starch/iodine during follow-up, no cases of Frey's were encountered (Bonanno et al. 2000). Other reported barriers have been the use

of parotid gland fascia (Zumeng, Zhi, Gang et al. 2006) and sternocleidomastoid muscle flaps, with mixed results (Filho et al. 2004; Kerawala, McAloney, and Stassen 2002).

It would appear that Frey's syndrome is preventable in most cases, and perhaps the use of the SMAS layer is the most convenient for the surgeon.

Hollowing

This is a complication seen in patients following parotidectomy rather than trauma and can be managed in a variety of ways. Reconstruction at the time of surgery to prevent the defect occurring is preferable to secondary reconstruction, when scarring and the superficial position of the facial nerve post-parotidectomy increase the risk of nerve damage. Various techniques have been used, some of which have been discussed in this chapter in relation to Frey's syndrome and in chapter 8. Techniques include the use of layered acellular dermis, free fat grafts (Figure 8.4), use of the SMAS layer, temporalis, and sternocleidomastoid flaps, as well as microvascular free flaps including fascial forearm flaps for larger defects. Choice of technique will depend on the size of the defect, the surgeon's own experience, and the wishes of the patient.

TRAUMA TO SALIVARY GLAND DUCTS

Transection

As has already been discussed above in the sections on fistulae and sialoceles related to parenchymal trauma, conservative management is usually satisfactory except in those cases where the injury involves partial or complete transection of the duct. Under these circumstances most papers have indicated that resolution is less certain and takes longer, with active management frequently required. There are studies that support conservative measures in duct injuries and in one report, of 19 patients with duct injury confirmed by methylene blue dye injection who were treated non-operatively, 9 patients (47%) healed without complications. Although 7 patients (36.8%) developed salivary fistulae and 4 (21%) sialoceles, these were described as short-term and resolved without the need for surgery (Lewis and Knottenbelt 1991). However, in most cases current management is

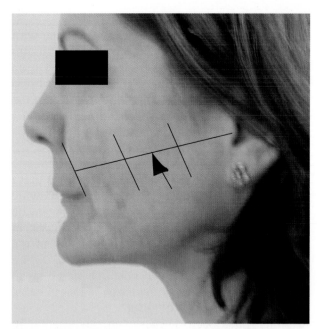

Figure 12.12. Surface markings of the parotid duct are shown by a line drawn from the tragus of the ear to bisect a line drawn from the alar base to the commissure. The middle third of this line (arrow) is surface marking of the parotid duct.

directed toward primary repair and the clinician must therefore have a high level of suspicion for injuries involving the region of the parotid duct. The anatomic surface markings of the duct are illustrated in Figure 12.12. Confirmatory evidence for transaction is obtained by cannulating the distal portion of the duct through Stenson's papilla and observing the catheter in the wound (Figure 12.13), or by injecting saline or a small (1 cc) amount of methylene blue through Stenson's papilla. Identification of the proximal end may be difficult, as it can retract into the gland substance. Milking the gland to obtain salivary flow is helpful in these circumstances, and the anesthesiologist must be cautioned preoperatively against the use of antiparasympathetic agents. If the proximal and distal ends of the duct are identified and can be coapted, then microsurgical repair can be carried out (Hallock 1992) (Figure 12.14).

The use of stents (usually indwelling catheters) for 10–14 days to prevent stenosis is advocated by some and appears a reasonable hypothesis, although no long-term studies of these injuries

with and without stenting have been published. A technique of using a 4 F Foley embolectomy catheter for identification of the transection and then leaving it in place as a stent has been described (Etoz, Tuncel, and Ozcan 2006). When the proximal and distal ends of the duct cannot be coapted due to tissue loss, repair using a vein graft has been reported (Heymans et al. 1999). Steinberg and Herréra (2005) recommended the use of sialography postoperatively to assess the result of duct repair, stating that this technique may not always be practical or possible in the acute setting. However, we have used sialography intraoperatively (Figure 12.13).

When the injury is too proximal, the wound is avulsive, or the duct cannot be identified, then the clinician can either create an intraoral fistula or ligate the proximal duct. A controlled fistula can be created by suturing the proximal duct through the buccinator into the oral cavity if enough length is present, or by placing a catheter or drain from the area of the wound into the mouth and leaving it to fistulize (Figure 12.15). Although tying off the proximal duct to cause eventual atrophy has been proposed (Van Sickels 1981), in our experience this is unpredictable and even with the use of pressure and antisialogogues these patients can have considerable swelling and pain. Chemical denervation using botulinum toxin A may help to achieve a good outcome in these circumstances (Arnaud et al. 2006).

In the case of the submandibular duct, transection is usually iatrogenic as a result of surgery on the sublingual gland, sialolithotomy from Wharton's duct, or resection of floor of the mouth cancer. In this case sialodochoplasty with repositioning of the duct posteriorly is all that is required. One of the authors formerly used a catheter as a stent (Ord and Lee 1996) following reposition of Wharton's duct in floor of the mouth cancer; however, now the duct lumen is identified and one blade of a sharp iris scissors is inserted and a vertical cut through one wall of the duct carried out. The duct is now "fish-tailed" and sutured to a newly created hole in the oral mucosa with 6-0 nylon sutures. Stenosis and stricture have not been a problem with this technique.

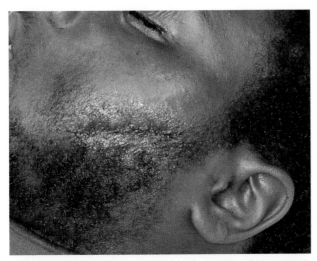

Figure 12.13a. Patient with cheek laceration that was primarily sutured and that now has developed sialocele due to missed duct injury.

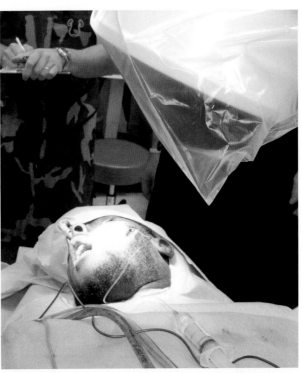

Figure 12.13c. Stenson's duct is approximated after finding the proximal end of the duct by milking the gland. The duct is cannulated and contrast dye injected for intraoperative sialogram.

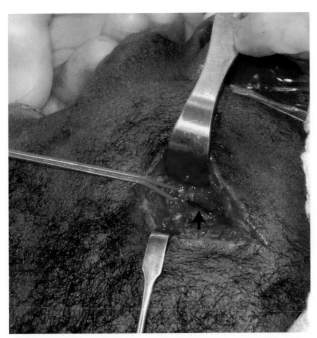

Figure 12.13b. Wound reopened for re-exploration; the duct is discovered to be transected. Vessel loop around distal end of duct. Lacrimal probe passed from intraoral through Stenson's duct into the wound (short arrow).

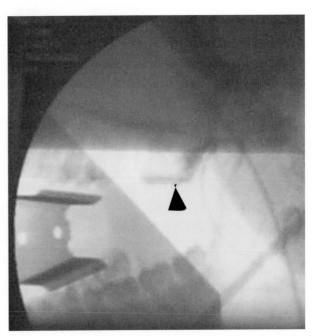

Figure 12.13d. Fluoroscopic image of intraoperative sialogram with repaired duct (arrow). Case treated by Dr. D. Coletti, Dept. OMS, University of Maryland.

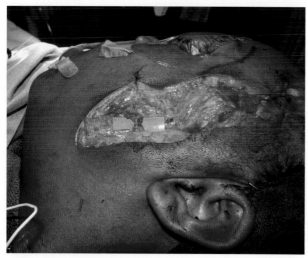

Figure 12.14a. Extensive slashing wound, with duct identified and repaired.

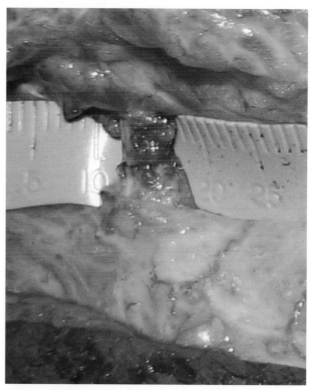

Figure 12.14b. High power of duct repair.

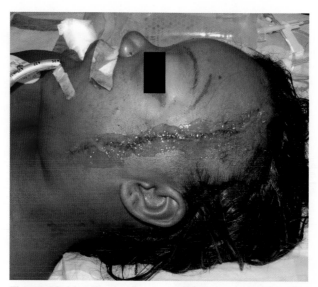

Figure 12.14c. Final skin repair. This case treated by Dr. J. Caccamese, Dept. OMS, University of Maryland.

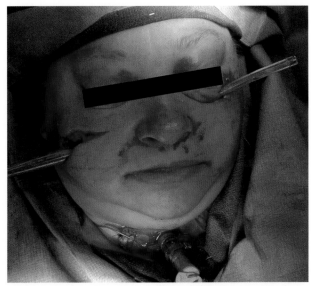

Figure 12.15a. Gunshot wound entering at right parotid region with exit at left infraorbital region as indicated by suction tubing.

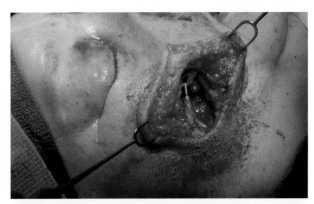

Figure 12.15c. The duct is diverted intraorally via the cannula. Note powder burn at entrance wound.

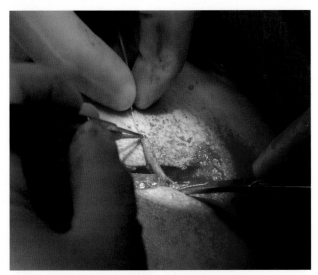

Figure 12.15b. The parotid duct is identified and dissected from the wound to be cannulated as shown.

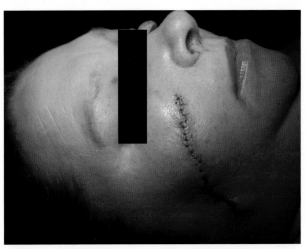

Figure 12.15d. Final repair. This case treated by Dr. J. Caccamese, Dept. OMS, University of Maryland.

Stenosis of the Duct

When ductal injuries are not surgically repaired immediately, complications such as fistulae and sialoceles may arise and their management has been discussed. If the duct has not been surgically repaired by 72 hours, conservative or medical therapy is recommended (Arnaud et al. 2006). In the long term, stricture of the duct may occur (Figure 12.16), although most strictures are sec-

ondary to inflammatory or infective conditions. In cases of intraductal salivary gland obstruction, 22.6% of 642 cases were due to strictures, which were more common in females (Ngu, Brown, and Whaites et al. 2007). When this occurs at the distal end of Stenson's duct, excision and diversion of the duct into the oral cavity may be feasible. When the main duct is involved with strictures, sialoendoscopy may be useful to dilate the strictures using

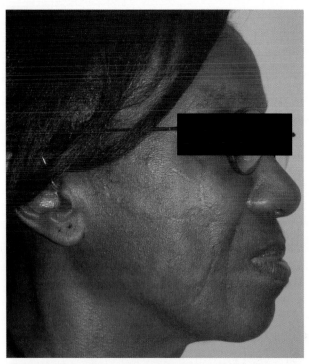

Figure 12.16a. Patient with soft tissue scarring from penetrating wounds caused by a road traffic accident 10 years previously; now has a 7-year history of parotid and cheek swelling.

saline pressure, balloon dilatation, or the miniforceps grasper and even the insertion of a stent to the duct lumen (Nahliel, Bar, and Shacham et al. 2004). Simple balloon angioplasty was successful in 7 of 9 patients, and 5 of these patients remained asymptomatic on follow-up (Salerno, Lo Casto, and Comparetto et al. 2007). If this is unsuccessful and the patient continues to have recurrent swelling and sialadenitis, denervation with botulinum toxin or even parotidectomy may be required.

In the submandibular gland the stricture can be excised and sialodochoplasty performed as described above.

Radiation Injury

EXTERNAL BEAM

Radiotherapy is commonly given for patients with head and neck cancer; however, the injurious effect that this treatment modality has on the salivary glands leading to profound xerostomia, which may be permanent, is well known. The serous cells (found in the parotid gland) are extremely sensitive to apoptotic death following even moderate doses of radiation. Indeed, permanent loss of sali-

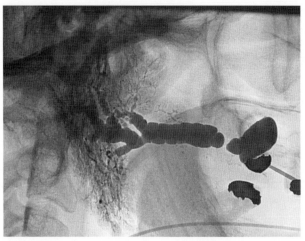

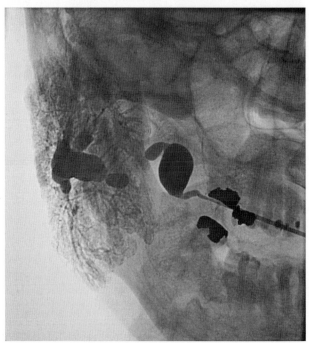

b   c

Figures 12.16b and 12.16c. Sialogram shows stricture of duct with proximal dilatation of Stenson's duct and secondary ducts and a large cystic swelling distal to the stricture.

vary function is seen after doses larger than approximately 3,500 cGy with little in the way of measurable parotid saliva, and 5% of patients will demonstrate a sialadenitis with gland swelling and raised amylase within 12 hours of their first treatment (Parsons 1994). However, although it is known that damage to the salivary glands will increase with radiation dose and volume of gland irradiated, there is no universal agreement over the dose required to produce xerostomia. Someya, Sakata, and Nagakura et al. (2003) found gradual recovery of function over time with doses of <5,000 cGy, while no significant recovery was seen in patients who had >5,800 cGy. The minor salivary/sublingual glands do not seem to play much of a role in the development of xerostomia, which seems to depend mainly on the mean dose to both the parotid and submandibular glands (Jellema, Doornaert, and Slotman et al. 2005). These authors also found that the stickiness of saliva post-radiation depended mainly on the mean dose to the submandibular glands.

The exact pathogenesis and mechanism of injury to the salivary glands as a result of radiation therapy is also controversial, with no universal agreement as to cause. Based on animal studies in the rat model, a mechanism of delayed serous cell death due to sublethal DNA damage, which results in death during a reproductive phase due to highly redox-reactive metal ions (e.g., iron, copper) associated with secretion granules has been proposed (Nagler 2002, 2003). Another study showed significant increase in cytotoxic T-cells in irradiated submandibular glands, suggesting cell-mediated mechanisms may be responsible for the sialadenitis with subsequent acinar cell destruction/atrophy (Teymoortash, Simolka, and Schrader et al. 2005).

Obviously once established the effects of radiation damage are difficult to treat or reverse, so much effort has been aimed at prevention. Important advances in the delivery of radiation therapy using 3-D conformal planning and intensity-modulated radiation therapy (IMRT), combined with drugs such as growth factors, cholinergic agonists, and cytoprotective agents (Amifostine), are currently the preferred modalities of prevention (Garden, Lewin, and Chambers 2006).

It has been shown with conventional radiation therapy that the ability to spare the contralateral major salivary glands or to spare the parotid by positioning of the portals can significantly increase salivary flow and reduce xerostomia (Beer et al. 2002; Malouf, Aragon, and Henson et al. 2003). The sophistication of 3-D conformal planning and IMRT allows the radiotherapist to give more radiation to the tumor target with increased sparing of normal tissue. In one study only 12% of patients developed xerostomia following IMRT for head and neck cancer, and there were no locoregional recurrences with a median follow-up of 24 months (Saarilahti, Kouri, and Collan et al. 2005). Jen, Shih, and Lin et al. (2005) compared 108 patients treated with conventional RT to 72 Gy treated with 3-D conformal RT, finding 3-D conformal RT delivered a higher dose to the tumor with better local control in T4 patients and improved survival with significantly better parotid function. IMRT has also been used to spare the submandibular glands to prevent radiation-induced xerostomia (Saarilahti, Kouri, and Collan et al. 2006). The ability to use 3-D conformal RT and IMRT to spare the opposite parotid by excluding the contralateral level II nodes from the field was not shown to be associated with any locoregional recurrence, and no recurrence occurred in the spared area (Bussels, Maes, and Hermans et al. 2004).

A number of drugs have been investigated for preventing radiation damage. A phase III prospective randomized trial of Amifostine (Ethyol) with 315 patients showed significant reduction in grade 2 or > xerostomia and chronic xerostomia with no effect on locoregional control, disease-free survival, or overall survival. In this study, however, 53% of patients experienced nausea and/or vomiting (Brizel, Wasserman, and Henke et al. 2000). A follow-up study to review results of this study after 2 years found the significant decrease in grade 2 or > xerostomia had been maintained, as well as an increase in the proportion of patients with meaningful unstimulated saliva and reduced mouth dryness. There was no compromise of locoregional control, progression-free, or disease-free survival (Wasseman, Brizel, and Henke et al. 2005). In this study the Amifostine was given intravenously, and a recent phase II study has shown a similar radioprotective benefit for Amifostine given subcutaneously as a simpler alternative (Anne, Machtay, and Rosenthal et al. 2007). Another approach has been to use pilocarpine, which has been used to treat xerostomia during radiotherapy as a chemopreventive agent. A randomized, double-blind, placebo-controlled trial of pilocarpine on 60 patients, only 39 of whom were evaluable, indicated that pilocarpine used with radiotherapy could lead to significant diminution in subsequent xerostomia (Haddad and Karimi 2002). Another randomized trial with 66 patients also concluded that patients with stimulated glands from pilocarpine during radiation had less decrease in salivary flow, which reduced radiation side effects (Nyarady, Nemeth, and Ban et al. 2006). However, the Radiation Therapy Oncology Group (RTOG) study 97-09, which was a phase III trial with 245 patients, showed that although there was a significantly increased unstimulated salivary flow in the pilocarpine group, there was no difference in parotid stimulated salivary flow, in the amelioration of mucositis, or in the quality of life between the two groups (Scarantino, LeVeque, and Swann et al. 2006). Other novel approaches to the problem have been the use of gene therapy, which has yielded promising results in animal models (Cotrim, Mineshiba, and Sugito et al. 2006; Thula et al. 2005).

Finally, a surgical approach to prevention of xerostomia has been the transfer of the submandibular glands into the submental triangle out of the radiation field prior to the commencement of radiation therapy. In a phase II trial of patients who had primary surgery for oro-pharyngeal cancer followed by adjuvant RT, with or without submandibular gland transfer 24 of 51 patients were evaluated for swallowing. The cohort with preservation of 1 gland (13 patients) had significantly increased saliva and swallowing function (Rieger, Seikaly, and Jha et al. 2005). Similar results were reported in a small series of patients undergoing chemoradiation (Al-Qahtani et al. 2006). Regarding long-term results in 26 patients followed for 2 years, normal amounts of saliva were reported in 83% (Seikaly, Jha, and Harris et al. 2004).

RADIOACTIVE IODINE

Radioactive iodine is used in the treatment of thyroid cancer but is also concentrated in the salivary glands, particularly the parotid, and may cause sialadenitis that is immediate or begins a few months after treatment (Mandel and Mandel 2003). In a prospective study of 76 patients receiving radioactive iodine, 20 (26%) developed salivary gland toxicity, 11 developed toxicity within 48 hours, and 9 not until 3 months post-therapy. A total of 16 patients had chronic toxicity, typically xerostomia, at 12 months (Hyer et al. 2007). In seeking to quantify salivary gland dysfunction using scintigraphy in 50 patients, 46% and 42%

were found to have decreased maximum secretion and uptake ratio, respectively (Raza et al. 2006). The damage was seen more in the parotid and was dependent on the radioiodine dose. The damage and symptoms may be permanent (Mandel and Mandel 1999). The damage is most likely related to an oxidation injury indicated by an increase in prostaglandin levels (Wolfram, Palumbo, and Chehne et al. 2004).

Current management is symptomatic as for sialadenitis and xerostomia from other causes. Animal studies using the rabbit model indicate that Amifostine can significantly reduce radioiodine-induced parenchymal damage (Kutta, Kampen, and Sagowski et al. 2005). The use of sialoendoscopic treatment in this condition for patients with partial duct stenosis has also been reported (Kim, Han, and Lee et al. 2007).

Barotrauma

Air can be forced in a retrograde fashion into the parotid duct by a rise in intraoral pressure and cause parotid emphysema or pneumoparotid. This condition may occur in glass blowers and musicians who play woodwind or brass instruments. It is usually a benign condition but can cause recurrent sialadenitis or even progress to subcutaneous emphysema. The condition has also been reported in conjunction with the use of an air syringe during routine dentistry (Takenoshite, Kawano, and Oka 1991), secondary to coughing with chronic obstructive airways disease (Cook and Layton 1993), and self-induced in children and adults (Goguen et al. 1995; Gudlaugsson, Geirsson, and Benediktsdottir 1998). The condition can be diagnosed by palpation of emphysema in the parotid and the escape of frothy saliva from the duct. Sialography and CT scans have been used for diagnosis (Gudlaugsson, Geirsson, and Benediktsdottir 1998; Maehara, Ikeda, and Ohmura et al. 2005). In one case with subcutaneous emphysema extending to the mediastinum parotid duct ligation was used for cure (Han and Isaacson 2004).

Summary (Figures 12.17 and 12.18)

- Most parenchymal penetrating injuries of the parotid gland will resolve with conservative treatment.

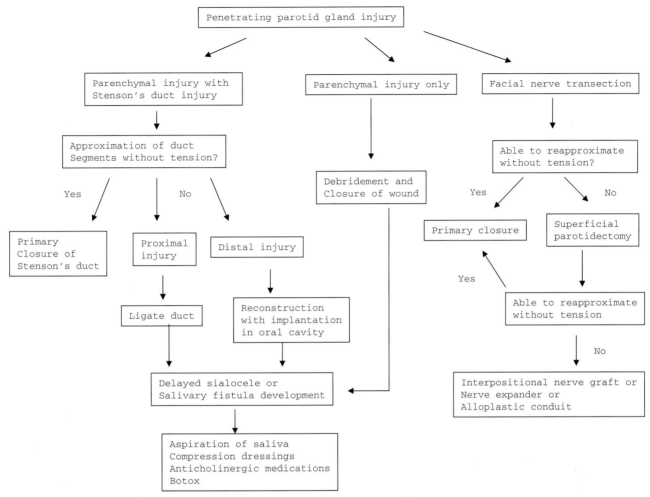

Figure 12.17. Algorithm for management of penetrating trauma to the parotid gland.

- Parotid fistulae and sialoceles due to parenchymal injury will also resolve with conservative therapy.
- Chemical denervation of the gland with botulinum A toxin injected subcutaneously appears to be a safe way of treating fistulae and sialoceles.
- It is important to recognize the possibility of duct injury early, as immediate repair is indicated.
- Microneural repair of facial nerve injuries primarily without tension is the ideal management for a transected facial nerve or its branches.
- At present the use of tissue glues for nerve repair does not appear to improve results.

- Most cases of Frey's syndrome following parotidectomy are subclinical.
- Botulinum toxin is useful in the treatment of Frey's.
- A variety of barrier techniques to prevent Frey's syndrome have been described with the use of the SMAS layer appearing to give good results.
- IMRT and 3-D conformal planning show great promise in preventing radiation damage to the salivary glands.
- Amifostine and pilocarpine used during radiation may act as radioprotectants.

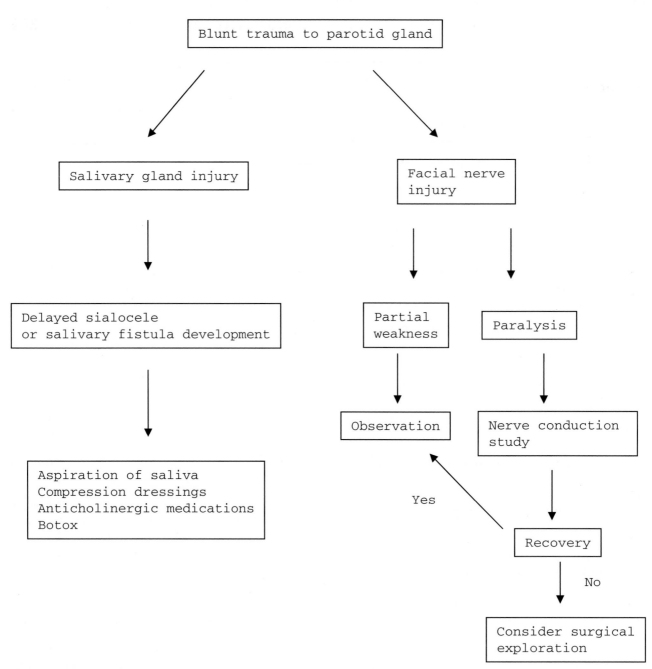

Figure 12.18. Algorithm for management of blunt trauma to the parotid gland.

References

Al-Qahtani K, Hier MP, Sultanum K, Black MJ. 2006. The role of submandibular salivary gland transfer in preventing xerostomia in the chemoradiotherapy patient. *Oral Surg Oral Med Oral Pathol Oral Radiol Endod* 101(6):753–756.

Ananthakrishnan N, Parkash S. 1982. Parotid fistulas: A review. *Br J Surg* 69:641–644.

Anne PR, Machtay M, Rosenthal DI et al. 2007. A phase II trial of subcutaneous amifostine and radiation therapy in patients with head and neck cancer. *Int J Radiat Oncol Biol Phys* 67(2):445–452.

Arnaud S, Batifol D, Goudot P, Yachouh J. 2006. Nonsurgical management of traumatic injuries of the parotid gland using type a botulinum toxin. *Plast Reconstr Surg* 117(7):2426–2430.

Beer KT, Zehnder D, Lussi A, Greiner RH. 2002. Sparing of contralateral major salivary glands has a significant effect on oral health in patients treated with radical radiotherapy of head and neck tumors. *Strahlenther Onkol* 178(12):722–726.

Berini-Aytes L, Gay-Escoda C. 1992. Morbidity associated with removal of the submandibular gland. *J Craniomaxillofac Surg* 20(5):216–219.

Bonanno PC, Palaia D, Rosenberg M, Casson P. 2000. Prophylaxis against Frey's syndrome in parotid surgery. *Ann Plast Surg* 44(5):498–501.

Breuer T, Ferrazzini A, Grossenberger R. 2006. Botulinum toxin A as a treatment of traumatic salivary gland fistulas. (Article in German.) *HNO* 54(4):385–390.

Brizel DM, Wasserman TH, Henke M et al. 2000. Phase III randomized trial of amifostine as a radioprotector in head and neck cancer. *J Clin Oncol* 18(19):3339–3345.

Bussels B, Maes A, Hermans R et al. 2004. Recurrences after conformal parotid sparing radiotherapy for head and neck cancer. *Radiother Oncol* 72(2):119–127.

Canosa A, Cohen MA. 1999. Post-traumatic parotid sialocele: Report of two cases. *J Oral Maxillofac Surg* 57(6):742–745.

Cant PJ, Campbell JA. 1991. Management of traumatic parotid sialoceles and fistulae: A prospective study. *Aust N Z J Surg* 61(10):742–743.

Capaccio P, Cuccarini V, Benicchio V et al. 2006. Treatment of iatrogenic submandibular sialocele with botulinum toxin Case report. *Br J Oral Maxillofac Surg*, epub March 31, 2006.

Captier G, Canovas F, Bonnel F, Seignarbieux F. 2005. Organization and microscopic anatomy of the adult human facial nerve: Anatomical and histological basis for surgery. *Plast Reconstr Surg* 115:1457–1465.

Cesteleyn L, Helman J, King S, Van de Vyvere G. 2002. Temporoparietal fascia flaps and superficial musculoaponeurotic system plication in parotid surgery reduces Frey's syndrome. *J Oral Maxillofac Surg* 60(11):1284–1297.

Cholankeril JV, Scioscia PA. 1993. Post-traumatic sialoceles and mucoceles of the salivary glands. *Clin Imaging* 17(1):41–45.

Chow TL, Kwok SP. 2003. Use of botulinum type A in a case of persistent parotid sialocele. *Hong Kong Med J* 9(4):293–294.

Cook JN, Layton SA. 1993. Bilateral parotid swelling associated with chronic obstructive pulmonary disease. A case of pneumoparotid. *Oral Surg Oral Med Oral Pathol* 76(2):157–158.

Cotrim AP, Mineshiba F, Sugito T et al. 2006. Salivary gland gene therapy 2006. *Dent Clin North Amer* 50(2):157–173.

Dulguerov P, Marchal F, Gusin C. 1999. Frey syndrome before Frey: The correct history. *Laryngoscope* 109(9):1471–1473.

Eckardt A, Kuettner C. 2003. Treatment of gustatory sweating (Frey's syndrome) with botulinum toxin A. *Head Neck* 25(8):624–628.

Etoz A, Tuncel U, Ozcan M. 2006. Parotid duct repair by use of an embolectomy catheter with a microvascular clamp. *Plast Reconstr Surg* 117(10):330–331.

Farrag TY, Lehar M, Verhaegen P et al. 2007. Effect of platelet rich plasma and fibrin sealant on facial nerve regeneration in a rat model. *Laryngoscope* 117(1):157–165.

Faussat JM, Ghiassi B, Princ G. 1993. Rhinnorrhea of parotid origin. Apropos of a case. *Rev Stomatol Chir Maxillofac* 94(6):363–365.

Ferraro G, Altieri A, Grella E, D'Andrea F. 2005. Botulinum toxin: 28 patients affected by Frey's syndrome treated with intradermal injections. *Plast Reconstr Surg* 115(1):344–345.

Filho WQ, Dedivitis RA, Rapoport A, Guimaraes AV. 2004. Sternocleidomastoid muscle flap in preventing Frey's syndrome following parotidectomy. *World J Surg* 28(4):361–364.

Frey L. 1923. Le Syndrome du nerf auriculo-temporal. *Rev Neurol* 2:97.

Garden AS, Lewin JS, Chambers MS. 2006. How to reduce radiation-related toxicity in patients with cancer of the head and neck. *Curr Oncol Rep* 8(2):140–145.

Gardetto A, Kovacs P, Piegger J et al. 2002. Direct coaptation of extensive facial nerve defects after removal of the superficial part of the parotid gland: An anatomic study. *Head Neck* 24(12):1047–1053.

Goguen LA, April MM, Karmody CS, Carter BL. 1995. Self induced pneumoparotitis. *Arch Otolaryngol Head Neck Surg* 121(12):1426–1429.

Govindaraj S, Cohen M, Genden EM et al. 2001. The use of acellular dermis in the prevention of Frey's syndrome. *Laryngoscope* 111(11 Pt 1):1993–1998.

Gudlaugsson O, Geirsson AJ, Benediktsdottir K. 1998. Pneumoparotitis: A new diagnostic technique and a case report. *Ann Otol Rhinol Laryngol* 107(4):356–358.

Guntinas-Lichius O, Straesser A, Streppel M. 2007. Quality of life after facial nerve repair. *Laryngoscope* 117(3):421–426.

Guntinas-Lichius O, Streppel M, Stennert E. 2006. Postoperative functional evaluation of different reanimation techniques for facial nerve repair. *Am J Surg* 191(1):61–67.

Haddad P, Karimi M. 2002. A randomized, double-blind, placebo-controlled trial of concomitant pilocarpine with head and neck irradiation for prevention of radiation-induced xerostomia. *Radiother Oncol* 64(1):29–32.

Hallock GG. 1992. Microsurgical repair of the parotid duct. *Microsurgery* 13(5):243–246.

Han S, Isaacson G. 2004. Recurrent pneumoparotid: Cause and treatment. *Otolaryngol Head Neck Surg* 131(5):758–761.

Heymans O, Nelissen X, Medot M, Fissette J. 1999. Microsurgical repair of Stenson's duct using an interposition vein graft. *J Reconstr Microsurg* 15(2):105–107.

Hyer S, Kong A, Pratt B, Harmer C. 2007. Salivary gland toxicity after radioiodine therapy for thyroid cancer. *Clin Oncol (R Coll Radiol)* 19(1):83–86.

Jellema AP, Doornaert P, Slotman BJ et al. 2005. Does radiation dose to the salivary glands and oral cavity predict patient-rated xerostomia and sticky saliva in head and neck cancer patients treated with curative radiotherapy? *Radiother Oncol* 77(2):164–171.

Jen YM, Shih R, Lin YS et al. 2005. Parotid gland-sparing 3-dimensional conformal radiotherapy results in less severe dry mouth in nasopharyngeal cancer patients: A dosimetric and clinical comparison with conventional radiotherapy. *Radiother Oncol* 75(2):204–209.

Junior EDP, Valmaseda-Castellon E, Gay-Escoda C. 2004. Facial nerve repair with epineural suture and anastomosis using fibrin adhesive: An experimental study in the rabbit. *J Oral Maxillofac Surg* 62(12):1524–1529.

Kerawala CJ, McAloney N, Stassen LF. 2002. Prospective randomized trial of the benefits of a sternocleidomastoid flap after superficial parotidectomy. *Br J Oral Maxillofac Surg* 40(6):468–472.

Kim JW, Han GS, Lee SH et al. 2007. Sialoendoscopic treatment for radioiodine induced sialadenitis. *Laryngoscope* 117(1):133–136.

Kutta H, Kampen U, Sagowski C et al. 2005. Amifostine is a potent radioprotector of salivary glands in radioiodine therapy. Structural and ultrastructural findings. *Strahlenther Onkol* 181(4):237–245.

Kyrmizakis DE, Pangalos A, Papadakis CE et al. 2004. The use of botulinum toxin type A in the treatment of Frey and crocodile tears syndromes. *J Oral Maxillofac Surg* 62(7):840–844.

Laage-Hellman J-E. 1957. Gustatory sweating and flushing after conservative parotidectomy. *Acta Otolaryngol (Stokh)* 48:234–252.

Landau R, Stewart M. 1985. Conservative management of post-traumatic parotid fistulae and sialoceles: A prospective study. *Br J Surg* 72:42–44.

Lewis G, Knottenbelt JD. 1991. Parotid duct injury: Is immediate surgical repair necessary? *Injury* 22:407–409.

Lewkowicz AA, Hasson O, Nablieli O. 2002. Traumatic injuries to the parotid gland and duct. *J Oral Maxillofac Surg* 60(6):676–680.

Maehara M, Ikeda K, Ohmura N et al. 2005. Multislice computed tomography of pneumoparotid: A case report. *Radiat Med* 23(2):147–150.

Malik TH, Kelly G, Ahmed A et al. 2005. A comparison of surgical techniques used in dynamic reanimation of the paralyzed face. *Otol Neurotol* 26(2):284–291.

Malouf JG, Aragon C, Henson BS et al. 2003. Influence of parotid-sparing radiotherapy on xerostomia in head and neck cancer patients. *Cancer Detect Prev* 27(4):305–310.

Mandel SJ, Mandel L. 1999. Persistent sialadenitis after radioactive iodine therapy: Report of two cases. *J Oral Maxillofac Surg* 57(6):738–741.

Mandel SJ, Mandel L. 2003. Radioactive iodine and the salivary glands. *Thyroid* 13(3):266–271.

Marchese-Ragona R, Marioni G, Restivo DA, Staffieri A. 2006. The role of botulinum toxin in post-parotidectomy fistula. A technical note. *Am J Otolaryngol* 27(3):221–224.

Morestin M. 1917. Contribution a l'etude du traitement des fistules salivaires consecutives aux blessures de guerre. *Bull Mém Soc Chir Paris* 43:845.

Nagler RM. 2002. The enigmatic mechanism of irradiation induced damage to the major salivary glands. *Oral Dis* 8(3):141–146.

Nagler RM. 2003. Effects of head and neck radiotherapy on major salivary glands—animal studies and human implications. *In Vivo* 17(4):369–375.

Nahliel O, Bar T, Shacham R et al. 2004. Management of chronic recurrent parotitis: Current therapy. *J Oral Maxillofac Surg* 62(9):1150–1155.

Navissano M, Malan F, Carnino R, Battiston B. 2005. Neurotube for facial nerve repair. *Microneurosurgery* 25(4):268–271.

Ngu, Brown JE, Whaites EJ et al. 2007. Salivary duct strictures: Nature and incidence in benign salivary obstruction. *Dentomaxillofac Radiol* 36(2):63–67.

Nolte D, Gollmitzer I, Loeffelbein DJ et al. 2004. Botulinum toxin for treatment of gustatory sweating. A prospective randomized study. (Article in German.) *Mund Kiefer Gesichtschir* 8(6):369–375.

Nyarady Z, Nemeth A, Ban A et al. 2006. A randomized study to assess the effectiveness of orally administered pilocarpine during and after radiotherapy of head and neck cancer. *Anticancer Res* 26(2B):1557–1562.

Ord RA, Lee VA. 1996. Submandibular duct repositioning after excision of mouth cancer. *J Oral Maxillofac Surg* 54:1075–1078.

Parkeh D, Glezerson G, Stewart M et al. 1989. Post-traumatic parotid fistulae and sialoceles. A prospective study of conservative management in 51 cases. *Ann Surg* 209(1):105–111.

Parsons JT. 1994. The effect of radiation on normal tissues of the head and neck. In: Million RR, Cassisi NJ (eds.), Management of Head and Neck Cancer: A Multidisciplinary Approach. Philadelphia: Lippincott, pp. 247–250.

Piza-Katzer H, Balough B, Muzika-Herczeg E, Gardetto A. 2004. Secondary end to end repair of extensive facial nerve defects: Surgical technique and postoperative functional results. *Head Neck* 26(9):770–777.

Ragona RM, Blotta P, Pastore A et al. 1999. Management of parotid sialocele with botulinum toxin. *Laryngoscope* 109(8):1344–1346.

Raza H, Khan AU, Hameed A, Khan A. 2006. Quantitative evaluation of salivary gland dysfunction after radioiodine therapy using salivary gland scintigraphy. *Nucl Med Commun* 27(6):495–499.

Rieger J, Seikaly H, Jha N et al. 2005. Submandibular gland transfer for prevention of xerostomia after radiation therapy: Swallowing outcomes. *Arch Otolaryngol Head Neck Surg* 131(2):140–145.

Saarilahti K, Kouri M, Collan J et al. 2005. Intensity modulated radiotherapy for head and neck cancer: Evidence for preserved salivary gland function. *Radiother Oncol* 74(3):251–258.

Saarilahti K, Kouri M, Collan J et al. 2006. Sparing of the submandibular glands by intensity modulated radiotherapy in the treatment of head and neck cancer. *Radiother Oncol* 78(3):270–275.

Salerno S, Lo Casto A, Comparetto A et al. 2007. Sialodochoplasty in the treatment of salivary duct stricture in chronic sialadenitis: Technique and results. *Radiol Med (Torino)* 112(1):138–144.

Scarantino C, LeVeque F, Swann RS et al. 2006. Effect of pilocarpine during radiation therapy: Results of RTOG 97-09, a phase III randomized study in head and neck cancer patients. *J Support Oncol* 4(5):252–258.

Scher N, Poe DS. 1988. Post-traumatic prandial rhinorrhea. *J Oral Maxillofac Surg* 46(1):63–64.

Seikaly H, Jha N, Harris JR et al. 2004. Long term outcomes of submandibular gland transfer for prevention of post radiation xerostomia. *Arch Otolaryngol Head Neck Surg* 130(8):956–961.

Singh B, Shaha A. 1995. Traumatic submandibular salivary gland fistula. *J Oral Maxillofac Surg* 53(3):338–339.

Someya M, Sakata K, Nagakura H et al. 2003. The changes in irradiated salivary gland function of patients with head and neck tumors treated with radiotherapy. *Jpn J Clin Oncol* 33(7):336–340.

Steinberg JM and Herréra AF. 2005. Management of parotid duct injuries. *Oral Surg Oral Med Oral Pathol Oral Radiol Endodont* 99(2):136–141.

Takenoshite Y, Kawano Y, Oka M. 1991. Pneumoparotitis an unusual occurrence of parotid gland swelling during dental treatment. Report of a case with a review of the literature. *J Craniomaxillofac Surg* 19(8):362–365.

Teague A, Akhtar S, Phillips J. 1998. Frey's syndrome following submandibular gland excision: An unusual post operative complication. *ORL J Otorhinolaryngol Relat Spec* 60(6):346–348.

Teymoortash A, Simolka N, Schrader C et al. 2005. Lymphocyte subsets in irradiation-induced sialadenitis of the submandibular gland. *Histopathology* 47(5):493–500.

Thula TT, Schultz G, Tran-Soy-Tay R, Batich C. 2005. Effects of EGF and bFGF on irradiated parotid glands. *Ann Biomed Eng* 33(5):685–695.

Van Sickels JE. 1981. Parotid duct injuries. *Oral Surg Oral Med Oral Pathol* 52(4):364–367.

Vargas H, Galati LT, Parnes SM. 2000. A pilot study evaluating the treatment of post parotidectomy sialoceles with botulinum toxin type A. *Arch Otolaryngol Head Neck Surg* 126(3):421–424.

Wasseman TH, Brizel DM, Henke M et al. 2005. Influence of intravenous amifostine on xerostomia, tumor control, and survival after radiotherapy for head-and-neck cancer: A 2-year follow up of a prospective, randomized phase III trial. *Int J Radiat Oncol Biol Phys* 15(4):985–990.

Wolfram RM, Palumbo B, Chehne F, et al. 2004. (iso) Prostaglandins in saliva indicate oxidation injury after radioiodine therapy. *Rev Esp Med Nucl* 23(30):183–188.

Ya Z, Gao Z, Wang J. 2007. Primary clinical study on using end to end neurorrhaphy following rapid nerve expansion to repair facial nerve defect. (Article in Chinese.) *Zhongguo Xiu Fu Chong Jian Wai Ke Za Zhi* 21(1):23–25.

Zumeg Y, Zhi G, Gang Z et al. 2006. Modified superficial parotidectomy: preserving both the greater auvicular nerve and the parotid gland fascia. *Arch Otolaryngol Head Neck Surg* 135(3): 458–62.

Chapter 13
Miscellaneous Pathologic Processes of the Salivary Glands

Outline

Introduction

This chapter will review a heterogenous group of salivary diseases that are not covered in other sections of this book. Hereditary and developmental conditions of the glands are rare, such that the most common branchial arch anomalies will be emphasized. Under the heading of saliva most clinical emphasis will be given to the treatment of drooling. This condition is not uncommon and there are a wide variety of treatment approaches that will be discussed.

Hereditary and Congenital Conditions

APLASIA

Aplasia of one or all of the major salivary glands is a rare condition that may present with severe xerostomia, rampant caries, candidiasis, pharyngitis, and laryngitis. In addition, "dental chipping"

(Mandel 2006) and recurrent herpes labialis (Heath, McCleod, and Pearce 2006) have been described as presenting signs of salivary gland aplasia. The condition may occur as part of a recognized syndrome, associated with other congenital anomalies, or as an isolated phenomena. Aplasia of the lacrimal and salivary glands (ALSG) presenting with irritable eyes and xerostomia is an autosomal dominant condition that appears to be related to mutations in FGF10 (Entesarium, Dalqvist, and Shashi et al. 2007). In lacrimo-auriculo-dento-digital syndrome (LADD), agenesis of salivary glands as well as lacrimal glands can be seen and is an autosomal dominant condition with variable expressivity (Inan, Yilmaz, and Demir et al. 2006). A case of submandibular agenesis with parotid gland hypoplasia in association with ectodermal dysplasia is reported (Singh and Warnakulasuriya 2004). In addition, aplasia in association with hypoplasia of the thyroid (D'Ascanio et al. 2006) and accessory parotid tissue (Antoniades et al. 2006) are described. Management of these cases is symptomatic and directed toward the xerostomia and other oral health care issues.

DUCT ATRESIA

Duct atresia is rare and in a 2001 review (Hoffrichter, Obeid, and Soliday) only 8 previous cases of submandibular duct atresia were found, with 6 unilateral and 2 bilateral. The condition usually presents in babies or infants as a "ranula" and is thought to be due to failure of the duct to penetrate the oral mucosa during development. The diagnosis can be made by the presence of dilated Wharton's duct(s) on CT scan. Management is by sialodochoplasty to create a new duct orifice.

ABERRANT GLANDS

Accessory glands are ectopic in position but possess a duct that usually opens into another main duct, for example, the accessory parotid gland, whereas aberrant glands have no duct system. Some of these aberrant glands can form fistulae and secrete while the patient is eating; others do not secrete but form choristomas. The commonest sites for these aberrant glands are the lateral neck, pharynx, and middle ear (Enoz and Suoglu 2006), presumably from their proximity to the first two branchial arches during development. These aberrant glands may be involved in neoplastic change and may account for the central salivary tumors of the jaws (usually the mandible).

POLYCYSTIC DISEASE OF THE SALIVARY GLANDS

This is a rare disease that may be a hereditary condition, as familial cases have been reported (Smyth, Ward-Booth, and High 1993). It is thought to be due to a developmental abnormality of the intercalated duct system. Seifert, Thomsen, and Donath (1981) reviewed 5,739 cases of salivary gland disease and found 360 cases of cystic disease, of which 2 patients were classified with dysgenetic polycystic parotid disease. Although it is usually bilateral, unilateral cases have been described (Seifert, Thomsen, and Donath 1981) (Figure 13.1). It is said to be always seen in females; however, a case of the condition in the submandibular glands in a male patient has been reported (Garcia, Martini, and Caces et al. 1998). Histologically the gland is replaced with multiple cysts that may contain spheroliths or microliths. There is a marked absence of inflammatory change. Parotidectomy may be carried out for aesthetic reasons.

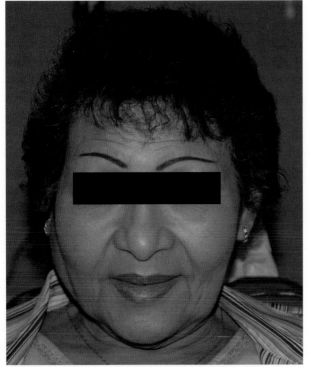
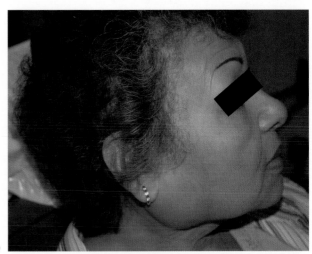

a   b

Figures 13.1a and 13.1b. Middle-aged woman with right parotid swelling for "many" years. Patient is concerned regarding her appearance, as she has no symptoms.

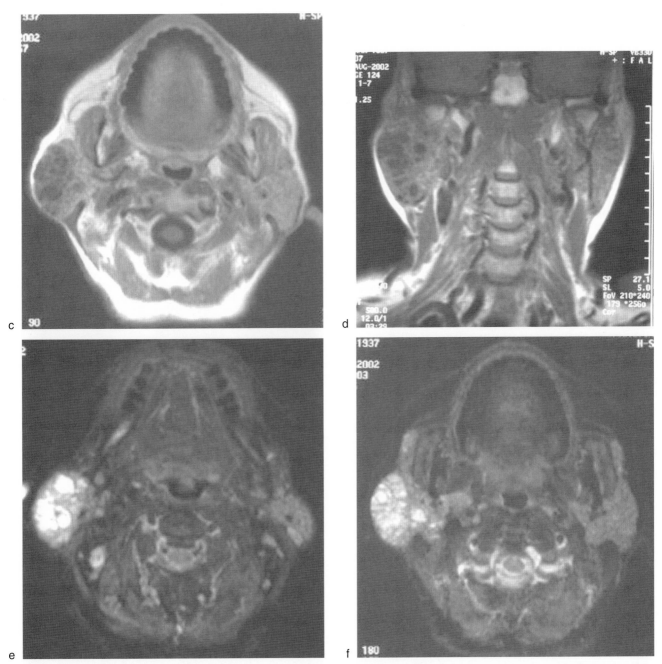

Figures 13.1c, 13.1d, 13.1e, and 13.1f. MR films show multiple cysts within the gland. At the time of surgery multiple microliths were seen.

FIRST BRANCHIAL CLEFT CYSTS, FISTULAE, AND SINUSES

Anomalies of the first brachial arch are intimately associated with the parotid gland and the periauricular structures. They are less common than second branchial arch anomalies. In a survey of 183 patients with branchial cleft cysts and fistulae, 148 patients (80.8%) had branchial cysts of which 35 (23.6%) arose from the first arch and 35 (23.6%) had fistulae of which 11 (31.4%) arose from the first arch (Agaton-Bonilla and Gay-Escoda 1996). The usual figure for the incidence of first branchial arch anomalies is 10% (Olsen, Maragos, and Weiland 1980).

Although Work (1972) classified type I cystic lesions containing only squamous epithelium and type II lesions, which contained squamous epithelium with adnexal skin structures plus cartilage, the presence of infection may make it impossible to classify these lesions using these criteria. Olsen, Maragos, and Weiland (1980) simplified this classification, dividing the type II anomaly into cysts, fistulae, and sinuses. Cysts are tracts with no opening, sinuses are a tract with a single opening usually from the external auditory canal, and fistulae are tracts with two openings usually from the external auditory meatus to the anterior neck above the hyoid bone. In their series of 39 cases, Triglia, Nichollas, and Ducroz et al. (1998) found 20 (51%) sinuses, 11 (28%) fistulae, and 8 (21%) cysts. Similarly, in the series of 10 patients by Solares, Chan, and Koltal (2003), 5 (50%) were sinuses, 3 (30%) fistulae, and 2 (20%) cysts.

Presentation is usually with recurrent infection, with discharge of pus or abscess in the anterior neck, a chronic purulent discharge from the ear, or an infected swelling of the parotid region (Figure 13.2). The usual age of presentation is between birth and 20 years, with most cases diagnosed at age 2.5 years.

Unfortunately the infection is often not recognized as a manifestation of a first branchial arch abnormality and is treated with drainage or inadequate limited exploration, which will complicate subsequent surgery. In the series of Triglia, Nichollas, and Ducroz et al. (1998), 44% of patients had undergone prior surgery, while 65% of patients had incomplete surgery before referral in another paper (Martinez et al. 2007). As the fistulae and sinuses communicate with the external auditory canal, and their relationship to the facial nerve is variable, a wide parotidectomy exposure with dissection of the nerve is essential for complete removal. In fistulae to the auditory meatus removal of the cartilage surrounding the fistulous tract is recommended (Figure 13.3). If the fistula or sinus tract is not completely removed the lesion will recur, and although the recurrence rate is small,

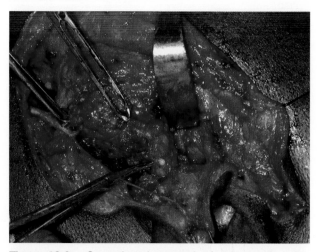

Figure 13.3a. Operative photograph of patient with a discrete mass thought to be a parotid tumor. (Patient's ear at lower right of image.) While dissecting down the external auditory meatus a fistulous tract to the cartilage was identified and the clamp points to a bead of pus from the fistulous tract.

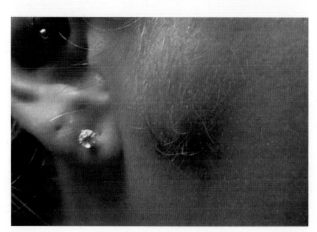

Figure 13.2. Twenty-year-old girl with recurrent localized infection of the parotid and a periparotid sinus.

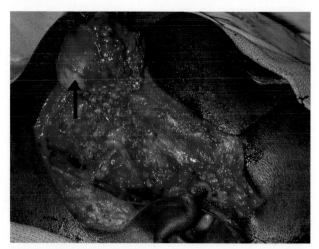

Figure 13.3b. The fistula was removed with a rim of the cartilage from the ear canal and a superficial parotidectomy carried out to remove the branchial cyst (arrow).

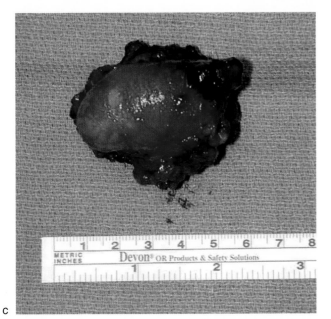

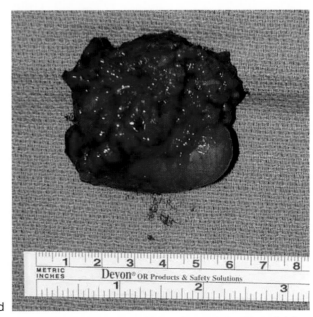

c   d

Figures 13.3c and 13.3d. The parotidectomy specimen shows the cyst deep in the parotid, but it was lying superficial to the facial nerve.

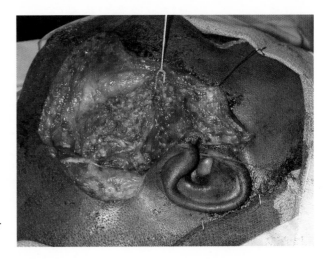

Figure 13.3e. Following superficial parotidectomy (the ear lobe is sutured up for surgical retraction).

3–5% (Stulner et al. 2001), this may increase in patients with previous infection or inadequate surgery. Branchial cysts will usually appear as parotid masses and are usually clinically diagnosed as cystic parotid tumors (Figure 13.4).

The first branchial lesions are usually superficial to the nerve, and Triglia, Nichollas, and Ducroz et al. (1998) reviewed 73 cases including their 39 and found that 63% were superficial, 29% deep, and 8% between the nerve. In the Solares, Chan, and Koltal (2003) small series, however, 7 of 10 lesions were deep to the nerve and 1 lay between the branches. Larger cysts deep to the nerve may be difficult to remove, as the nerve may be adherent to them (Figure 13.5), and dissection can be slow and tedious.

It is very important to recognize the first arch abnormality, as its complexity and anatomical variety necessitates wide exposure through a parotidectomy incision and dissection of the facial nerve to minimize the chances of subsequent facial nerve damage.

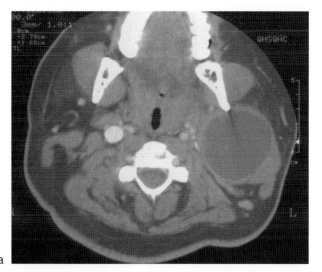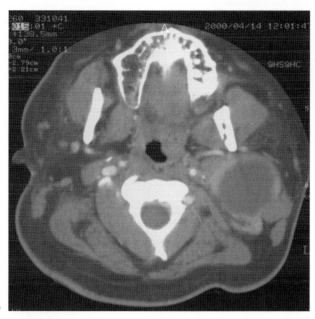

a   b

Figures 13.4a and 13.4b. CT scans of large branchial cyst in the parotid gland.

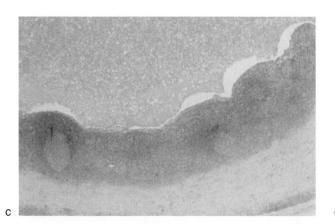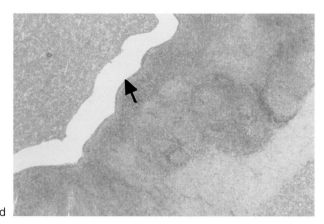

c   d

Figures 13.4c and 13.4d. Histology of the branchial (lymphoepithelial cyst). The proteinaceous cyst contents are superior and the arrow points to the squamous epithelial lining and its associated lymphoid follicles.

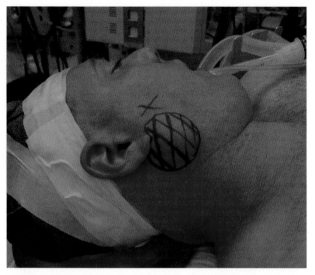

Figure 13.5a. A 27-year-old man with a large cystic lesion in his right parotid. The FNAB showed benign disease.

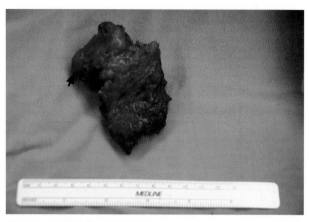

Figure 13.5d. Parotidectomy specimen with deep lobe branchial cyst.

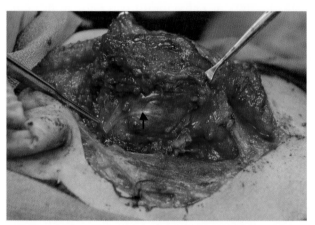

Figure 13.5b. Initial superficial parotidectomy (superficial lobe retracted by an Allis clamp) reveals the cyst lying deep to the cervico-mandibular branch of the facial nerve (arrow).

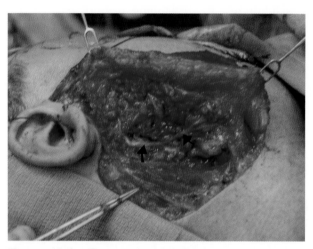

Figure 13.5e. The cervico-mandibular trunk (arrow) is stretched over the defect that the deep lobe branchial cyst occupied.

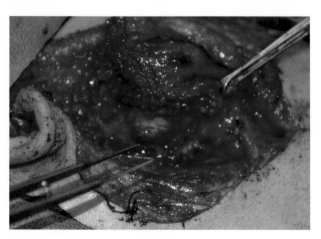

Figure 13.5c. The cervico-mandibular branch is carefully dissected off the cyst capsule and retracted toward the ear.

321

CYSTIC FIBROSIS

The composition of saliva is changed in cystic fibrosis and the formation of viscous mucus may lead to cystic dilations of the ducts and acini, especially in the sublingual gland. The calcium concentration in saliva is also raised and microliths of calcium complexes with the viscous mucus can be seen.

Saliva

SALIVA AS A DIAGNOSTIC FLUID

In many ways saliva represents an ideal fluid for diagnostic analysis, being readily available and not requiring invasive techniques. Currently there is much interest in developing technologies to use saliva to diagnose, monitor progress, and assess treatment and recurrence of oral cancer. However, its mucous nature has made it difficult to analyze. In addition there is evidence to suggest that the methods of processing saliva prior to analysis may have a significant effect on the results obtained for proteins in proteome analysis (Ohshiro, Rosenthal, and Koomen et al. 2007). In seeking to analyze the proteome of saliva, researchers are hoping to find specific diagnostic biomarkers and develop techniques to discriminate between these biomarkers using proteomic and genomic technologies (Wong 2006). Several different research groups have examined varying aspects of salivary composition and have demonstrated significant differences between saliva in healthy subjects and those with oral cancer. Studies have examined biochemical and immunological parameters (Shpitzer et al. 2007), salivary endothelin levels (Pickering, Jordan, and Schmidt 2007), and reactive nitrogen species and antioxidant profile (Bahar, Feimesser, and Shpitzer et al. 2007). Using genomic analysis, four mRNAs (OAZ, SAT, IL8, IL1b) were identified that collectively had a discriminatory power of 91% sensitivity and specificity for detecting oral cancer (Zimmerman, Park, and Wong 2007). Nonetheless, despite these promising initial results this technique remains a research tool at the present time.

DROOLING

The term "drooling" is often used synonymously with sialorrhea; however, virtually all patients who drool do not have an increase in the amount of saliva they produce. Patients with Parkinson's disease with a reduced saliva production can often suffer from drooling. Drooling is the result of a lack of coordinated swallowing with pooling of saliva in the anterior floor of the mouth with subsequent drooling as exemplified in conditions such as cerebral palsy and amyotrophic lateral sclerosis. This condition can have a severe impact on the patient's quality of life. Many different methods of managing this condition have been proposed and were summarized in an excellent review by Meningaud et al. in 2006. These patients benefit from a multidisciplinary team approach and both medical and surgical treatments are used in their management. Medical therapy includes oral motor therapy, orofacial regulation therapy, and behavioral modification via biofeedback. In an analysis of studies from 1970 to 2005 of behavioral treatments of drooling only 17 articles with 57 patients met the inclusion criteria. The evidence base found 15 studies that used a single participant design and 2 that used an experimental comparison group design. Some studies were poorly designed and methodological flaws were identified. Conclusions were that it was not possible to assess the efficacy of behavioral therapy and that further research is needed (Van der Burg et al. 2007). Drug therapy may be by the use of anticholinergics given orally or by botulinum toxin injections. Certain conditions such as glaucoma preclude the use of these oral drugs, and side effects are not uncommon. In a systematic review of the literature only 7 papers were found to meet the inclusion criteria and the authors concluded that there was some evidence benztropine, glycopyrrolate, and bezhexol hydrochloride were effective in children with drooling (Jongerius, van Tiel, and van Limbeek et al. 2003). Botulinum toxin A has been injected into the parotid glands solely or with the submandibular glands with good results. However, the effect is only temporary. In a double-blind placebo-controlled study on 20 patients with Parkinsonism, botulinum toxin A injection into the parotid and submandibular glands was found to be an effective and safe treatment for drooling (Mancini, Zangaglia, and Cristina et al. 2003). In another prospective, double-blind, placebo-controlled trial of different doses of botulinum toxin A (18.75, 37.5, and 75 MU per parotid), the primary end point was achieved with the highest dose of 75 MU without side effects (Lipp, Trottenberg, and Schink et al. 2003). Similarly, in a controlled trial of botulinum against scopolamine in children with cerebral palsy and drooling, botulinum toxin was found to have a significant effect (Jongerius, van den Hoogen, and van Limbeek et al. 2004). Although botulinum showed fewer and less severe side effects than transdermal scopolamine, general anesthesia was required for the injections. Despite the fact that treatment by botulinum toxin A can improve drooling for up to 6 months, there is currently no data in the literature for optimum or maximum dosage, frequency of injections, and duration of action (Lal and Hotaling 2006).

Radiation therapy has been used to reduce saliva production but is obviously contraindicated in children due to its effects on growth and the possibility of radiation-induced sarcoma. Even in adults its long-term side effects preclude its use. An exception may be in patients such as those with poor life expectancy, including those with amyotrophic lateral sclerosis, where radiation may be of benefit in reducing salivary production.

Surgery encompasses both sectioning of secretory nerves and also operations on the glands and ducts. Sectioning of Jacobson's nerve in the middle ear has fallen out of favor and sectioning of the chorda tympani will cause loss of taste. Many different surgical techniques have been described since Wilkie's classic paper advocating excision of the submandibular glands combined with posterior positioning of the parotid ducts (Wilkie 1967). These methods have included duct ligation, duct repositioning, and gland excision of one or more of the major glands. At the present time excellent permanent results have been reported with submandibular duct repositioning and sublingual gland excision. Although submandibular gland excision with parotid duct ligation has been reported as 87% successful (Manrique, do Brasil Ode, and Ramos 2007), it does give rise to temporary parotid edema that can be significant, and Greensmith et al. (2005) reported that bilateral submandibular duct repositioning gland with sublingual gland excision was superior to this technique. However, some authors have questioned the need for excision of the sublingual glands. In a study to assess submandibular duct reposition alone against duct reposition and sublingual gland removal, a 3% postoperative hemorrhage and 12% of parents expressing concerns of pain were found for the duct reposition only procedure, while 13.7% hemorrhage and 36% concern over postoperative pain were found in the group with sublin-

gual gland excision (Glynn and O'Dwyer 2007). As both procedures were equally effective in controlling drooling, the authors state that they no longer carry out sublingual gland excision.

Due to the number of different causes of drooling and the multiple treatment choices available, these patients are best assessed by a multidisciplinary team. As in many other aspects of pediatrics and medicine, simple non-invasive methods of management are attempted first before suggesting surgical management.

SALIVA IN THE MANAGEMENT OF XEROPHTHALMIA

Although dry eyes may occur in relation to dry mouth in conditions such as Sjogren's syndrome, keratoconjunctivitis sicca can occur in isolation. Isolated keratoconjunctivitis sicca is not an uncommon condition and currently there is no satisfactory treatment. Transfer of the submandibular gland duct into the lacrimal basin was first undertaken in 1986 (Murube-Del-Castillo 1986). The largest series of cases with micro-anastomosis of the submandibular gland vessels to the temporal vessels in the temporal fossa and insertion of Wharton's duct into the upper eyelid is 38 (Yu, Zhu, and Mao et al. 2004). In this series only 5 cases failed, 8 cases had epiphora, which required reduction of the size of the submandibular gland, and 2 cases had ductal reconstruction secondary to blockage. The authors stress the use of scintigraphy preoperatively to assess the salivary gland function and rule out a Sjogren's disease, and also postoperatively to assess revascularization and function. Paniello (2007) reported success in 6 of 7 transfers (86%). Four of 5 patients had keratoconjunctivitis sicca secondary to Stevens-Johnson syndrome.

Ischemic/Degenerative Changes
NECROTIZING SIALOMETAPLASIA

Necrotizing sialometaplasia can be seen in any of the salivary glands but is most commonly diagnosed in the minor salivary glands of the palate (Figure 13.6).

It is thought to be secondary to local ischemia with secondary necrosis of the gland and may be secondary to trauma or surgery but is usually

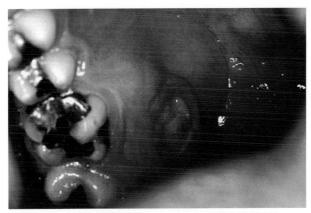

Figure 13.6a. Necrotizing sialometaplasia of palate with rolled edge and granular base clinically resembling squamous cell carcinoma.

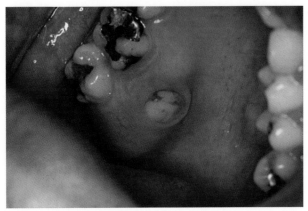

Figure 13.6b. Necrotizing sialometaplasia at a later stage with exposed palatal bone.

spontaneous. Initially there is swelling quickly followed by ulceration, which may be deep down to the bone. Healing may take 2–3 months. Biopsy may be necessary to distinguish this lesion from a malignancy and the histology may be misinterpreted. There is lobular necrosis of the salivary gland with squamous metaplasia of the ducts, and this can be misdiagnosed as mucoepidermoid carcinoma or squamous cell carcinoma. In addition the epithelium adjacent to the ulcer can display pseudo-epitheliomatous hyperplasia, which can also be mistaken for squamous cell carcinoma. If the patient keeps the lesion clean with mouthwashes, healing will occur and recurrence is not seen. Biopsy will often be required to rule out malignancy and histologic interpretation by an experienced pathologist is essential.

AGE CHANGES IN SALIVARY GLANDS

Generalized acinar atrophy can occur in the major salivary glands with age. Frequently the glandular tissue is replaced with fat. In addition, oncocytic metaplasia increases in older patients. Oncocytes are large granular eosinophilic cells. Their granular cytoplasm appears to be secondary to numerous mitochondria. A diffuse oncocytosis of the salivary glands can occur. These changes are not clinically relevant, although oncocytes can give rise to an oncocytoma, which is usually benign but may occasionally be a malignant type. Oncocytomas are of interest as they are similar to Warthin's tumor in appearing as "hot" spots on technetium scans.

Summary

- Fistulae and sinuses above the hyoid bone in the periparotid region should be suspected of being first arch anomalies.
- In managing first branchial arch anomalies, wide exposure with complete dissection of the facial nerve is mandatory because of the complex and unpredictable relationship of the sinuses, fistulae, and cysts to the nerve.
- In managing drooling a multidisciplinary team is optimum.
- Surgery for drooling is used when other less invasive therapies have been tried and failed. Posterior repositioning of the submandibular ducts with or without sublingual gland excision appears to give good results.
- Necrotizing sialometaplasia should be considered in the diagnosis of ulcerative palatal lesions and may be mistaken clinically and histologically for a malignancy.

References

Agaton-Bonilla FC, Gay-Escoda C. 1996. Diagnosis and treatment of branchial cleft cysts and fistulae: A retrospective study of 183 patients. *Int J Oral Maxillofac Surg* 25:449–452.

Antoniades DZ, Markopoulos AK, Deligianni E, Andreadis D. 2006. Bilateral aplasia of the parotid glands correlated with accessory parotid tissue. *J Laryngol Otol* 120(4):327–329.

Bahar G, Feimesser R, Shpitzer T et al. 2007. Salivary analysis in oral cancer patients: DNA and protein oxidation, reactive nitrogen species and anti oxidant profile. *Cancer* 109(1):54–59.

D'Ascanio L, Cavuto C, Martinelli M, Salvinelli F. 2006. Radiological evaluation of major salivary gland agenesis: A case report. *Minerva Stomatol* 55(4):223–228.

Enoz M, Suoglu Y. 2006. Salivary gland choristoma of the middle ear. *Laryngoscope* 116(6):1033–1034.

Entesarium M, Dalqvist J, Shashi V et al. 2007. FGF10 missense mutations in aplasia of major salivary gland agenesis: A case report. *Minerva Stomatol* 55(4):379–382.

Garcia S, Martini F, Caces F et al. 1998. Polycystic disease of the salivary glands: Report of an attack on the submandibular glands. (Article in French.) *Ann Pathol* 18(1):58–60.

Glynn F, O'Dwyer TP. 2007. Does the addition of sublingual gland excision to submandibular duct relocation give better overall results in drooling control? *Clin Otolaryngol* 32(2):103–107.

Greensmith AL et al. 2005. Prospective analysis of the outcome of surgical management of drooling in the pediatric population: A 10 year experience. *Plast Reconstr Surg* 116(5):1233–1242.

Heath N, McCleod I, Pearce R. 2006. Major salivary gland agenesis in a young child: Consequences for oral health. *Int J Pediatr Dent* 16(6):431–434.

Hoffrichter MS, Obeid G, Soliday JT. 2001. Bilateral submandibular duct atresia: Case report. *J Oral Maxillofac Surg* 59:445–447.

Inan UU, Yilmaz MD, Demir Y et al. 2006. Characteristics of lacrimo-auriculo-dento-digital (LADD) syndrome: Case report of a family and literature review. *Int J Pediatr Otorhinolaryngol* 70(7):1307–1314.

Jongerius PH, van Tiel P, van Limbeek J et al. 2003. A systematic review for evidence of efficacy of anticholinergic drugs to treat drooling. *Arch Dis Child* 88:911–914.

Jongerius PH, van den Hoogen FJ, van Limbeek J et al. 2004. Effect of botulinum toxin in the treatment of drooling: A controlled clinical trial. *Pediatrics* 114(3):620–627.

Lal D, Hotaling J. 2006. Drooling. *Curr Opin Otolaryngol Head Neck Surg* 14(6):381–386.

Lipp A, Trottenberg T, Schink T et al. 2003. A randomized trial of botulinum toxin A for treatment of drooling. *Neurology* 61(9):1279–1281.

Mancini F, Zangaglia R, Cristina S et al. 2003. Double-blind, placebo-controlled study to evaluate the efficacy and safety of botulinum toxin type A in the treatment of drooling in Parkinsonism. *Mov Disord* 18(6):685–688.

Mandel L. 2006. An unusual pattern of dental damage with salivary gland aplasia. *J Am Dent Assoc* 137(7):984–989.

Manrique D, do Brasil Ode O, Ramos H. 2007. Drooling: Analysis and evaluation of 31 children who underwent bilateral submandibular gland excision and parotid duct ligation. *Rev Bras Otorhinolaryngol* (Eng ed.) 73(1):40–44.

Martinez DP, Majumdar S, Bateman N, Bull PD. 2007. Presentation of first branchial cleft anomalies: The Sheffield experience. *J Laryngol Otol* 121(5):455–459.

Meningaud JP, Pitak-Arnnop P, Chikhani L, Bertrand JC. 2006. Drooling of saliva: A review of the etiology and management options. *Oral Surg Oral Med Oral Pathol Oral Radiol Endod* 101(1):48–57.

Murube-Del-Castillo J. 1986. Transplantation of salivary gland to the lacrimal basin. *Scand J Rheumatol Suppl* 61:264–267.

Ohshiro K, Rosenthal DI, Koomen JM et al. 2007. Preanalytic saliva processing affects proteomic results and biomarker screening of head and neck squamous carcinoma. *Int J Oncol* 30(3):743–749.

Olsen KD, Maragos NE, Weiland LH. 1980. First branchial cleft anomalies. *Laryngoscope* 90:423–435.

Paniello RC. 2007. Submandibular gland transfer for severe xerophthalmia. *Laryngoscope* 117(1):40–44.

Pickering V, Jordan RC, Schmidt BL. 2007. Elevated salivary endothelin levels in oral cancer patients—a pilot study. *Oral Oncol* 43(1):37–41.

Seifert G, Thomsen ST, Donath K. 1981. Bilateral dysgenetic polycystic parotid glands: Morphological analysis and differential diagnosis of a rare disease of the salivary glands. *Virchows Archives (Pathol Anat)* 390:273–288.

Shpitzer T, Bahar G, Feinmesser R, Nagler RM. 2007. A comprehensive salivary analysis for oral cancer diagnosis. *J Cancer Res Clin Oncol*, epub May 4, 2007, ahead of print.

Singh P, Warnakulasuriya S. 2004. Aplasia of submandibular glands associated with ectodermal dysplasia. *J Oral Pathol Med* 33(10):634–636.

Smyth AG, Ward-Booth RP, High AS. 1993. Polycystic disease of the parotid glands: Two familial cases. *Br J Oral Maxillofac Surg* 31(1):38–40.

Solares CA, Chan J, Koltal PJ. 2003. Anatomical variations of the facial nerve in first branchial cleft anomalies. *Arch Otolaryngol Head Neck Surg* 129(3):351–355.

Stulner C, Chambers PA, Telfer MR, Corrigan AM. 2001. Management of first branchial cleft anomalies: Report of two cases. *Br J Oral Maxillofac Surg* 39(1):30–33.

Triglia J-M, Nichollas R, Ducroz V et al. 1998. First branchial cleft anomalies: A study of 39 cases and a review of the literature. *Arch Otolaryngol Head Neck Surg* 124(3):291–295.

Van der Burg JJ, Didden R, Jogerius PH, Rotteveel JJ. 2007. A descriptive analysis of studies on behavioral treatment of drooling (1975–2005). *Dev Med Child Neurol* 49(5):390–394.

Wilkie TF. 1967. The problem of drooling in cerebral palsy: A surgical approach. *Can J Surg* 10:60–67.

Wong DT. 2006. Salivary diagnostics powered by nanotechnologies proteomics and genomics. *J Am Dent Assoc* 137(3):313–321.

Work WP. 1972. Newer concepts of the first branchial cleft defects. *Laryngoscope* 106:137–143.

Yu GY, Zhu ZH, Mao C et al. 2004. Microvascular submandibular gland autologous transfer in severe cases of keratoconjunctivitis sicca. *Int J Oral Maxillofac Surg* 33(3):235–239.

Zimmerman BG, Park NJ, Wong DT. 2007. Genomic targets in saliva. *Ann N Y Acad Sci* 1098:184–191.

Index

Page references in *italics* refer to figures.
Page references in **bold** refer to tables.